ATLAS OF
CLINICAL DIAGNOSIS

Dedication

To the memory of my dear mother, TAJ, who said to me,
'Get knowledge from whoever has it, and give it freely to
anyone who asks for it, for learning is the noblest form of
begging'.

Commissioning Editor: Laurence Hunter
Project Development Manager: Siân Jarman
Project Manager: Nancy Arnott
Design Direction: Erik Bigland
Illustration Manager: Bruce Hogarth

ATLAS OF
CLINICAL DIAGNOSIS

M. Afzal Mir DCH FRCP

Former Senior Lecturer and Consultant Physician
University Hospital of Wales, Cardiff

SECOND EDITION

SAUNDERS

EDINBURGH LONDON NEW YORK PHILADELPHIA ST LOUIS SYDNEY TORONTO 2003

SAUNDERS
An imprint of Elsevier Science Limited

First published 1995
Second edition 2003

ISBN 0-7020-2668-9

British Library Cataloguing in Publication Data
A catalogue record for this book is available from the British Library

Library of Congress Cataloging in Publication Data
A catalog record for this book is available from the Library of Congress

Notice
Medical knowledge is constantly changing. Standard safety precautions
must be followed, but as new research and clinical experience broaden
our knowledge, changes in treatment and drug therapy may become
necessary or appropriate. Readers are advised to check the most current
product information provided by the manufacturer of each drug to be
administered to verify the recommended dose, the method and duration
of administration, and contraindications. It is the responsibility of the
practitioner, relying on experience and knowledge of the patient, to
determine dosages and the best treatment for each individual patient.
Neither the Publisher nor the editors assumes any liability for any injury
and/or damage to persons or property arising from this publication.
The Publisher

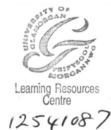

Learning Resources
Centre

12541087

your source for books,
journals and multimedia
in the health sciences
www.elsevierhealth.com

The
publisher's
policy is to use
**paper manufactured
from sustainable forests**

Printed in China
S/1

Preface

The traditional teaching of clinical medicine by the bedside, by lectures, tutorials and through textbooks is mainly system- and disease-oriented. Diseases are presented under their relevant system headings and all the clinical manifestations, irrespective of their regional and anatomical diversity, are presented under each disease. This discipline of learning clinical medicine is contrary to how it is practised in real life, where the history and examination may have to be constructed on a single symptom or an asymptomatic sign. The patient presents with one or more symptoms and the examiner, during history-taking and clinical examination, takes note of various signs that are present and constructs a diagnosis from these.

In this book I have endeavoured to mirror life and have presented signs as they are likely to be seen on a visual survey of a patient, starting at the face and moving down step-by-step to the feet. A brief description of each disease is given as the part of the body it affects is covered in the sequence of the scalp-to-sole survey, and with each mention of a condition a few more details are added. The book explores the visual content of clinical medicine and covers both pathognomonic and fundamental signs as well as non-specific signs. These clinical features presented in an anatomical context will, hopefully, offer an iterative stimulus to the student's memory and thereby help the retentive ability of the reader. Thus, this atlas presents the synthesis of a clinical diagnosis from the features scattered around the body and encourages the student to look for these.

In this age of 'superspecialization', it is becoming increasingly difficult for undergraduates as well as postgraduate students anywhere in the world to see the full spectrum of clinical signs. The increasing demands on the clinical curriculum from the advancing old specialities and emerging new ones have reduced the time available to students to experience the full breadth of clinical medicine. Today it is quite usual to find students graduating from various medical schools in this and other countries with no clinical instruction in, for example, dermatology, rheumatology or neurology! This problem is compounded by the fact that many diseases are often treated early, more effectively and now, more often, in the community. There are fewer opportunities for students to see the usual and less common signs, and yet they are likely to be confronted with these signs in examination and in their subsequent clinical practice. In this book I have addressed this problem by covering as much neurology, dermatology, rheumatol-ogy and ophthalmology as may confront a hospital doctor and a general practitioner. In addition to the colour pictures of the clinical signs of each condition presented here, anatomical sketches and line diagrams have been included, wherever appropriate, both to improve the understanding of clinical features and to cover some important, but non-visual signs.

This book presents a structured approach to clinical diagnosis from a single sign, suggests other areas to look at for relevant supplementary signs and, at appropriate places, gives the critical 'chairside' tests to confirm a diagnosis. This approach makes some repetition inevitable, but this has been kept to a minimum and the clinical signs have been cross-referenced for easy revision.

When I started work on the first edition of this book my main objective was to present a pictorial guide for the inspection part of the clinical assessment. Some of my well-wisher colleagues had expressed understandable doubt about the success of such a venture in an age when technology makes it possible to see the condition of almost any internal organ. Contemporary clinical practice tends to suggest that the budding clinician of today would much rather get an ultrasound of the abdomen than spend time at looking at its external contours. I felt that my modest effort would at least serve those students whose self-esteem would not allow them to dispense with what their eyes could do before calling technology to their aid. It is pleasing to note that in the UK and USA 12,000 copies have been sold and the book was translated into seven languages. Bedside medicine is not dead after all! I am grateful to all those who have found this book of some use and have encouraged me to produce the second edition.

In introducing some embellishments I have taken advice mainly from students who have generously given their comments to me. In the first edition, I had omitted the legends because I thought that students would have a chance to make their own observations before reading the text to look for the diagnosis. I am told that it would be preferable to have the legends giving the telling feature of each picture, and that it would also help students to apply appropriate descriptive terms. In addition to providing the legends, I have made some amendments and additions to the text. I have withdrawn seven pictures that were either repetitive or unsatisfactory, replaced eight others with those with more expressive visual content, and introduced 39 pictures with additional signs. I hope the students will find these changes useful.

Once again I would like to thank all staff of the Media Resource Centre, University of Wales College of Medicine, for their continued cooperation in producing the images shown in this book. I would like to thank my wife, Lynda, who has always encouraged and helped me in these ventures.

Cardiff   A.M.
                                                                                          2003

Acknowledgements

Although more than one-half of the illustrations used in this book come from my personal collection, I needed help from many other colleagues in covering the broad range of clinical medicine, including some rare and unusual conditions. My largest source was the archives of the Department of Medical Illustrations and Audiovisual Services at the University of Wales College of Medicine. I am grateful to Professor Ralph Marshall who was the director of the department and has now retired. My thanks also go to Rachael Konten for helping me search for the appropriate slides. I an indebted to Mrs Joe Dunlop-Rowles from the Medical Illustration Department at the Cardiff Royal Infirmary for providing me with the slides of some rare conditions. I gratefully acknowledge the help and advice of Dr Anne Freeman who read the entire manuscript at an earlier stage. I am grateful to all those listed below who have generously helped me by lending their slides and giving me their valuable advice:

Professor M Addy (Bristol); Mrs L Beck (Cardiff); Mr K Bellamy (Cardiff); Professor L K Borysiewicz (London); Professor D A S Compston (Cambridge); Dr A C Douglas (Edinburgh); Mrs J Dunlop-Rowles (Cardiff); Professor G Elder (Cardiff); the late Mr R W Evans (Cardiff); Professor A Y Finlay (Cardiff); Dr A Freeman (Cardiff); Dr J G Graham (Cardiff); Dr M Hall (Cardiff); the late Professor R Hall (Cardiff); Professor L E Hughes (Cardiff); Dr J D Jessop (Cardiff); Dr M K Jones (Swansea); Dr A G Knight (Cardiff); Mrs R Konten (Cardiff); Mrs C Lane (Cardiff); Professor J H Lazarus (Cardiff); Mr S McAllister (Cardiff); Professor R Marks (Cardiff); Professor R J Marshall (Cardiff); Dr R Mattley (Cardiff); Professor T S Maughan (Cardiff); Dr R Mills (Cardiff); Professor D Owen (Cardiff); Mr M Puntis (Cardiff); Professor J Rhodes (Cardiff); Professor A K Saeed (Pakistan); Professor M F Scanlon (Cardiff); Professor D J Shale (Cardiff); Dr P Smith (Cardiff); Dr J M Stansbie (Coventry); Dr J P Thomas (Cardiff); Professor A P Weetman (Sheffield); the late Dr C Wells (Cardiff); Dr J A Whittaker (Cardiff); Professor M Wiles (Cardiff); Mr S Young (Cardiff).

Contents

1 THE FACE

The visual scan

The face is the most revealing area of the body, showing the features of its physical and psychological well-being and disease. In no other part of the body can one find so many signs of clinical disorders. Face-to-face contact is often the first interaction with the patient and thus forms an essential part of the clinical examination. Although looking at someone's face is considered to be friendly, staring is not. For this reason it is important to develop an unobtrusive method of scanning a face that takes just a few seconds. The objectives of this first look should be to decide whether there is anything abnormal and whether a further assessment is necessary. Although a detailed scrutiny may be required to confirm an initial impression, this should be broken into several brief sections thereby covering the various subsections of the face, and recalling the possible abnormalities associated with them (Tables 1.1 and 1.2).

At first sight one should establish eye contact and decide whether the face and head look normal or whether there are characteristic features suggestive of an endocrine, neuromuscular or a dermatological disorder.

The apparently normal face

There are two situations when an apparently normal-looking face has to be scrutinized carefully before accepting it as normal. First, from other circumstantial evidence it may be suspected that the patient has a systemic disorder, in which facial abnormalities occur but none is obvious at first sight. Second, one may be called upon to make a 'spot' diagnosis of a subtle abnormality, either in an examination setting or on a clinical ward round.

It is a good habit to inspect the face in separate parts, with the objective of excluding an abnormality from each part. Thus, if from initial scanning of the eyes nothing obvious is seen, all the individual structures that make up the eyes should be scrutinized sequentially (see Table 1.1). There may be a mild degree of ptosis or a heliotrope rash on the upper eyelids (**dermatomyositis**); the eyelashes may be sparse or absent (**alopecia**); there may be an arcus around a part or whole of the cornea (normal in the elderly, but possibly seen at an early age in **diabetes mellitus** and **hypercholesterolaemia**); the cornea may be opaque with a ground-glass appearance (**congenital syphilis**); the sclerotics may be mildly icteric (**haemolytic or hepatic disorders**), or may have a bluish tint (**osteogenesis imperfecta**); the pupils may be small, irregular, large or asymmetrical; the lens may be opaque or dislocated (**Marfan's syndrome**); the iris may have lost its distinct features ('muddy iris' in **iritis**); and the conjunctiva may be dry (**keratoconjunctivitis sicca**), pale, particularly in the gutterings (**anaemia**), icteric or congested (**superior vena caval obstruction, polycythaemia**).

More detailed examples of the signs listed in Table 1.1 are given in relevant chapters. Suffice it here to say that some of these abnormalities are hardly obvious unless specifically looked for. For example, a mild degree of ptosis with unequal pupils (1.1), a yellowish (1.2) or bluish tint to the sclerotics (1.3), or even fairly obvious xanthelasmata may all be missed unless the observer, however briefly,

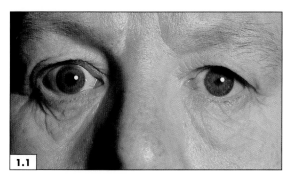

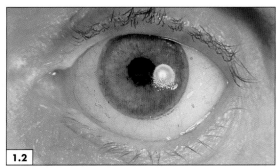

1.1
Miosis (<2 mm) and partial ptosis of the left eye

1.2
Yellow sclera

Table 1.1 Substructure scrutiny of the eyes

Structures	Signs	Conditions
Eyelids	Ptosis, lid retraction, puffiness, heliotrope rash	Hemiparesis, myopathy, Graves' disease, allergy, hypothyroidism, dermatomyositis
Eyelashes	Scanty/absent	Alopecia
Cornea	Calcification (band keratopathy)	Hyperparathyroidism
	Arcus	Senescence, hypercholesterolaemia, diabetes mellitus
	Opacity	Old keratitis, congenital syphilis
Sclera	Yellowish	Jaundice
	Bluish	Osteogenesis imperfecta
Lens	Opaque	Cataract from any cause
	Dislocation	Marfan's syndrome
Pupils	Unequal, small	Holmes–Adie, Argyll Robertson pupils, third cranial nerve palsy
Iris	Shimmering	Dislocated or absent lens
	'Muddy'	Iritis
Conjunctiva	Pale	Anaemia, low perfusion state
	Icteric	Jaundice
	Congested	Conjunctivitis, polycythaemia rubra vera, superior vena cava obstruction

1.3
Thin, blue sclerae

1.5
Left external rectus palsy

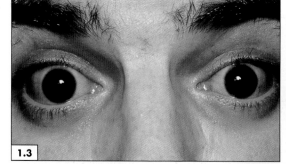

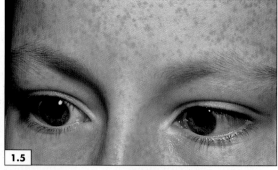

1.4
Xanthelasma

1.6
Droopy left side

1.7
Immobile left face

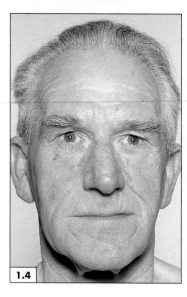

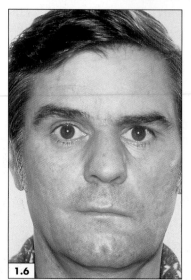

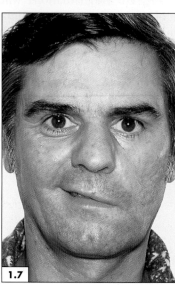

focuses on the eyes (1.4). Similarly, asymmetry of the eyeballs will be easily missed by an observer who does not look at both eyes and follow the patient's gaze (1.5).

After inspecting the eyes, a purposeful glance over the rest of the face will reveal any asymmetry, erythema, scarring or plaques. A slight asymmetry of the face and the angles of the mouth (1.6) may escape notice unless the observer is looking for it. Some normal faces are asymmetrical and the temptation to diagnose a facial nerve palsy should be resisted until the facial muscles are seen in action (1.7).

The mouth should be viewed for circumoral wrinkling (**systemic sclerosis**) and for the fine, angular wrinkling of **gonadotrophin failure**. Angular cheilitis caused by dribbling from ill-fitting dentures or **deficiency states of iron** or **riboflavin** may not be obvious unless specially looked for. The inside of the mouth and the tongue should be inspected for telangiectasia (**Osler–Weber–Rendu syndrome**), cyanosis and pigmentation (**Addison's disease**). The whole face can be covered rapidly in this manner. In most cases, having spotted an abnormality and formed an initial impression, the examiner can carry out further 'chairside' clinical tests to confirm or refute the suspected diagnosis.

Abnormal facies

If the face looks abnormal then a logical way to proceed further would be to characterize the appearance so that it can be placed in one of the four groups of abnormal facies (Table 1.2).

Endocrine facies
Acromegaly

The face may show one or more of the many characteristic features associated with **acromegaly** (1.8). The patient may have prominent and thickened supraorbital and nuchal ridges, exaggerated wrinkles with thickened facial features, a *wide and fleshy nose*, full and plump lips and a *large and protuberant lower jaw*. Such a patient with acromegaly may be hirsute with thickened and greasy skin.

Alternatively, none of these features may be gross or exaggerated: the subject may, for example, simply be a well-built, burly rugby player or a boxer with rugged features (1.9). A patient with **Paget's disease** (1.10) or

---

Table 1.2 Abnormal facies

- **Endocrine facies**
  Acromegaly
  Cushing's syndrome
  Graves' disease
  Hypothyroidism
  Addison's disease
  Hypopituitarism
  Pseudohypoparathyroidism
- **Neuromuscular facies**
  Ptosis
  Ocular palsies
  Proptosis
  Pupillary abnormalities
  Facial muscular atrophy/weakness
- **Skin and mucosal lesions**
  Dermatoses
  Systemic disorders
- **Miscellaneous group**
  Characteristic facies not included in the other groups (e.g. mongolism)
  Enlargement or underdevelopment of an area (e.g. Paget's disease, parotid swelling, maxillary hypoplasia, etc.)

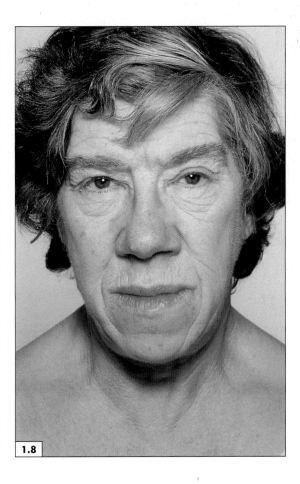

1.8

1.8
Fleshy, plump nose and lips

hypothyroidism may be mistaken, at first sight, as having acromegaly. Occasionally, there may be one or more of the characteristic features of acromegaly such as thickened supraorbital ridges, a fleshy nose and thickened skin, as seen in **pachydermoperiostosis** (1.11); in this case a false impression of acromegaly may be formed. A side-view of a patient with acromegaly (1.12), against that of a patient of comparable age with pachydermoperiostosis (1.13), will show that, in the former, the nose is not only bulkier but

its contours are also rounded and the contours of the nose and ear are less distinct than in the latter. As expected, the lower jaw looks somewhat protuberant in the acromegalic patient. Similarly, **hypothyroidism** with an increased soft-tissue mass (1.14) may cause confusion and further clinical tests may be required to distinguish the two. The **insulin-resistance syndrome** with associated *lipodystrophy* (1.15, 1.16), with or without acanthosis nigricans, may be confused with acromegaly.

1.9
Large but distinct
features

1.10
Prominent frontal
bones

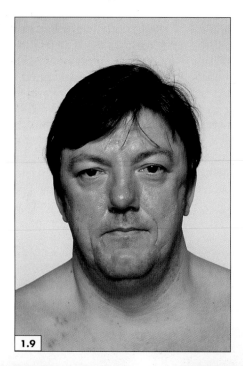

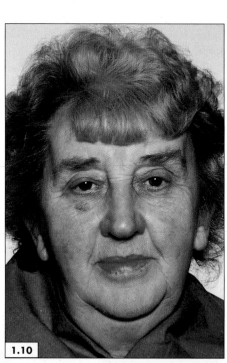

1.11
Thickened skin with
indistinct folds

1.12
Large and rounded
contours of the nose
and ear

1.13
Pachydermoperiostosis:
distinct contours of
nose and ear

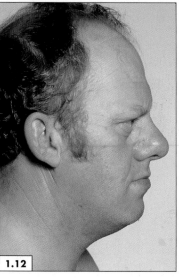

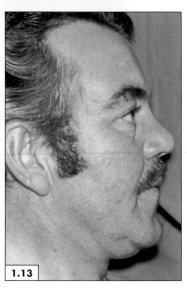

In **HIV-associated lipodystrophy syndrome** there is lipoatrophy over the face and proximal muscles, and excessive deposition of subcutaneous fat around the neck (buffalo hump), breast and abdomen (axial obesity). This complication occurs in HIV patients treated with a protease inhibitor but the exact pathogenesis is unknown.

Clinical confirmation

To make the diagnosis in a patient with the characteristic features, and to exclude it in a patient with some mimicking signs, particular attention should be paid to the patient's history. They may have required progressively larger sizes of shoes, hats, gloves and rings. This is a condition with a variety of clinical features (1.17) that should be sought. The patient should be asked if there is an old photograph available for comparison. In this patient (1.18), the current picture shows a striking contrast with the one taken at her wedding. In addition, a few chairside clinical tests will be required to make the clinical diagnosis.

When asked, patients often volunteer that their relatives and close friends have noticed a major change in the size

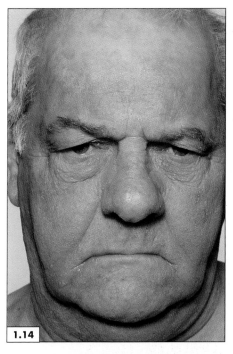

1.14
Hypothyroidism: large nose and facial folds. Note a noncommunicative affect

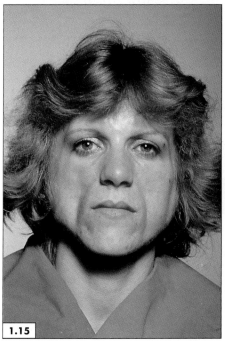

1.15

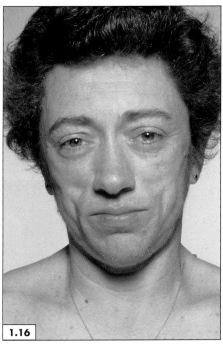

1.16

1.15 and 1.16
Lipodystrophy: prominent muscular contours due to deficient subcutaneous fat

of the patient's nose, which has gradually become bulkier and fleshy (1.19). In some patients this is the only characteristic feature of acromegaly on the face (1.20). The lower jaw gradually increases in size and becomes large, bulky and overgrown, producing *prognathism* (1.21). The change is so striking and arresting that the clinical diagnosis of acromegaly is hardly in doubt (1.22).

Macroglossia is an accessible manifestation of visceromegaly in this disease. It can be demonstrated by asking patients to protrude their tongue out as far as possible. The acromegalic tongue (1.23) is thick and wide and has lost its normal triangular shape (1.24). It fills nearly the whole of the mouth and there is only a rim, or sometimes no space at all, between the tongue and the cutting line of the upper teeth (1.23). When viewed in profile, such a tongue (1.25) looks thicker and bulkier (1.26); it also reaches far further down towards the chin, which itself is longer than normal. The spaces between the teeth are also increased. Although this appearance may also be seen in **lipodystrophy** (1.27), and sometimes in normal subjects, a steady increase of the spaces between the teeth is characteristic of acromegaly.

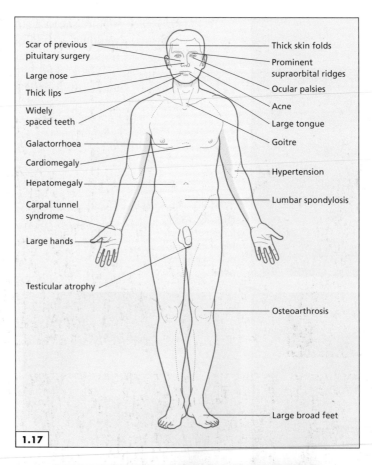

Scar of previous pituitary surgery
Large nose
Thick lips
Widely spaced teeth
Galactorrhoea
Cardiomegaly
Hepatomegaly
Carpal tunnel syndrome
Large hands
Testicular atrophy

Thick skin folds
Prominent supraorbital ridges
Ocular palsies
Acne
Large tongue
Goitre
Hypertension
Lumbar spondylosis
Osteoarthrosis
Large broad feet

1.17
Clinical features of acromegaly

1.17

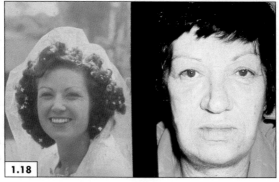

1.18
Before and after acromegaly

1.18

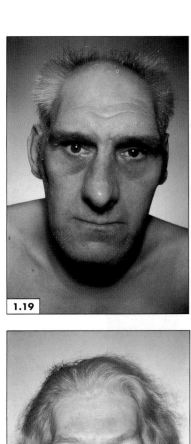

1.19

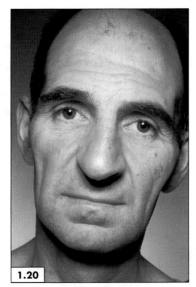

1.20

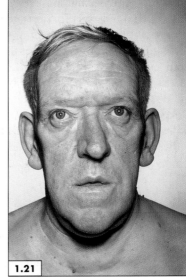

1.21

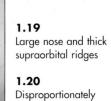

1.19
Large nose and thick supraorbital ridges

1.20
Disproportionately large nose

1.21
Overgrown lower jaw

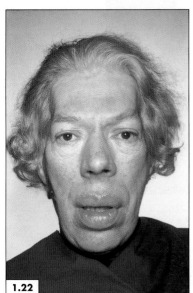

1.22

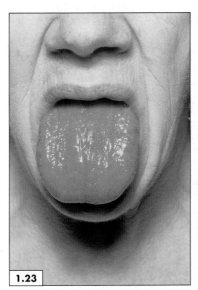

1.23

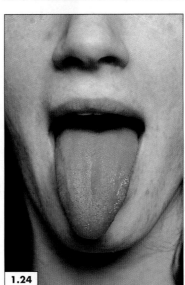

1.24

1.22
Large, fleshy lips with prognathism

1.23
Large, square tongue

1.24
Normal, triangular tongue

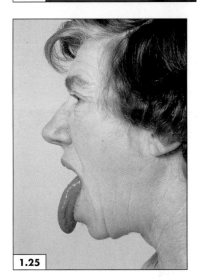

1.25

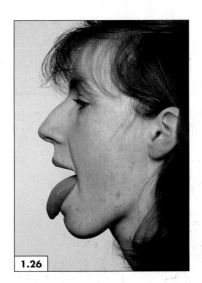

1.26

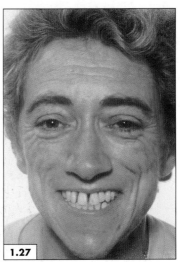

1.27

1.25
Thickened, bulky tongue

1.26
Normal tongue

1.27
Lipodystrophy

Malocclusion of the teeth is by far the most reliable sign and this can be demonstrated by asking patients to clench their teeth. In an acromegalic patient, the lower teeth overbite the upper teeth owing to the prognathism of the lower jaw (1.28, 1.29). A comparison between 1.27 and 1.28 will demonstrate this.

Both the hands (1.30) and feet (1.31) are square, wide and enlarged. The massive and spade-like hands and the *increased skin thickness* are characteristic clinical signs of acromegaly. All of these features can be assessed conve-

niently by inspection; in addition, a skinfold can be raised on the back of the hand and then compared with that from a normal subject of comparable age (1.32, 1.33).

Visual field defects occur whenever the associated pituitary tumour extends outside the pituitary fossa and compresses the optic chiasma. The most commonly encountered visual field defects are a bitemporal upper quadrantanopia or a *bitemporal hemianopia*. These defects can be demonstrated by the confrontation method at the chairside (1.34, 1.35).

1.28
Overbiting lower
teeth

1.29
Prognathism

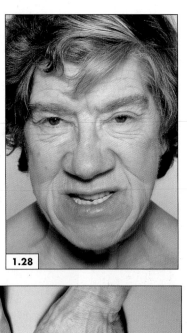

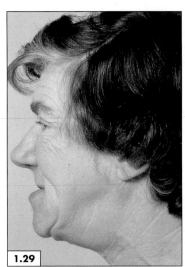

1.30
Normal and
acromegalic hands

1.31
Large, square feet

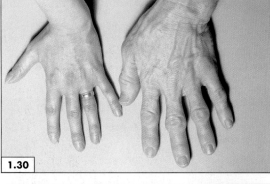

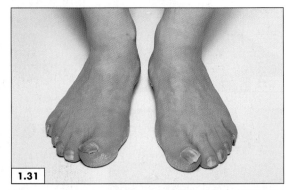

1.32
Acromegalic skin
fold

1.33
Normal skinfold

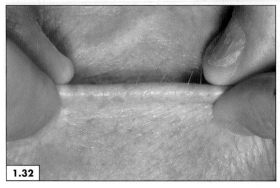

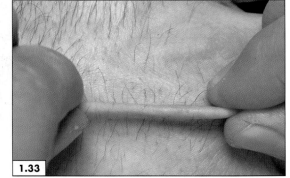

The definitive diagnosis of acromegaly can be made by demonstrating an elevated serum growth hormone level that is not suppressed by the rising plasma glucose during a glucose tolerance test. Single estimations of the hormone are unreliable since growth hormone secretion is pulsatile in short bursts.

Cushing's syndrome

Cushing's syndrome is easy to suspect but can be difficult to diagnose, since the visible clinical signs of obesity, hirsutism, plethora, easy bruising and acne are all also very common in the general population. Most patients referred to endocrinologists with these features have simple obesity. A careful look at some of the principal features will enable the clinician to identify those patients who are most likely to have Cushing's syndrome.

In a fully developed case, the most striking facial features are rounding of the face (*moon face*), plethora with telangiectasis, hirsutism, loss of scalp hair, acne and pigmentation (1.36–1.38). Facial rounding and plethora are usually present, even in milder cases where the disease has not yet developed fully (1.39). These features are particularly striking in younger subjects (1.40). As in most endocrine disorders, examination of an earlier photograph can be useful. In this lady's current photograph (1.41, left) there is a marked plethora and facial rounding compared with that in the photograph taken 3 years earlier (1.41, right). Increased fat deposition occurs in all the likely fat depots, from the face to the buttocks. The obesity is axial (like a *lemon on matchsticks*) owing to excessive fat deposition in the supraclavicular fossae, over the back of the neck (*buffalo hump*), the breasts, abdominal wall and the buttocks, and from the relative wasting of the limb muscles.

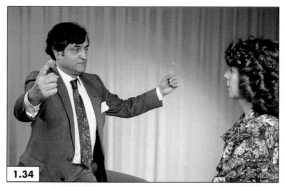

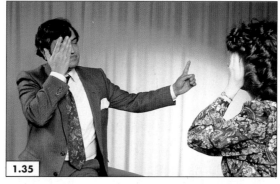

1.34
Testing peripheral visual fields

1.35
Testing right temporal visual field

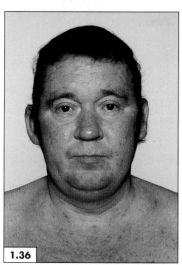

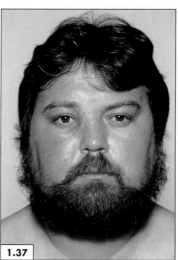

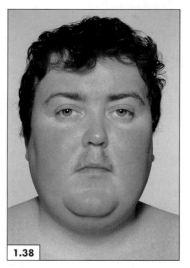

1.36
Facial plethora

1.37
A rounded, moon face and plethora

1.38
Moon face and plethora

1.39
Facial rounding and
plethora

1.40
Moon face –
Cushing's syndrome

1.41
After and before
Cushing's syndrome

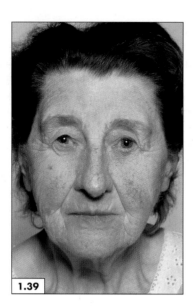

1.39

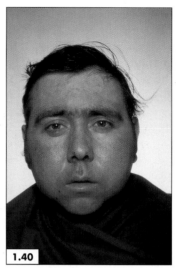

1.40

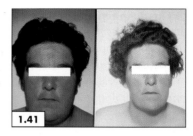

1.41

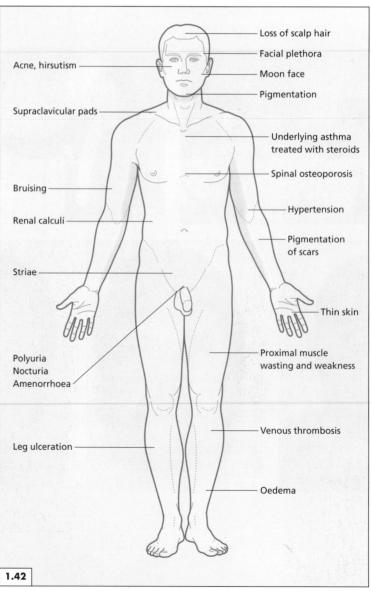

Loss of scalp hair

Facial plethora

Moon face

Pigmentation

Acne, hirsutism

Supraclavicular pads

Underlying asthma
treated with steroids

Spinal osteoporosis

Bruising

Renal calculi

Hypertension

Pigmentation
of scars

Striae

Thin skin

Polyuria
Nocturia
Amenorrhoea

Proximal muscle
wasting and weakness

Leg ulceration

Venous thrombosis

Oedema

1.42

1.42
Clinical features of
Cushing's syndrome

Clinical confirmation

The initial impression can be changed into a firm clinical diagnosis by seeking the characteristic clinical features (1.42). Moderate obesity presents a major problem, not only because it shares some of the characteristics with Cushing's syndrome but also because most obese patients insist that they have some 'gland' trouble! In simple obesity, fat deposition does not spare the arms and thighs (1.43) in comparison with Cushing's syndrome where thin extremities appear in striking contrast with truncal obesity (1.44). These characteristic differences between the appearances of the two conditions can be appreciated

better with the frontal views of these partially undressed patients (1.45, 1.46). Both views provide an opportunity to look for some additional features, such as the characteristic *purple striae* in Cushing's syndrome, caused by the stretching of the thin, protein-depleted skin over rapidly fattening areas. Apart from the abdomen (1.44, 1.46), purple striae are also seen over the buttocks (1.47) and the thighs (see also 11.38, 11.39). Hirsutism can be a marked feature in some patients (1.48).

Fat deposition over the supraclavicular areas raises banana-shaped folds, which look prominent in both the frontal (1.49) and the lateral views (1.50). Unlike simple obesity, fat deposition is excessive over the lower

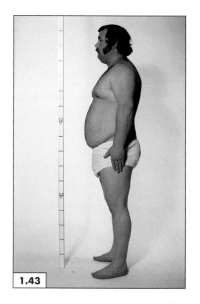

1.43

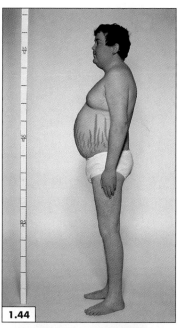

1.44

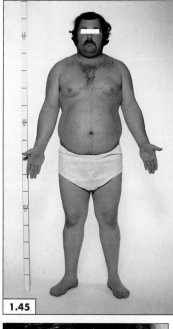

1.45

1.43
Obesity

1.44
Axial obesity, thin extremities and striae

1.45
Simple obesity

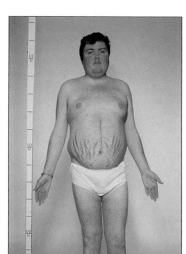

1.46

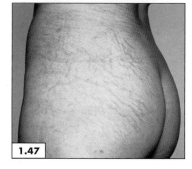

1.47

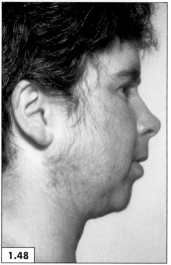

1.48

1.46
Cushing's syndrome with truncal obesity and striae

1.47
Purple striae

1.48
Hirsutism with facial plethora

cervical vertebrae, giving the back a characteristic *buffalo hump* appearance (1.51). This is also seen in the **pseudoCushing's syndrome** of **alcoholism** (1.52). This geographical predilection of fat deposition is characteristic of Cushing's syndrome (also occurs in HIV-associated lipodystrophy syndrome, see p. **5**) and is seen even in younger subjects (1.53).

Two chairside tests are of particular importance and should always be performed to complete the clinical assessment. First, the skin of patients with Cushing's syndrome is paper-thin and transparent so that the underlying capillaries and veins look prominent, particularly in the antecubital fossa (1.54). This excessive thinning of the skin can be demonstrated readily by compressing the antecubital fossa

1.49
The adipose 'necklace' of Cushing's syndrome

1.50
Supraclavicular adipose deposits

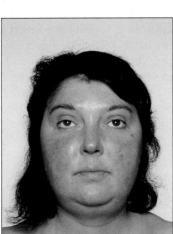
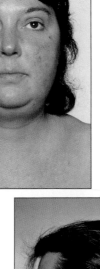

1.51
Cushing's syndrome

1.52
PseudoCushing's syndrome

1.53
Iatrogenic Cushing's syndrome

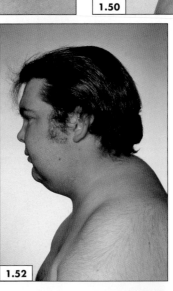
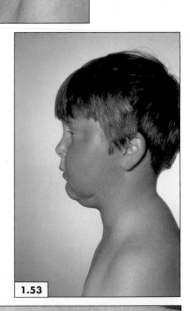

1.54
Transparent and thin skin with visible underlying veins

1.55
Paper-thin skin folds

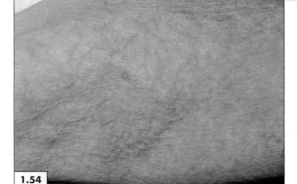
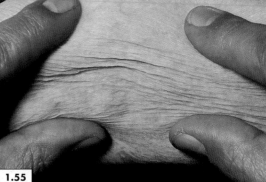

between the thumb and the middle finger, thereby raising multiple thin and transparent skin folds (1.55). Similarly, it can also be assessed by raising a skin fold on the back of the patient's hand and comparing it (1.56) with that of a normal hand (1.57). Second, proximal muscular weakness commonly associated with Cushing's syndrome (caused by muscle catabolism and compounded by hypokalaemia) can be demonstrated by asking the patient to stand up from a squatting position (1.58). Most patients with Cushing's syndrome are unable to do this without touching the floor (1.59), their thighs (1.60) or any other prop.

Excessive bruising and ecchymoses are usually seen on the back of the hands (1.61), shins and invariably on venesection sites (1.62).

The appearances of the various forms of Cushing's syndrome do not differ markedly from one another. A probing history will be required to diagnose the pseudoCushing's syndrome caused by alcoholism (1.63).

The distinctive facial appearances of Cushing's syndrome (1.64) usually revert to normal after treatment (1.65).

The diagnosis of **Cushing's disease** (spontaneous hypercortisolism from excessive pituitary adrenocorticotrophic hormone (ACTH) production) is confirmed by demonstrating hypercortisolism, loss of circadian rhythm of cortisol secretion, raised 24 h urinary free cortisol level, with a modest elevation of ACTH concentration. Dynamic tests are required to establish the aetiological diagnosis of Cushing's syndrome.

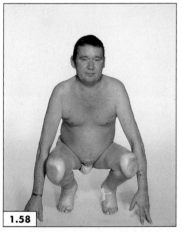

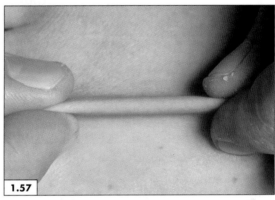

1.56
Thin skinfold of Cushing's syndrome

1.57
Normal skinfold

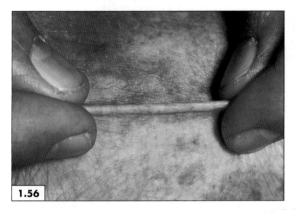

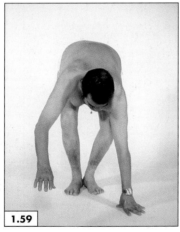

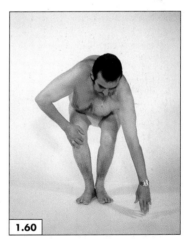

1.58
Attempting to stand up

1.59 and 1.60
Needing a prop to stand up

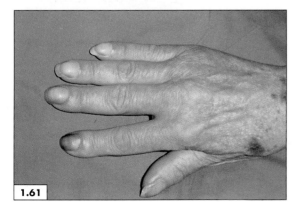

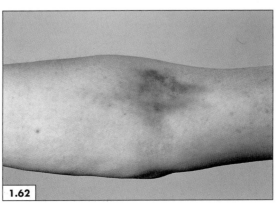

1.61
Spontaneous bruising and purpura

1.62
Postvenesection bruising

Graves' disease

Graves' disease is essentially recognizable by its eye signs, which direct one's attention to the other accompanying features (1.66). Exophthalmos (proptosis), periorbital swelling, upper lid retraction, chemosis and ophthalmopathy occur in various combinations. **Proptosis**, or the forward, axial protrusion of the globe, results from enlarge-ment of the muscles and fat within the orbit. It is easy to recognize, particularly when associated with other signs such as periorbital oedema (1.67). Both these features are better appreciated if the eye is inspected from the side (1.68). Compared with the normal eye and the valleys above and below it (1.69), the globe in exophthalmos looks protuberant with puffed-up and discoloured skin around it.

1.63
Facial plethora in pseudoCushing's syndrome

1.64
Cushing's syndrome: before treatment

1.65
Cushing's syndrome: after treatment

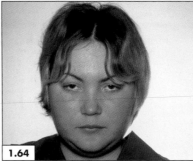

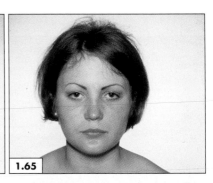

1.63

1.64

1.65

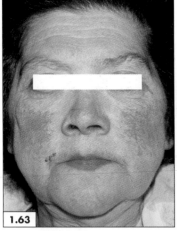

Loss of scalp hair

Hyperphagia
Polydipsia

Eye signs

Lypodystrophy

Diffuse goitre

Gynaecomastia
(in males)

Tachycardia
Systolic
flow murmur

Systolic
hypertension

Lymphadenopathy
Splenomegaly

Atrial
fibrillation

Weight loss

Acropachy
Onycholysis

Polyuria
Diarrhoea

Warm,
moist skin

Proximal muscle
weakness

Tremor

Brisk reflexes

Pretibial
myoedema

Oedema

1.66

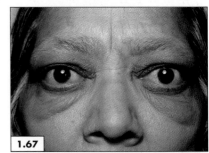

1.67

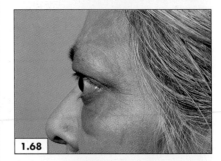

1.68

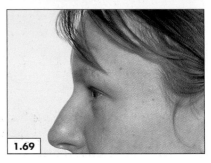

1.69

1.66
Clinical features of Graves' disease

1.67
Proptosis with periorbital oedema

1.68
Axial protrusion of the eyeball

1.69
Normal orbit

Upper lid retraction is a common eye sign in Graves' disease; it can be recognized by a rim of sclera, visible between the lower margin of the upper lid and the cornea in the relaxed position of forward gaze (1.70). Sometimes the lid retraction is so marked that the eyelashes are buried under the retracted lid (1.71). Chemosis (congestion of the conjunctivae) frequently occurs in Graves' ophthalmopathy and often the medial caruncle is red and enlarged (1.72).

Of the other clinical features, *thyroid acropachy* (1.73) and *pretibial myxoedema* (1.74) are visually impressive. The former resembles clubbing of the fingers (1.75) but, unlike clubbing, the swelling is found more often around and over the root of the nail and much less under the nail bed (1.76). *Onycholysis* is sometimes seen when the nails separate from the nail beds and become thin and discoloured (1.77). It also occurs in a variety of dermatological disorders, particularly in psoriasis (see **The Nails**).

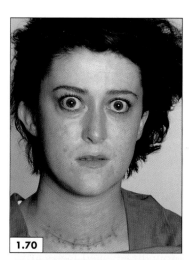

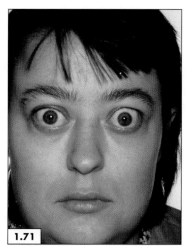

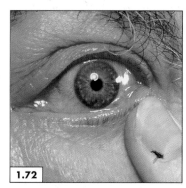

1.70
Upper lid retraction

1.71
Lid retraction with buried eyelashes

1.72
Enlarged medial caruncle and congestion

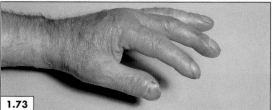

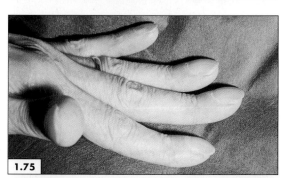

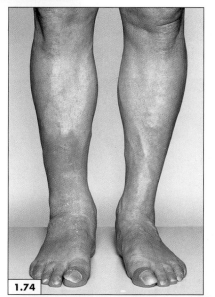

1.73
Acropachy

1.74
Pretibial myxoedema

1.75
Clubbing of the fingers

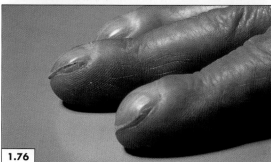

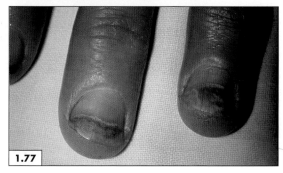

1.76
Thyroid acropachy: convex nails with periungal swelling

1.77
Onycholysis

Pretibial myxoedema is a localized violaceous induration that usually occurs on the shins and, in many cases, appears several months after a patient has been rendered euthyroid with surgery or radioiodine.

Clinical confirmation

A careful history is sufficient to establish the clinical diagnosis in most cases with *thyrotoxic facies*. Loss of weight despite a good appetite (with an *increased dietary intake*), heat intolerance, irritability, restlessness, palpitations, diarrhoea and undue fatiguability are among the usual presenting features. A few chairside tests can be used to confirm the clinical impression. The patient is usually lightly clad, thin, nervous and fidgety. The hands are warm and moist (*cold* and sweaty in simple anxiety) and, when outstretched, exhibit a fine rhythmic tremor. The resting pulse rate is rapid and there may be atrial fibrillation.

Sometimes the thyroid gland is only slightly enlarged and the patient may have to be given a sip of water to swallow, in order to fully reveal the enlargement of an upwardly moving gland. The bell of the stethoscope should be placed lightly on the gland to listen for a *bruit*, which is a reliable sign of increased vascularity and hyperactivity.

Lid retraction can be elicited by asking the patient to follow the examiner's index finger as it moves slowly downwards. The upper lids lag behind the downwardly moving eyeballs (1.78, 1.79). Exophthalmic ophthalmopathy can be demonstrated by revealing the inability of the patient to converge his eyes (1.80) and to look up and outwards (1.81).

Laboratory diagnosis can be made by demonstrating an increased level of free serum T_4 or T_3, or both, and a low thyroid-stimulating hormone (TSH) level by a sensitive assay. In difficult cases, the thyrotrophin-releasing hormone (TRH) provocative test can be undertaken to establish the diagnosis.

Hypothyroidism

The typical **hypothyroid** facies showing all the characteristic features (1.82) is easy to recognize but is seldom encountered nowadays. The patient is usually excessively clothed, mentally and physically slow, obese with nonpitting oedema of the legs and face, and has some of the characteristic facial features. There is often some degree of periorbital oedema, thickening of the nose and lips, malar flush with a yellowish tinge, sparse hair, and dull eyes with noncommunicative looks (1.83). The example of advanced myxoedema shown in 1.83 is seldom seen today. More often patients have less profoundly affected facies (1.84) and the diagnosis is made by a combination of a careful history, physical examination and laboratory investigation.

1.78
Marked lid retraction

1.79
Lid lag

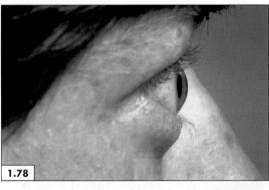
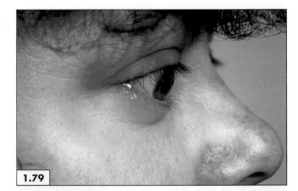

1.80
Unable to converge

1.81
The tethered left eye fails to move up and outwards

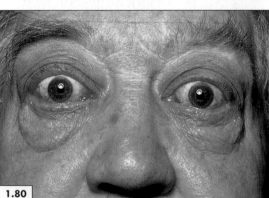
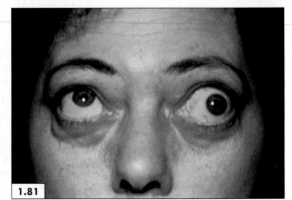

Clinical confirmation

The skin is *cold*, *dry*, pale, thick and inelastic, with the hair being coarse and sparse (1.85). There is sometimes a prominent malar flush when other features of myxoedema are less striking (1.84, 1.86). The patients are uninterested in their surroundings and slow to respond to enquiries. The patient's voice is thick and croaky, the *pulse is slow* and the *relaxation* of the tendon jerks is *slow*, as demonstrated easily on the ankle jerk. In an office situation this can be tested by asking the patient to kneel on a chair (1.87). The diagnosis should always be confirmed by laboratory investigations by demonstrating a low serum free T_4 and *elevated* TSH levels. A few cases are detected by laboratory methods alone, usually by routine thyroid function tests requested for patients attending a lipid or geriatric outpatient clinic.

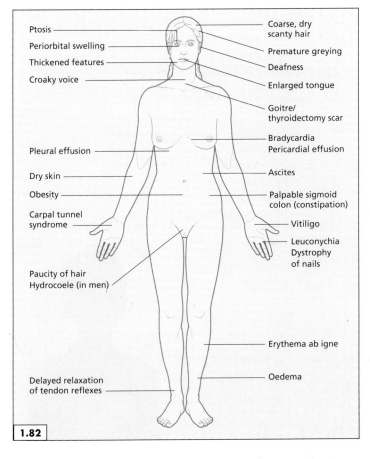

Ptosis
Periorbital swelling
Thickened features
Croaky voice

Coarse, dry scanty hair
Premature greying
Deafness
Enlarged tongue
Goitre/ thyroidectomy scar

Pleural effusion
Dry skin
Obesity
Carpal tunnel syndrome

Bradycardia Pericardial effusion
Ascites
Palpable sigmoid colon (constipation)
Vitiligo
Leuconychia Dystrophy of nails

Paucity of hair Hydrocoele (in men)

Erythema ab igne
Oedema

Delayed relaxation of tendon reflexes

1.82

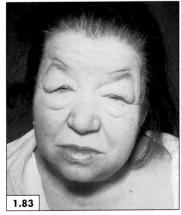

1.83

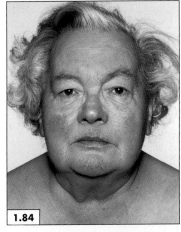

1.84

1.82
Clinical features of hypothyroidism

1.83
Myxoedema

1.84
Hypothyroidism: malar flush

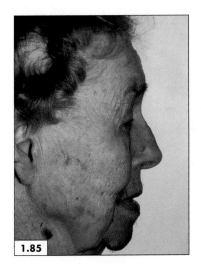

1.85

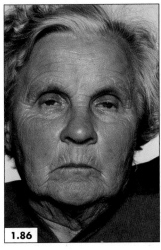

1.86

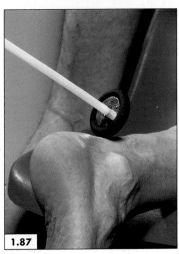

1.87

1.85
Hypothyroidism: hair loss

1.86
Hypothyroidism: malar flush and noncommunicative affect

1.87
Testing ankle jerk on a kneeling leg

Addison's disease

Unlike the endocrine disorders discussed so far, **Addison's disease** and hypopituitarism do not produce strikingly diagnosable facies. The diagnosis is suspected by the presence of other associated features (1.88) along with the facial appearance. For example, *pigmentation*, the hallmark of Addison's disease, may be racial, constitutional or the result of some other disease (Table 1.3). Progressive darkening is more significant than long-standing pigmentation. Clinical diagnosis can be established with a competent history and physical examination.

Clinical confirmation

Although the symptoms of tiredness, dizziness, anorexia, weight loss, cramps, depression, nausea and vomiting may seem vague and nonspecific, they can be very meaningful if considered together with the thin, apathetic and pigmented patient (1.89). Apart from the face, which looks dark (1.90), marked pigmentation may also be found on the exposed areas of the skin such as the fingers (1.91), palmar creases (1.92), elbows (1.93) and around or

Table 1.3 Some causes of hyperpigmentation

■ **Localized**
Freckles
Lentigines – Peutz–Jeghers syndrome
Chloasma
Café-au-lait spots – neurofibromatosis
Postinflammatory phenomenon

■ **Generalized**
Excessive melanocyte-stimulating hormone (MSH) or
 adrenocorticotrophic hormone (ACTH)
Addison's disease
Nelson's syndrome (bilateral adrenalectomy for Cushing's
 syndrome)
Ectopic ACTH
Malignancy
Chronic infections (especially tuberculosis)
Hyperthyroidism
Systemic sclerosis
Primary biliary cirrhosis
Haemochromatosis
Chronic arsenic poisoning

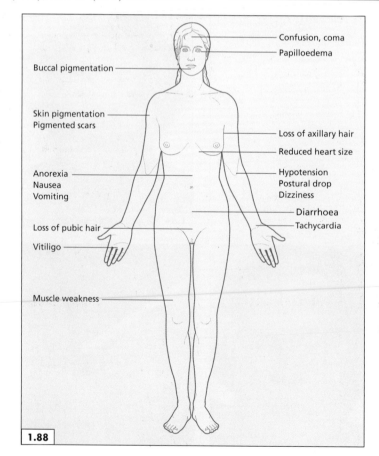

Confusion, coma
Papilloedema
Buccal pigmentation
Skin pigmentation
Pigmented scars
Loss of axillary hair
Reduced heart size
Anorexia
Nausea
Vomiting
Hypotension
Postural drop
Dizziness
Diarrhoea
Tachycardia
Loss of pubic hair
Vitiligo
Muscle weakness

1.88
Clinical features of Addison's disease

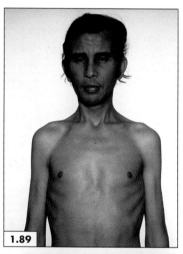

1.89
Loss of weight and pigmentation

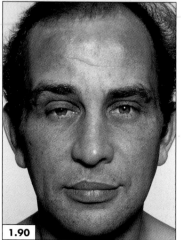

1.90
Pigmentation

in scars (1.94). The inside of the mouth should be examined for the presence of pigmentation on the gums and buccal mucosa (1.95). There is often a loss of pubic hair in females.

Laboratory diagnosis is made by demonstrating impaired production of adrenal cortical hormones, principally cortisol. Plasma cortisol levels may be normal under resting conditions but fail to rise after the administration of ACTH. A short *synacthen test* can be performed as a screening procedure on an ambulant patient.

Hypopituitarism

Many endocrinologists would admit that although the facies of **hypopituitarism** have some distinct features, these are often only appreciated if taken in conjunction with the other clinical findings (1.96), or if the presence of an aetiological factor is suspected. The changes are often subtle and their emergence into the eventual picture depends on the degree of pituitary failure, the pattern of individual hormone deficiencies and the underlying pathology.

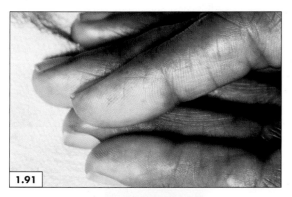

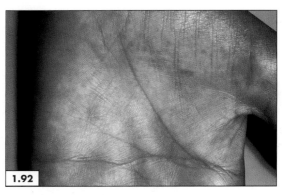

1.91
Addison's disease: hyperpigmentation of the fingers

1.92
Dark palmar creases

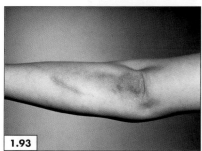

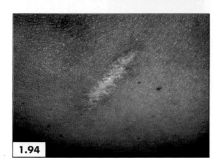

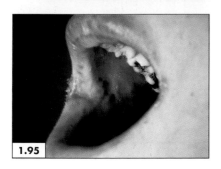

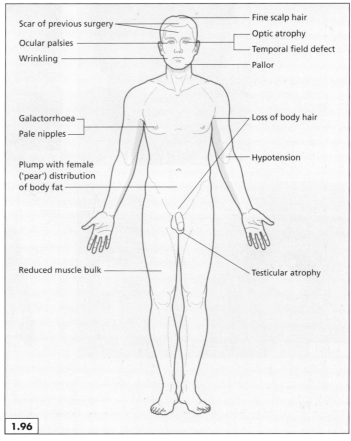

Scar of previous surgery
Ocular palsies
Wrinkling
Galactorrhoea
Pale nipples
Plump with female ('pear') distribution of body fat
Reduced muscle bulk

Fine scalp hair
Optic atrophy
Temporal field defect
Pallor
Loss of body hair
Hypotension
Testicular atrophy

1.93
Pigmented skin creases

1.94
Pigmentation in and around a scar

1.95
Pigmentation of the buccal mucosa

1.96
Clinical features of hypopituitarism

Clinical confirmation

The face has an ageing, pale, waxy appearance (1.97), and fine wrinkles can be seen at the angles of the mouth and eyes (gonadotrophin failure) (1.98). Thyrotrophin deficiency adds its own features including dryness of the skin, dull and lustreless eyes, neutral looks and sparse hair (1.99), but these are seldom as gross as in primary thyroid failure.

The pallor of the skin (1.100, 1.101) is out of proportion to the degree of the anaemia (haemoglobin usually about 10–11 g/dl), contrasting with the pinkish conjunctiva. The nutritional state of the patient is good but there is generalized pallor, loss of hair and gonadal atrophy (1.102).

1.97
Pale, waxy
complexion

1.98
Periorbital angular
wrinkling

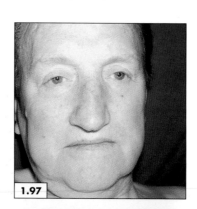

1.97

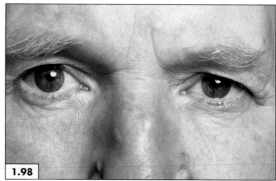

1.98

1.99
Pituitary
hypothyroidism

1.100
Pale skin

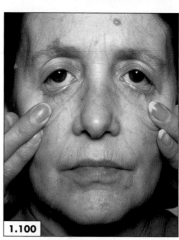

1.99

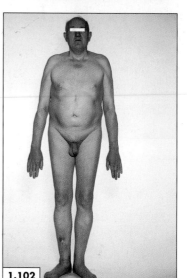

1.100

1.101
Pinkish conjunctiva,
pale skin

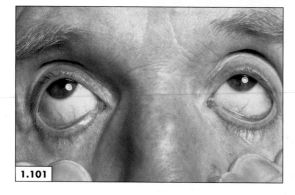

1.101

1.102
Hypopituitarism with
loss of hair, gonadal
atrophy

1.102

In men, hair loss involves the chest (1.103) and the axillae (1.104) and there is loss of pubic hair in both sexes. A closer look shows empty follicle pits unassociated with any dermatological disorder (1.105).

Laboratory diagnosis is essential since the patient will be committed to replacement therapy for life. The diagnostic work-up includes the measurement of end-organ and pituitary hormones, their inadequate response to insulin-induced hypoglycaemia and neuroanatomical studies. Computerized tomography (CT) and magnetic resonance imaging (MRI) scans are often necessary to define the underlying disorder.

Neuromuscular facies

Although facial expressions originate in the cerebral cortex, their shape, substance and communicability depend on the content and overall integrity of the anatomical structures of the face. The eyes are by far the most important among these structures and give life, meaning and direction to any expression. All clinical assessments start at the eyes of the patient even by those clinicians who profess to begin their examination by looking at a patient's hands! Physicians maintain eye contact with their patients, not only to get behind their verbal and facial expressions but also to look for any anatomical and functional abnormalities. Any abnormality in one part often affects, and cannot be entirely separated from, the other structures of the face.

The eyes

Ptosis

Of the various abnormalities in the eyes and eyelids, ptosis is the one that can be detected by a single look and from a distance. It is also the one that is often missed by the unwary clinician. The various causes of ptosis are given in Table 1.4 and it is obvious that this easily detectable sign can often direct one's attention to a serious disorder of the central nervous system. Ptosis may be mild and unilateral

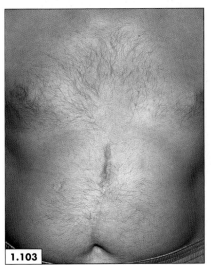

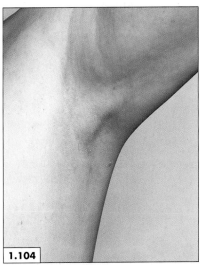

1.103
Hair loss

1.104
Axillary hair loss

1.105
Empty follicle pits

Table 1.4 Causes of ptosis

Type	Cause
Congenital	Levator muscle/oculomotor nerve maldevelopment may be unilateral or bilateral
Local disease	Dehiscence of levator aponeurosis, inflammatory (e.g. chalazion, stye), infiltrative (e.g. amyloidosis, lymphoma, etc.)
Myopathic	Myasthenia, botulism, myotonic dystrophy, chronic progressive external ophthalmoplegia
Neuropathic	Horner's syndrome, oculomotor paresis, tabes dorsalis, Guillain–Barré syndrome, mid-brain lesion, facial paresis, frontal lobe lesions

when a part of the eyeball can be seen (1.106), or it may be complete, which is usually caused by a third cranial nerve palsy (1.107). The diagnosis can be made by carrying out a few clinical tests. Bilateral ptosis is almost always incomplete and may affect one eye more than the other; indeed, there may not be any other additional neuromuscular signs in the face (1.108). In the absence of any muscular disorder, the frontalis muscle is usually wrinkled over the forehead, in an effort to compensate for the droopy eyelids (1.109).

Differential diagnosis of ptosis

The clinical diagnosis of ptosis and an understanding of its underlying pathology both depend on answering several questions. First it must be established whether the ptosis is real by asking the subject to look upwards without tilting the head, since some normal subjects, particularly of Asian origin, have droopy upper eyelids that they can lift when

1.106
Partial and unequal ptosis

1.107
Complete right ptosis

1.108
Partial ptosis

1.109
Ptosis with overaction of frontalis

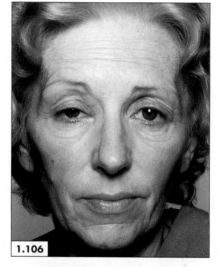
1.106

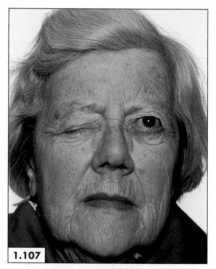
1.107

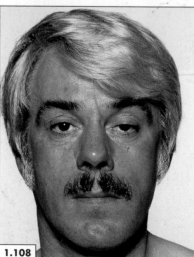
1.108

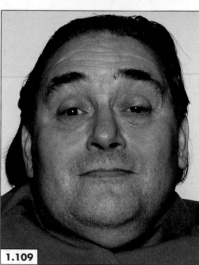
1.109

so required. This procedure also provides an opportunity to distinguish the ptosis of a *sympathetic paresis* (**Horner's syndrome**) from that of a third cranial nerve palsy, since in patients with a smooth muscle paresis the upper lid *lifts* when the patient tries to stare or look upwards. This patient with a right Horner's syndrome (1.110) can lift his right eyelid up to the limbus when he tries to stare (1.111), whereas the patient with a right third cranial nerve palsy is unable to do so (1.112). Note the smaller pupil on the right in 1.111.

This method may seem too difficult for a proper interpretation by those not trained in the subtleties of neurol-

ogy. An easier method is to look at the eyes and answer the following three questions:

1. Is the pupil on the side of the ptosis small? If so **Horner's syndrome** (1.111, 1.113) is suspected.
2. Is the pupil of normal size (1.112) or large (1.114)? If large, the **probable** diagnosis is **third cranial nerve palsy**.
3. Is there an associated ocular palsy? If so **third cranial nerve palsy** or **myasthenia gravis** is suspected.

To answer these questions satisfactorily the eye must be examined carefully for any abnormalities of the lids or

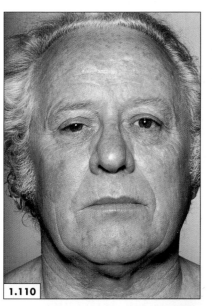

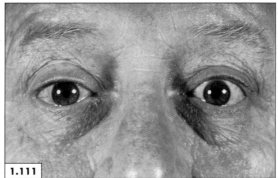

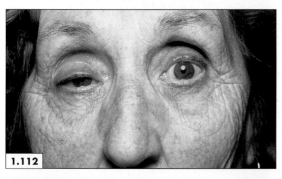

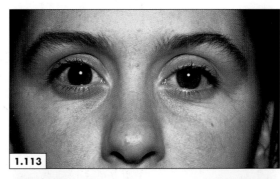

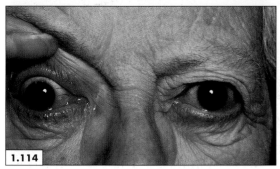

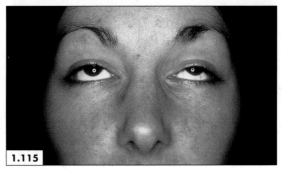

1.110
Right Horner's syndrome

1.111
Able to stare! Note smaller right pupil

1.112
Right third cranial nerve palsy: unable to stare!

1.113
Left Horner's syndrome

1.114
Right third cranial nerve palsy: complete ptosis and large pupil

1.115
Myotonic dystrophy: ptosis with unwrinkled face

globe and for any ocular palsies (see Table 1.1). Finally, one needs to consider whether the ptosis is a part of a neuromuscular disorder such as **myasthenia gravis**, **myotonia dystrophica** and **mitochondrial myopathy**.

Patients with a myotonic dystrophy tend to have a long, lean, expressionless face and they can neither lift their upper eyelids nor create any wrinkles on their forehead (1.115). Bilateral ptosis with *overaction of the frontalis* may be **congenital** and be present since birth, as in this patient (1.116), or acquired as in **tabes dorsalis** (1.117). The ptosis of myasthenia gravis tends to get worse as the day progresses or if the patient is asked to open and close the eyes

repeatedly; in this situation it improves after an intravenous injection of edrophonium (1.118, 1.119).

Ocular palsies

Complete or partial ptosis associated with a dilated pupil on the affected side is always the result of a third cranial nerve palsy (1.120). Deviation or strabismus of the eyeball can also be caused by a fourth or sixth cranial nerve palsy as in this patient (1.121), whose right eye is turned inwards because of the weakness of the right lateral rectus muscle, thereby permitting unopposed adduction by the medial

1.116
Congenital ptosis

1.117
Acquired ptosis with overaction of frontalis

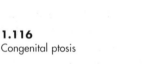

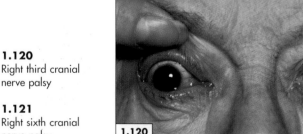

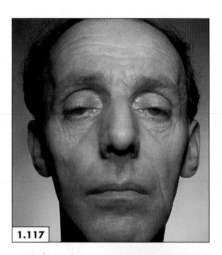

1.118
Before and 30 s after intravenous edrophonium

1.119
Before and 1 min after intravenous edrophonium

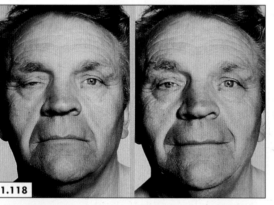

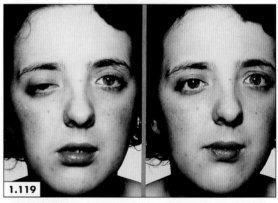

1.120
Right third cranial nerve palsy

1.121
Right sixth cranial nerve palsy

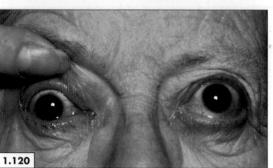

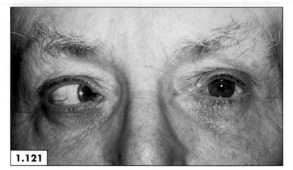

rectus. Apart from a strabismus, one should ascertain whether the patient experiences diplopia and whether there is any proptosis. The former confirms that there is an ocular palsy and its direction is suggestive of the particular cranial nerve involved. Proptosis suggests the presence of a local pathology.

If the fifth cranial nerve is also involved as part of **mononeuritis multiplex**, then the ptosis may be associated with inflammation of the eyelids and loss of the soft portion of the nose (1.122), due to sensory deprivation and consequent failure of protection from recurrent trauma.

Ocular myopathy begins with a progressive bilateral ptosis (1.123). There is often a myopathy of other external ocular muscles and sometimes there is evidence of other concomitant lesions in the central nervous system (e.g. paraplegia, retinitis pigmentosa, ataxia). Mitochondrial abnormalities have been reported both in ocular and skeletal muscles.

Differential diagnosis of ocular palsies

The diagnosis of a third, fourth, or sixth cranial nerve palsy can be made by testing the eye movements in nine directions – straight in front, to the right, to the left, up, down, to the right and up, to the left and up, down to the right and down to the left. Apart from the full movement of the eyeball in each direction, the patient should be asked to report the appearance of any diplopia, which suggests weakness of the muscle that acts in that direction. Figures 1.124–1.129 were obtained from a patient with a right **cavernous sinus thrombosis** affecting the right third, fourth and sixth cranial nerves. These pictures illustrate the usefulness of testing the eye movements.

Right third cranial nerve palsy is suggested by a complete ptosis (1.130), dilatation of the pupil (1.124) and the inability to elevate (1.128) and adduct the eyeball (1.126); this is because the third cranial nerve supplies the levator of the upper lid, the constrictor of the pupil, all the extrinsic muscles of the eye except the lateral rectus (the sixth cranial nerve) and the superior oblique muscle (the fourth cranial nerve). The patient is unable to look to the right because of the right lateral rectus (sixth cranial nerve) palsy (1.125), or downwards and inwards (1.129) because of right third and fourth cranial nerve palsy. Often it is difficult to test the integrity of the fourth cranial nerve (downward gaze of the adducted eyeball) when there is a coexistent third cranial nerve palsy, as this renders adduction of the eyeball incomplete or altogether impossible. However, if one looks carefully at the affected eyeball, it will be seen to *intort* when a patient with right third cranial nerve palsy but with an intact fourth cranial nerve attempts to look down and to the left.

Figure 1.131 shows an example of an **internuclear ophthalmoplegia**; the top and the bottom panels show the left lateral gaze, which reveals paresis of the right internal rectus. When the patient tries to look in the opposite direction (to the right, see middle panel) it is the left internal rectus that now fails to follow. The *failure of adduction* is a pathognomonic sign of the internuclear ophthalmoplegia caused by a lesion in the medial longitudinal fasciculus. This patient had **multiple sclerosis**.

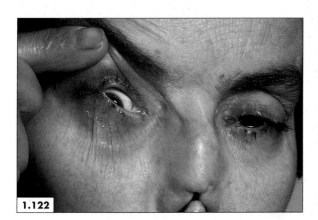

1.122

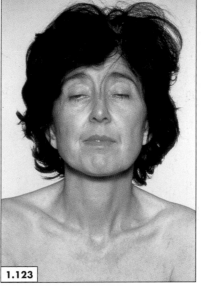

1.123

1.122
Mononeuritis multiplex: bilateral third, fourth, fifth and sixth cranial nerve palsy

1.123
Bilateral ptosis

1.124
Looking straight in front

1.125
Looking to the right

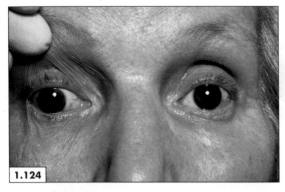
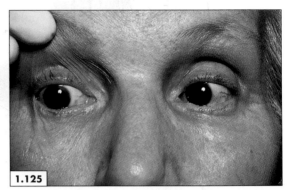

1.126
Looking to the left

1.127
Looking down

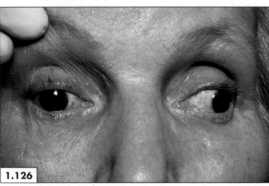
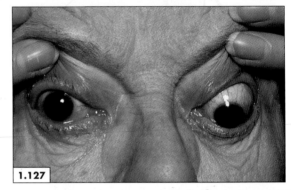

1.128
Looking up

1.129
Looking down and inwards

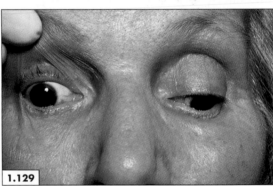

1.130
Complete ptosis

1.131
Internuclear ophthalmoplegia: failure of adduction

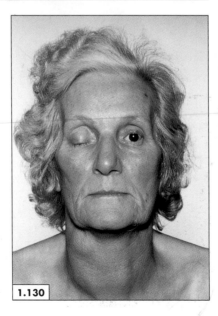
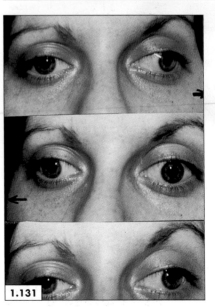

Proptosis

Proptosis associated with an ocular palsy may point to a cavernous sinus thrombosis with the involvement of one or more of the ocular nerves as they traverse the sinus. Proptosis of a moderately severe degree can confuse the diagnosis since a protruding eyeball does not move freely in various directions and falsely suggests an ocular palsy.

A **unilateral proptosis** of any degree is easy to recognize so long as one remembers to compare it with the normal side (1.132). Many clinical teachers advocate that patients with a suspected proptosis should be observed from above. This procedure, when performed properly, can be successful in showing the bulge of the proptosed eye above the level of the normal eye, both in gross proptosis (1.133) and when there is only a moderate degree of proptosis (1.134, 1.135). However, a careful look at the protuberant eyeball, the periorbital furrows that are filled out, and at the lateral view of the eyeball compared with the normal side, is all that one needs to distinguish a protruding eyeball from a normal one (1.136, 1.137).

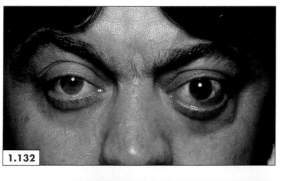

1.132
Left proptosis

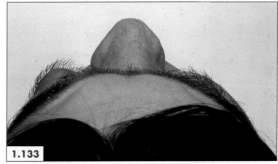

1.133
Viewed from above

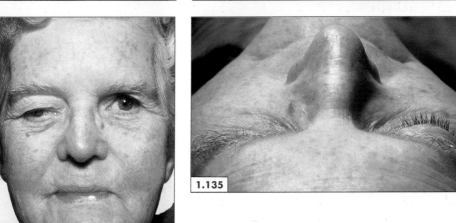

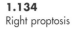

1.134
Right proptosis

1.135
Viewed from above

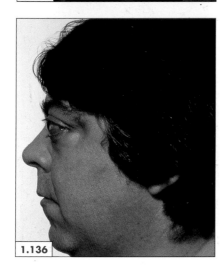

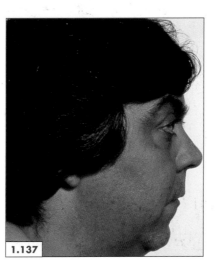

1.136
Proptosed eye

1.137
Normal eye

This procedure can be successful even when there is only a modest degree of proptosis, which can be suspected first by looking at a patient's face (1.138). Comparing the eyes with each other and by looking at each eye carefully, the superior periorbital sulcus clearly seen above the right eye (1.139) is obscured by the bulging eyeball on the left side (1.140). The lower eyelid also looks a little fuller on the left side and the left eye does not look so comfortably housed in the orbit, unlike the right eye with room to spare.

The examination of proptosis should be completed by determining its direction, whether it is pulsatile and reducible (by gently pressing on the eyeball) as it was in this patient with a **carotid-cavernous fistula** (1.138), or whether it is fixed and irreducible as in Figure 1.132.

Pupillary abnormalities

Pupillary abnormalities may be bilateral, as in **neurosyphilis**, or unilateral, as in the **Holmes–Adie syndrome** (myotonic pupil). A clinician's task is not only to spot the asymmetry but also to identify the abnormal side. Often there are associated abnormalities in the eyeball or eyelids such as a partial ptosis in Horner's syndrome (1.141) or complete ptosis in a third cranial nerve palsy (1.142).

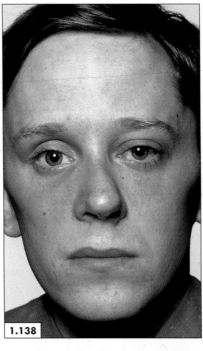

1.138
Left proptosis

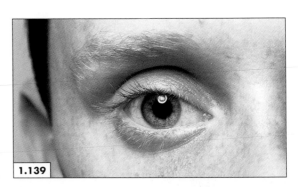

1.139

1.139
Normal orbital contours

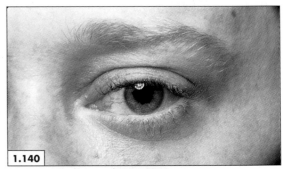

1.140

1.140
Obscured superior orbital furrow

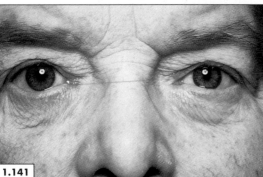

1.141
Left Horner's syndrome

1.142
Left third cranial nerve palsy

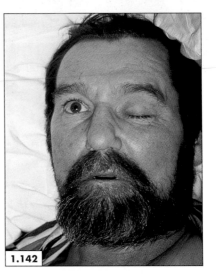

1.142

The absence of any ocular abnormalities associated with a dilated pupil (1.143) suggests a diagnosis of the myotonic pupil, a condition usually seen in young women and often associated with absent ankle and knee jerks. Such pupils are always regular but *react poorly* to light and on accommodation. The **Argyll Robertson pupils** are small (1.144), often irregular and unequal (although these changes may be very subtle), and their characteristic feature is that they are either non-reactive to light or react poorly but respond *better* on accommodation. Their reaction to light and accommodation is sometimes difficult to determine because of their small size but, on repeated testing, some reaction on accommodation can be detected in the pupils that are non-reactive even to intense light.

Facial muscles

Facial muscles make a major contribution to the contour and shape of the face. Any weakness or wasting of one or more muscles is betrayed by a resulting asymmetry and distortion of the facial features. Atrophy of one side of the face – **facial hemiatrophy** – may occur in otherwise healthy subjects (1.145). This is a rare disorder and is often heralded by the appearance of a dimple, which progressively enlarges and, within a few years, invovles all the structures on one side of the face. The abnormal side (1.146) with its infrazygomatic pit, thinned nose and hollow periorbital spaces shows a striking contrast to the normal side (1.147), which looks full and fleshy.

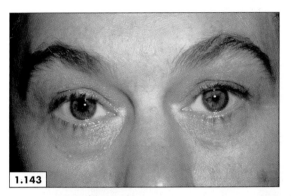

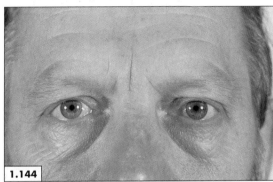

1.143
Holmes–Adie syndrome

1.144
Argyll Robertson pupils

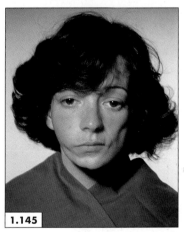

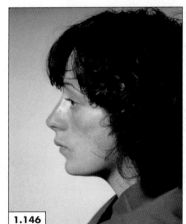

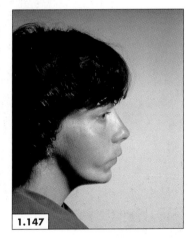

1.145
Facial hemiatrophy

1.146
Hollow side

1.147
Normal side

Myopathic facies are characteristically unwrinkled, expressionless and sad, with lax and pouting lips, as seen in this patient with **myotonia dystrophica** (1.148). This long, lean and expressionless face with gaping lips can be detected even in young subjects with the condition (1.149). An expressionless face may also be seen in association with the **facioscapulohumeral muscular dystrophy** (1.150). There is characteristic pouting of the lips, which, together with poverty of expression, is seen even in those patients in whom muscular wasting of the face is not very marked

and in whom there is no ptosis (1.151). This form has an autosomal dominant inheritance but there is substantial variation in the severity in affected members of the same family. In contrast, profound muscular wasting of the entire face, as in this patient with **bulbospinal muscular atrophy** (1.152), gives the face a characteristic appearance with wide, noncommunicative eyes, lax and open lips, an unlined face and a sagging lower jaw. Facial features are much less marked in the early stages of **myasthenia gravis** when ptosis may be the only abnormality (1.153).

1.148
Myopathic facies: bilateral ptosis with a smooth, unlined face

1.149
Long, lean face with pouting lips

1.150
Facial muscular atrophy: unwrinkled, expressionless face

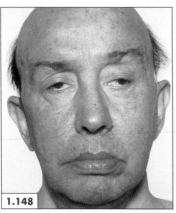

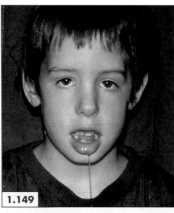

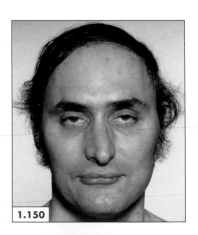

1.151
Mild facial muscular wasting

1.152
Severe facial muscular wasting: wide open eyes and a lax, partially open mouth

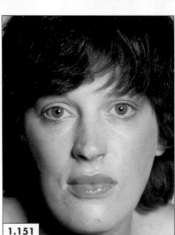

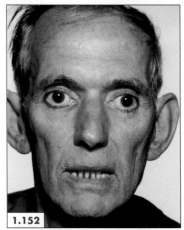

1.153
Ptosis in myasthenia gravis

1.154
Right Bell's palsy: wide open right eye, smooth right face

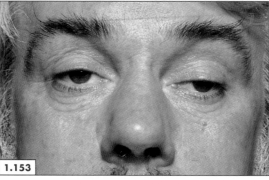

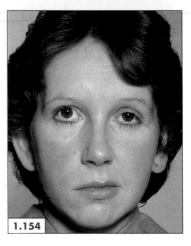

Facial nerve palsy is by far the commonest abnormal neuromuscular facies encountered in clinical practice. In its complete form, as in **Bell's palsy** (1.154), there is paralysis of the upper and lower parts of the face, the wrinkles on the affected side of the forehead and the nasolabial fold are smoothed out, both the eyelids look lax and somewhat retracted and the corner of the mouth appears to droop.

In the **upper motor neurone muscular weakness** (e.g. lesion in the internal capsule), the paralysis is less well marked and spares the upper part of the face if the lesion is supranuclear since there is bilateral innervation of the forehead from the corticobulbar fibres. This fact tends to be overemphasized by clinical teachers since, despite the bilateral innervation, there is often some widening of the eyebrows on the affected side. Emotional and involuntary movements such as spontaneous smiling may be much less affected. Voluntary effort to force a smile and retract the angles of the mouth reveals the weakness on the right side in this patient with weakness of the facial muscles of central origin (1.155).

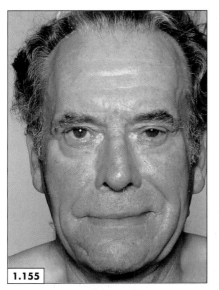

1.155

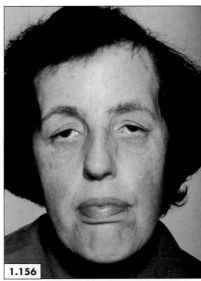

1.156

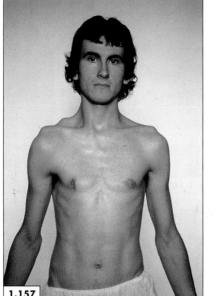

1.157

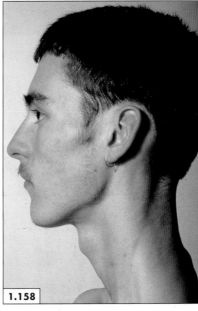

1.158

1.155
Right hemiparesis

1.156
Myotonia
dystrophica

1.157
Facioscapulohumeral
muscular atrophy

1.158
Attenuated facial
and neck muscles

Differential diagnosis

Both a family and personal past history of muscular weakness, details of the onset and of any associated symptoms, and a neurological examination all help to establish the diagnosis. Facioscapulohumeral (Landouzy and Dejerine) type and myotonia dystrophica are both inherited familial disorders, transmitted through an autosomal dominant gene. Other members of the family may be affected, although in a remarkably varying degree. Myotonia dystrophica occurs more commonly in males and is often heralded by myotonia whereby *relaxation* of a muscle after use is *slow and incomplete*, embarrassingly noticeable during a handshake! Other associated features are testicular atrophy, cataract, pre-mature senility and alopecia causing frontal baldness in both sexes (1.156).

The facioscapulohumeral type occurs equally in both sexes and affects the muscles of the face and shoulder girdles (1.157). Both the face and neck usually look thin and attenuated (1.158) and there is often profound wasting of the thoracic muscles with *winging of the scapulae* (1.159). This sign may be demonstrable even in patients with minimal muscle wasting (1.160). The weakness is often remarkably selective with bilateral prominence of the scapulae (1.159) and weakness of the pectoral muscles. The facial muscles are involved first and then the weakness descends to the scapular muscles and the muscles of the upper arms and anterior legs. Other muscles may be spared altogether or may be only minimally weak.

1.159
Winging of the scapulae

1.160
Winging with mild muscular wasting

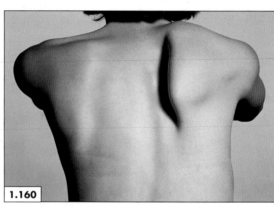

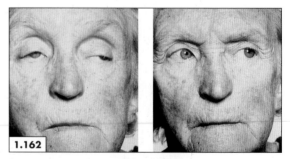

1.161 and 1.162
Improvement after intravenous edrophonium

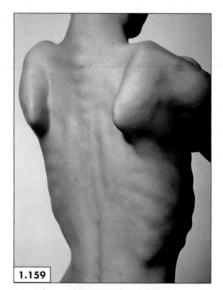

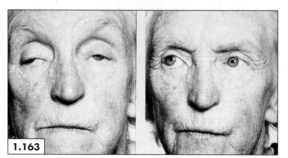

1.163 and 1.164
Myasthenia gravis: before and after intravenous edrophonium

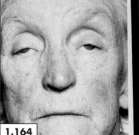

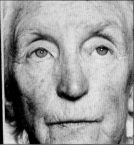

In a typical case, myasthenia gravis is easy to diagnose by its characteristic abnormal fatiguability that affects a diverse range of motor functions such as talking, combing, chewing, shaving, typing, walking, etc. The patient is better in the morning after a night's rest but the symptoms return as the day progresses when the patient may have diplopia, the voice may be hoarse and even smiling may become an effort. The *edrophonium test* can confirm the diagnosis and may be very useful in difficult cases. A good response is indicated by a marked improvement in the ptosis and by the restoration of free ocular movements in all directions (1.161–1.164). The improvement may be seen within a few seconds and the patient may lose his or her ptosis and be able to look upwards 30–60s after the injection, as illustrated in the three sequential panels in 1.165.

This patient with a complete Bell's palsy is unable to close her eye on the affected side (1.166), the eyeball rolls upwards on attempted closure (*Bell's phenomenon*) and the eyelids can be separated easily on the affected side (1.167). The patient with a partial palsy or the patient recovering from a complete palsy can close the eye but cannot bury the eyelashes (1.168). If asked to smile, the face contracts to the normal side (1.169) and the patient is unable to puff out her cheek on the affected side (1.170).

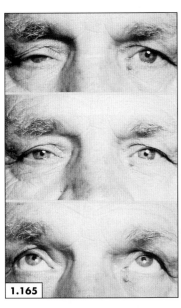

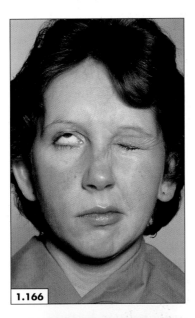

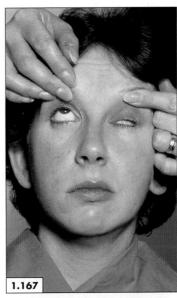

1.165
Myasthenia gravis: response to intravenous edrophonium

1.166
Bell's palsy: unable to close the eye

1.167
Bell's phenomenon

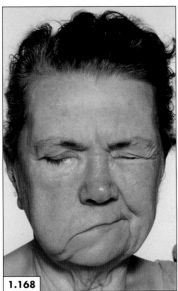

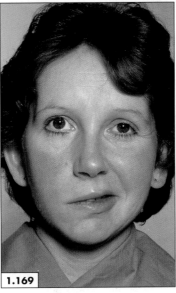

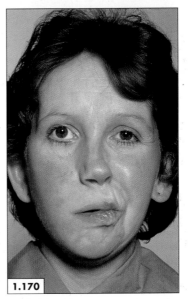

1.168
Unable to bury the eyelashes

1.169
Contraction towards the normal side

1.170
Unable to puff out the affected cheek

The external auditory meatus should be examined for the presence of a herpetic eruption (1.171), which is associated with herpes zoster of the geniculate ganglion in patients with the **Ramsay Hunt syndrome**. Taste is lost over the anterior two-thirds of the tongue.

Skin and mucosal lesions

Dermatology is a pictorial subject and skin lesions can be recognized by a careful inspection of the lesion, the skin around it, its distribution and the uniqueness of its pattern, followed by examination of the other expected systemic and cutaneous abnormalities. A generalist may usefully begin by deciding whether the lesion represents one of the **dermatoses** such as psoriasis, eczema, acne, etc., or is a manifestation of a **systemic disorder**, such as an endocrine, neoplastic, gastrointestinal or a metabolic disease.

Dermatoses

These comprise several conditions that affect the scalp and the skin of the face.

Common skin conditions

Psoriasis of the scalp usually results in reddish lesions on the hairline (1.172) or plaques with scaling, which often occur either behind or in front of the ear (1.173). The skin between the plaques is normal. Sometimes there is profuse scaling along the hairline (1.174) and the condition is indistinguishable from seborrhoeic dermatitis. This form of psoriasis is often difficult to treat and can result in loss of hair.

The face is not usually involved in psoriasis except in the **guttate** variety in which 'salmon pink' erythematous papules, 2 mm–1 cm in diameter may occur on the face (1.175) and elsewhere on the body (1.176). Guttate (from

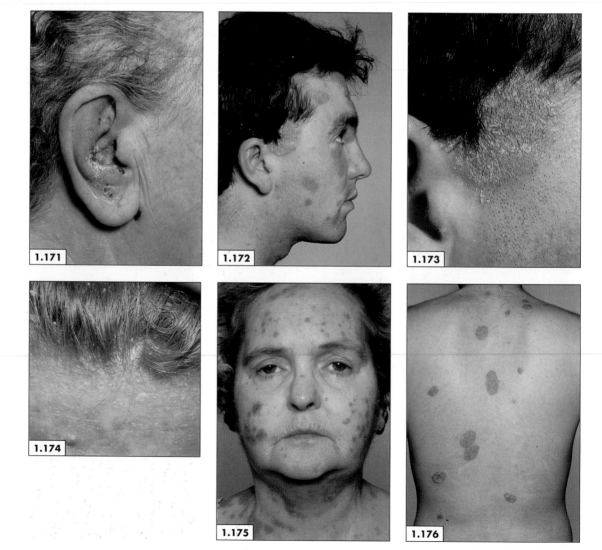

1.171
Resolving herpetic rash

1.172
Predilection for the hairline

1.173
Psoriatic plaque with scaling

1.174
Psoriasis: excessive scaling. Note the erythematous plaques with scaling

1.175
Guttate psoriasis: discrete, erythematous papules and plaques

1.176
Psoriasis: papules with scaling

the Latin meaning 'spots that resemble drops') psoriasis may be chronic but more often appears as an acute exanthem with a shower of papules that develop rapidly in young adults, often following a streptococcal pharyngitis. This form of psoriasis should be distinguished from a psoriasiform drug eruption.

As the name suggests, **contact dermatitis** is an acute (chronic cases also occur) inflammation of the skin caused by contact with an external toxic or antigenic agent. The lesions appear as ill-defined red patches with fine fissuring and nonumbilicated vesicles sometimes covered with crusts. The usual offending agents are plants, washing powders, hair dyes or make-up powder, as in this patient (1.177), and metals. In acute cases, the onset is rapid with erythema, oedema and exudative vesiculation. Pruritus and a burning sensation are the major presenting symptoms.

Atopic eczematous dermatitis affects between 2 and 20% of the population. It is probably even commoner as some patients learn to live with it without consulting their doctors. Histologically, eczema is characterized by a lymphohistiocytic infiltration around the upper dermal vessels, acanthosis and spongiosis. Clinically, the important features are *itching*, *redness*, *scaling* and *papulovesicles*. **Atopic dermatitis** is the commonest of its many variants.

In adults, atopic dermatitis is a chronic recurrent disorder with exacerbations often related to personal psychosocial adversities. There may or may not be a history of childhood atopic dermatitis, asthma and hay fever; nevertheless many patients have a positive family history of the *atopic triad* – dermatitis, asthma and allergic rhinitis. Serum levels of IgE are elevated. In acute cases there is erythema, oedema, exudation and intense *itching*, with resultant excoriations and erosions; there may also be clusters of papulovesicles (1.178). In chronic forms, there may be dryness, scaling and lichenification (thickening of the epidermis with deepening of the skin lines) (1.179), plaques, papulovesicles, excoriations, dry and wet crusts and cracks (1.180).

One of the serious complications associated with atopic dermatitis is the susceptibility to severe and generalized **herpes simplex type 1** infection (**eczema herpeticum**), and to **Kaposi's varicelliform eruption** after vaccination. In patients with atopic dermatitis, a few harmless-looking herpetic vesicles on the lips may soon develop into a generalized papulovesicular eczema herpeticum (1.181).

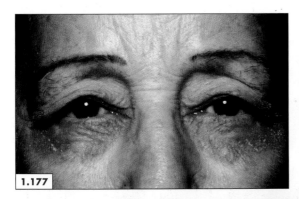

1.177

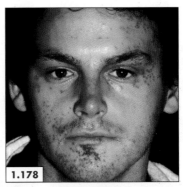

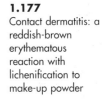

1.177
Contact dermatitis: a reddish-brown erythematous reaction with lichenification to make-up powder

1.178
Atopic dermatitis: papulovesicular lesions on erythematous skin

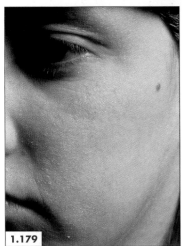

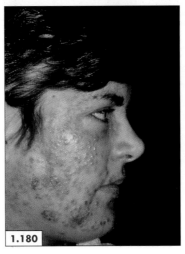

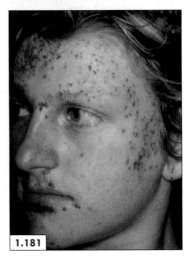

1.179
Chronic atopic dermatitis: lichenification over erythematous skin

1.180
Papulovesicular rash with crusting

1.181
Eczema herpeticum: scattered papulovesicular lesions

In **acne rosacea** there is widespread erythema on the face with red papules (1.182). The rash may also involve the eyelids. These patients have hyperreactive facial vessels, with flushing in response to various stimuli such as hot tea, spicy foods and alcohol. Over a period of years this transient and recurrent flushing produces persistent erythema and papules. In a well-developed case there is usually a purplish-red hue to the face with macules, papules and telangiectasia (1.183). Although called acne rosacea, unlike acne there are neither comedones nor seborrhoea (see 1.201, 1.202).

Urticaria is an intensely *itchy* condition with swelling of the dermis that raises the epidermis into weals (1.184). Acute rashes are often IgE-dependent in patients with an atopic background. In chronic cases the aetiology is mostly unknown. There are special varieties of **cold**, **solar** and **cholinergic urticaria** induced by cold, sunshine (action spectra 290–500 nm) and excessive sweating, respectively.

In **angioneurotic oedema**, the subcutaneous tissue rather than the dermis is swollen, usually affecting the lips, mouth, eyes (1.185) and genitalia. The name is misleading since the nerves and vessels are not involved. A rapid appearance of erythematous weals around the mouth should be regarded as a medical emergency; in this situation the patient should be monitored carefully for any signs of **respiratory obstruction**. The causes are multifactorial as in other urticarias. The hereditary variety is an autosomal dominant disorder and is characterized by life-threatening laryngeal oedema and acute abdominal pains caused by oedema of the bowel wall. During the acute episodes, the facial features are grossly distorted with erythema and swelling (1.186) but there is usually no itching.

1.182
Acne rosacea: erythema with papules

1.183
Maculopapular rash with lichenification

1.184
Urticaria: oedematous dermal weals of varying size

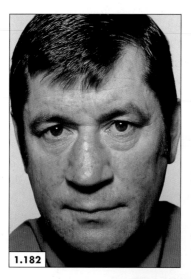

1.182

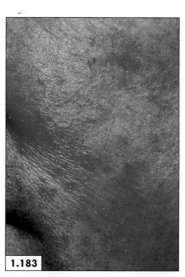

1.183

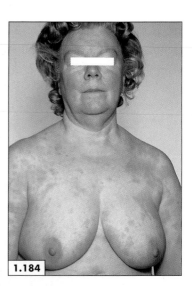

1.184

1.185
Angioneurotic oedema

1.186
Acute erythema and generalized oedema

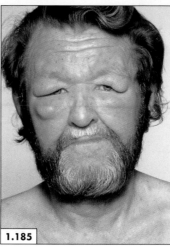

1.185

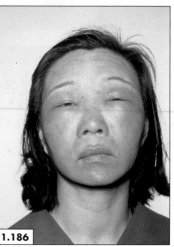

1.186

As the name **erythema multiforme** implies, the cutaneous reaction to circulating immune complexes (stimulated by infections, drugs, collagen diseases, etc.) is diverse, ranging from a maculopapular rash (1.187) to erythematous plaques (1.188), blisters and target lesions. The latter are diagnostic with a central, purplish area or a blister surrounded by a pale, oedematous zone, which in turn is surrounded by a rim of erythema (1.189). These lesions may be scattered all over the body (1.190 and 1.191). The mucous membranes of the eyes and mouth (1.188, 1.192) may also be affected; the condition is then referred to as the **Stevens–Johnson syndrome**. Recurrent herpes simplex infection is a common cause of recurrent erythema multiforme. Other provocating factors are bacterial infec-

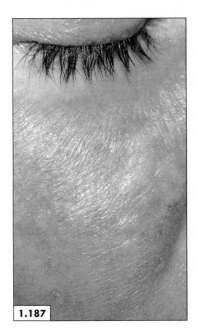

1.187

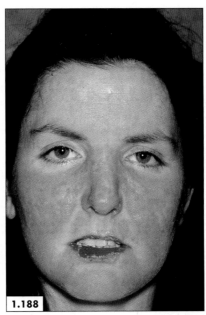

1.188

1.187
Erythema
multiforme:
maculopapular rash

1.188
Stevens–Johnson
syndrome. Note
labial involvement

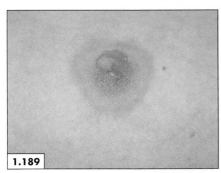

1.189

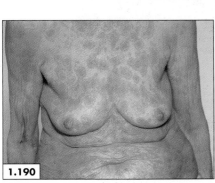

1.190

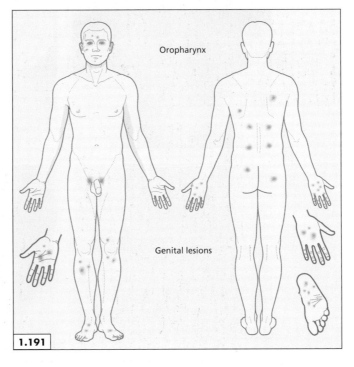

1.191

Oropharynx

Genital lesions

1.189
Target lesion

1.190
Scattered target
lesions

1.191
Distribution of
lesions in erythema
multiforme

tions and a variety of drugs. An association with *Mycoplasma pneumoniae* in young adults has been reported.

Basal cell carcinoma starts as a cluster of small nodules with telangiectasia (1.193) and early ulceration. It occurs mostly on exposed areas, commonly on the face or forehead as in the patient shown in Figure 1.194. It is the commonest form of cutaneous malignancy, grows slowly (the lesion has often been present for over a year before the patient seeks advice) and causes locally destructive changes, hence it is also called **rodent ulcer**.

Infections

Folliculitis results when the hair follicles become infected with *Staphylococcus* spp. On the face the infection may spread by shaving (**sycosis barbae**) (1.195). The hallmark of the lesion is the pustule confined to the ostium of the hair follicle (1.196). Papulopustules may coalesce to form indurated plaques.

Staphylococcal or streptococcal infection of the epidermis causes thin-roofed vesicles or pustules which often become crusted because of scratching – a condition known as **impetigo contagiosa** (1.197). This condition predominantly

1.192
Stevens–Johnson syndrome

1.193
Early basal cell carcinoma: coalescing cluster of reddish nodules

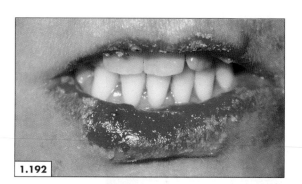
1.192

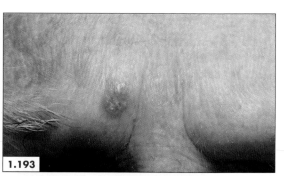
1.193

1.194
Basal cell carcinoma: common site

1.195
Sycosis barbae

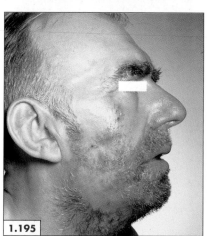
1.194

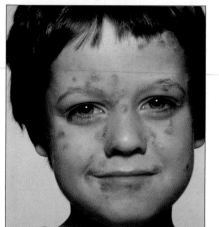
1.195

1.196
Pustules arising in the hair pits

1.197
Impetigo contagiosa

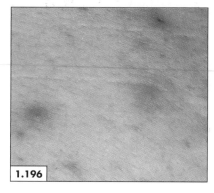
1.196

1.197

occurs in children and young adults with poor hygiene and crowded living conditions. The face and hands are the sites most commonly affected and the hallmark of impetigo is *honey-coloured crusting* (1.198, 1.199). Lesions develop rapidly and the infection can spread to those in close contact with the patient. It may complicate pre-existing atopic dermatitis and in some susceptible children a bullous form of impetigo occurs (1.200), which can be difficult to treat.

Acne vulgaris is essentially a disease of adolescence and affects the sebaceous glands, with an increase in sebum production and sebaceous duct blockage at puberty. Fol-licular papules appear and these often develop into pustules (**comedones**) with whiteheads (closed) or blackheads (open) (1.201). There may also be nodules, nodulo-ulcerative lesions, cysts, scars and considerable seborrhoea of the face and scalp (1.202).

In moderately severe cases, the entire face and forehead is affected with papules and pustules (1.203). Mild to moderate lesions heal without scarring. In severe cases, rupture of the follicles and inflammation lead to dermal damage leaving behind scarred pits (1.204). The condition deteriorates premenstrually in some women, while pregnancy has

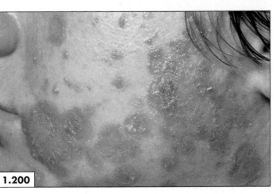

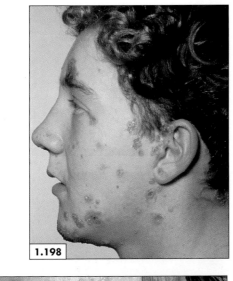

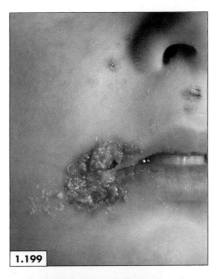

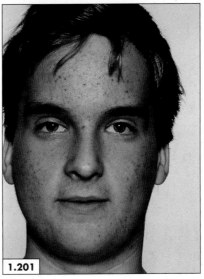

1.198
Impetigo: multiple small abscesses

1.199
Impetigo: honey-coloured crusting

1.200
Bullous impetigo: thin-walled, intraepidermal bullae

1.201
Acne: comedones with blackheads

a beneficial effect. **Tropical acne** (in young Caucasians living in the Far East), **steroid acne** (in patients with Cushing's syndrome or those on corticosteroids), and **chemical acne** (in patients exposed to chlorinated hydrocarbons) are some of the variants.

Erysipelas is an acute, spreading streptococcal infection of the dermal and subdermal tissues causing *tender*

erythematous induration with sharply defined, irregular borders (1.205). It may occur anywhere on the body but is often seen on the face and legs. **Immunocompromised states** such as **diabetes mellitus** and some **haematological malignancies** are the usual underlying risk factors but erysipelas may occur in otherwise healthy subjects. The organism gains entry through a minor abrasion (usually

1.202
Acne with
seborrhoea

1.203
Acne: multiple
papulopustular
lesions

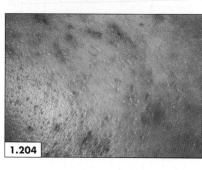

1.204
Acne: scarring

1.205
Erysipelas: cellulitis
with well-defined
borders

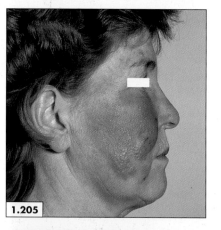

1.206
Widespread
erysipelas affecting
both sides of the
face

1.207
Shiny, reddish-
brown plaque with
scarring

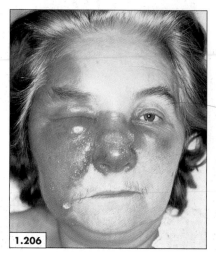

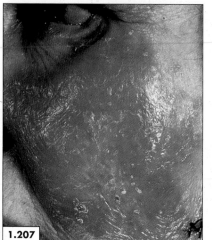

visible on the surface) and infects the superficial lymphatics. Erysipelas is usually unilateral but, in severe cases, the infection may spread to both sides of the face and the neck (1.206). Recurrent infection of the same site can lead to **chronic lymphoedema**.

Lupus vulgaris is a form of cutaneous tuberculosis and often evolves as clusters of flat, brownish-red papules with ulceration, scarring and disfigurement (1.207). In contrast, **lupus pernio** (cutaneous sarcoidosis) is a bluish-red granuloma that neither gives an appearance of translucency nor causes scarring (1.208; see also 1.282 and 1.283) despite diffuse granulomatous involvement of the nose in some cases (1.209). Lupus vulgaris has become rare since the advent of effective antituberculous treatment but cases are still seen in northern Europe – more commonly in females, children and the elderly.

The infection commonly affects the face and neck but may also occur on the arms (1.210) and legs. Initially, the lesions look like firm, translucent, brownish-red nodules (1.211). Ulcerative forms can present as serpiginous, punched-out ulcers surrounded by a brownish infiltrate, which is referred to as 'apple-jelly' (yellowish-brown) because of its appearance when a glass slide is pressed on the surface (diascopy).

Tinea capitis is caused by ringworm fungal infection of the scalp. There is excessive scaling, fracture of the hairs (*'dots' on the surface*) atrophy of the skin (1.212) and sometimes pustule formation with adherent yellowish crusts.

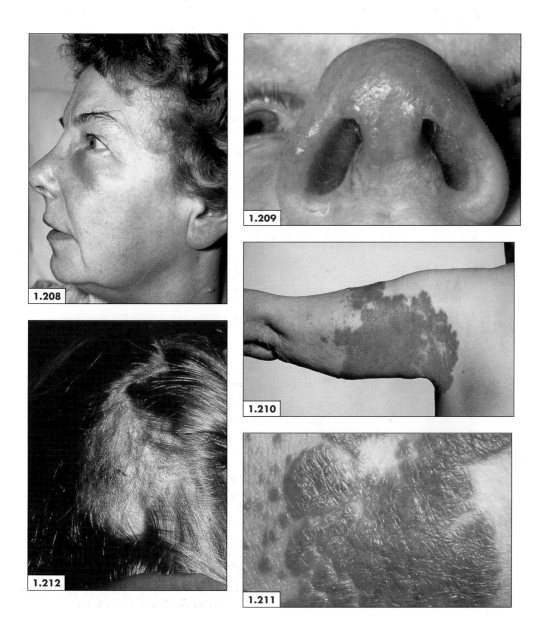

1.208
Lupus pernio

1.209
Cutaneous sarcoidisis with granulomatosis infiltration of the skin

1.210
Lupus vulgaris

1.211
Lupus vulgaris: reddish nodules and plaques

1.212
Tinea capitis: fractured hairs

These scaling papular lesions of **tinea corporis** occur in an annular formation, spreading peripherally and clearing centrally (1.213). The outer border is red and irregular with fine scaling. The lesions occur on the face, limbs and trunk.

Herpes zoster is a common and easily recognizable condition caused by the varicella virus and characterized by a localized vesicular or bullous eruption, usually limited to a dermatome (often the ophthalmic branch of the trigeminal nerve; 1.214), which is innervated by the corresponding sensory ganglion. Along the distribution of a cutaneous nerve there are usually clusters of vesicles with erythema, oedema and scabs (1.215). Intense pain can be a very distressing and chronic feature of this condition.

Blistering diseases

Of the common blistering disorders, erythema multiforme and herpes zoster have been mentioned already, and herpes simplex will be discussed in the next chapter. Dermatitis herpetiformis and porphyria are referred to later in this chapter (see Systemic Disorders). Since pemphigus often, and pemphigoid sometimes, can affect the face, these will be presented here briefly.

Pemphigus vulgaris usually starts in the oral mucosa and then many months later involves the skin of the face (1.216). Large, thin bullae occur usually on normal skin and on rupture leave non-healing, red erosions on the face (1.217) and scalp (1.218). The epidermis can be made to

1.213
Tinea corporis: advancing erythema with scaling

1.214
Herpes zoster: ruptured blisters with crusting

1.215
Clusters of vesicles with scabs

1.216
Pemphigus: ruptured bullae and mucosal lesions

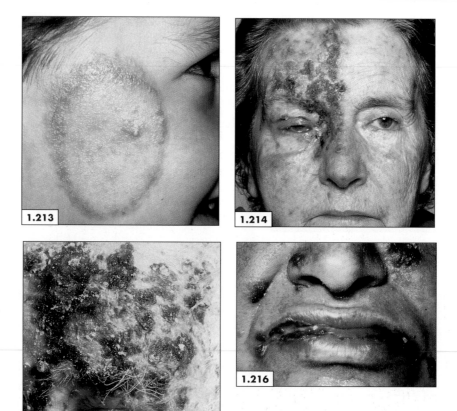

slide over the underlying dermis if lateral pressure is applied to the skin with the thumb (*Nikolsky sign*). Pruritus is not a feature but the ruptured, raw erosions are painful. Secondary infection and electrolyte imbalance are common complications of generalized pemphigus.

Pemphigoid involves the face much less commonly than pemphigus. Initially the lesions often appear as urticaria, eczema or erythema (1.219) and then evolve to form thick bullae, which may appear suddenly over various parts of the body (1.220). Unlike pemphigus, these lesions may itch but they are less painful and the bullae are thick and rupture less easily.

An important diagnostic feature between pemphigus and pemphigoid is that in the former the bullae arise from within the epidermis and are consequently thin and easily ruptured. In pemphigoid, on the other hand, the bullae are dermal–epidermal, thick and not easily ruptured. Thus, when one encounters a patient with many intact bullae then pemphigoid takes the top place in the diagnostic consideration. It is important to bear this in mind when considering the various blistering disorders (see Table 1.7).

The differential diagnosis of these conditions is further discussed on page **60**.

Infectious exanthemata

Since the advent of effective vaccination, the blotchy erythematous rash of **measles** (1.221) is seen less often today.

Table 1.5 Some causes of vesiculobullous diseases

Intradermal (thin) blisters	Dermal–epidermal (thick) blisters
Pemphigus	Pemphigoid
Herpes simplex	Dermatitis herpetiformis
	Herpes gestationis
Herpes zoster	Erythema multiforme
Toxic epidermal necrolysis	Porphyria cutanea tarda
Bullous impetigo	Bullous disease in diabetes mellitus

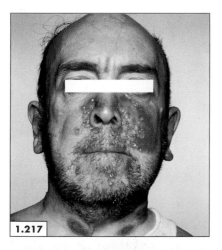

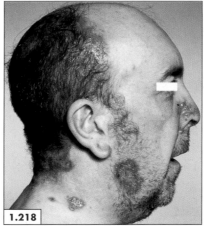

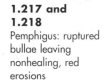

1.217 and 1.218 Pemphigus: ruptured bullae leaving nonhealing, red erosions

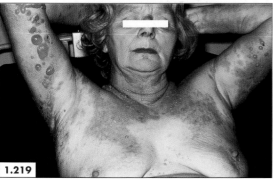

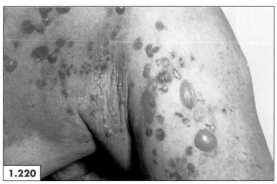

1.219 and 1.220 Pemphigoid: erythematous lesions and intact, thick bullae

The maculopapular rash, which rapidly coalesces to large, irregular blotches, appears on the face and trunk (1.222) approximately 2–4 days after the prodromal phase of fever, catarrh and conjunctivitis. *Koplik's spots* are white or greyish-white patches, 1–3 mm in size, found over the buccal mucosa (1.223) during the pre-eruptive stage and are highly characteristic of measles. These spots may persist even after the rash has faded.

The hallmark of **chicken pox (varicella)** is that macules, papules, vesicles and pustules appear simultaneously on the face and the trunk (1.224, 1.225). In adults, the lesions appear on an erythematous base. In children, varicella causes only a minor illness but adults may experience considerable malaise, headache and muscle pains. In immunocompromised patients the condition is very severe. Approximately one-third of children with lymphoma and leukaemia who acquire a varicella infection will develop 'progressive varicella' associated with deep vesicles.

Darier's disease (keratosis follicularis) is a rare autosomal dominant disorder of keratinization that is characterized by hyperkeratotic papules (1.226). It is not an infectious disease but is presented here because it has to

be considered in the differential diagnosis of a 'spotty face' and can cause confusion to a generalist. The distinctive lesion is a firm, crusted, skin-coloured or yellowish-brown papule appearing mostly on the face (1.227), scalp (1.228), hands, soles and on the flexural surfaces. Sometimes the early lesions on the face may be mistaken for acne (1.201–1.203), but the presence of greasy papules with crusted tops and the absence of comedones distinguish the two. In Darier's disease, the palms and soles may show punctate keratosis with minute pits (1.229), which are pathognomonic.

In considering various dermatoses of the face, the clinician should be aware of the possibility that the lesions may be self-inflicted (**dermatitis artefacta**). Such lesions vary from redness to ulceration, favour accessible (to the patient) areas, have a bizarre shape, may be linear or oddly grouped, and do not resemble any known pathological process (1.230). The same area may be repeatedly damaged and the treatment, left to the patient to carry out, may not lead to any improvement (1.231, see also 2.4). The patient is usually a young woman with some medical knowledge, who may be expecting some form of 'secondary gain' from having skin lesions.

1.221
Measles

1.222
Measles: diffuse, blotchy rash

1.223
Koplik's spots

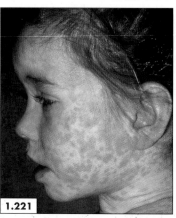
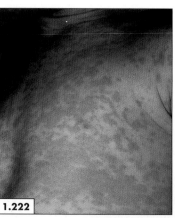
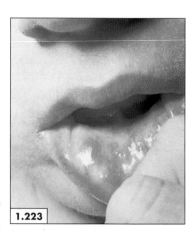

1.224
Varicella: macules, papules, vesicles and pustules

1.225
Varicella: maculopapular and vesicopustular lesions

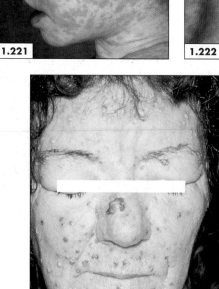
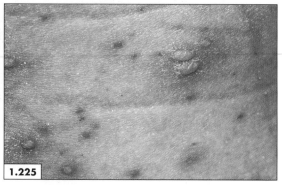

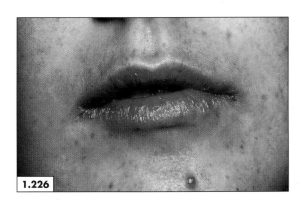

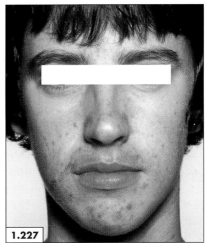

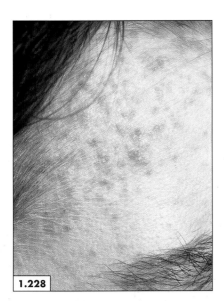

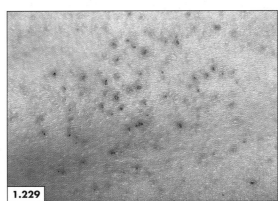

1.226
Darier's disease:
papules with
hyperkeratotic crusts

1.227
Hyperkeratotic
papules

1.228
Yellowish-brown
papules and
scattered pits

1.229
Punctate keratosis
with pits

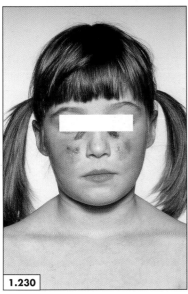

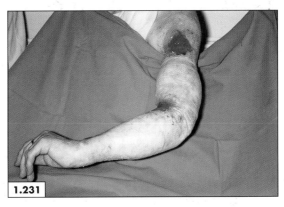

1.230
Dermatitis artefacta

1.231
Clean-cut, self-
inflicted ulcers

Cutaneous manifestations of systemic disorders

The skin as a system, or an organ, shares the manifestations of some diseases with other systems but it does so in its own special, pictorial way. It thereby provides a window through which one can see, suspect and, at times, identify the offending underlying disorder.

Gastrointestinal disorders

In the **Peutz–Jeghers syndrome** the orocutaneous pigmentation has a characteristic appearance of brownish-black spots (lentigines) around the mouth (1.232). The pigmented macules on the lips and oral mucous membranes (*periorificial lentiginosis*) may be present at birth or may develop during early childhood. These are usually associated with multiple hamartomatous polyposis in the small bowel, stomach and occasionally in the colon. Malignant transformation of the polyps is known to occur particularly in the Japanese with this syndrome. The condition is inherited as an autosomal dominant trait. Bowel polyposis and cutaneous lesions may not coexist in affected families.

A close look at a single **spider naevus** reveals a focal telangiectatic network of dilated capillaries, radiating from a central arteriole (punctum) (1.233). Although spider angiomas may be present occasionally in normal subjects (mostly females) without any reason, they are usually associated with hepatocellular disease (1.234) and with hyperoestrogenic states such as pregnancy and oral contraceptive therapy. On diascopy (pressing the skin against a glass slide), the central arteriole can be seen to pulsate.

Dermatitis herpetiformis is a chronic, recurring, intensely *pruritic* blistering eruption (1.235) seen in younger patients 30–40 years of age, with a high incidence of associated **coeliac disease**. Small vesicles, papules and urticarial weals (1.236) occur often in *symmetrical* groups (1.237). Erythematous papules, tiny vesicles and sometimes bullae are heralded by severe itching, which is a persistent symptom causing excoriation and crusting. Spotty pigmentation occurs in chronic cases. Anaemia from iron or folate deficiency may be seen in association with the coexisting malabsorption. A duodenal biopsy should be performed in all patients with dermatitis herpetiformis.

Connective tissue disorders

In this group **systemic lupus erythematosus** is the commonest condition with skin lesions on the face. Usually an

1.232
Perioral pigmented macules

1.233
Spider naevus

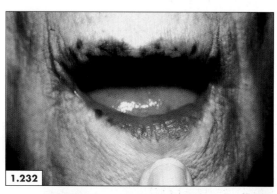

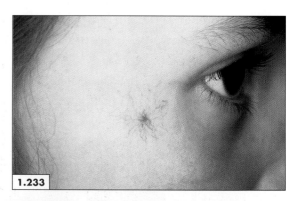

1.234
Portal cirrhosis: spider naevi and telangiectasia

1.235
Dermatitis herpetiformis: grouped erythematous papules and ruptured blisters

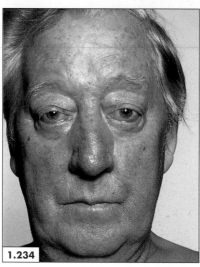
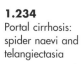

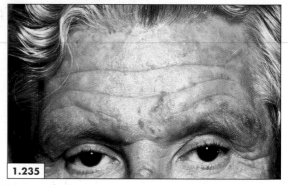

erythematous, confluent, macular and mildly oedematous eruption appears in a butterfly distribution (covering the cheeks and the bridge of the nose) predominantly in female (80%) subjects (1.238). The rash is itchy and may be maculopapular with some erosions and crusting (1.239). It may appear spontaneously but is sometimes induced, and often exacerbated, by exposure to the sun. Discoid papules, as in the discoid variety, occur on the face and there may also be scaling, hypopigmentation and vasculitic lesions (1.240, 1.241). A variety of drugs (Table 1.6) are known to induce a systemic erythematosus-like syndrome.

Atrophic contracture of the skin from fibrosis of the connective tissue is the hallmark of **systemic sclerosis**. Even in the early stages the thinned skin can be seen stretched over prominent bony parts such as the bridge of the nose, the larynx and the trachea (1.242), with furrows radiating from the laryngeal prominence and the mouth. Such a patient may also have telangiectasia on the face. The lips become thin with perioral furrowing (*rhagades*), and the tightening of the paper-thin skin may cause pitting over the bony ends of the nose (1.243).

As the condition progresses there is loss of the normal facial lines associated with any emotional expression (such

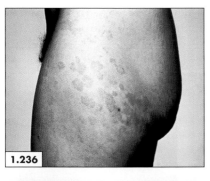

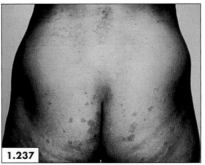

1.236
Papules, vesicles and weals

1.237
Symmetrical papulovesicular groups

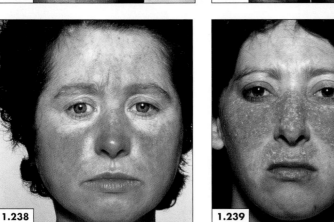

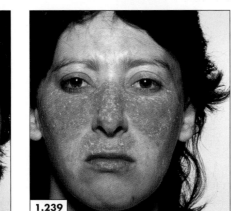

1.238
Systemic lupus erythematosus: butterfly distribution

1.239
Maculopapular rash with crusting and scales

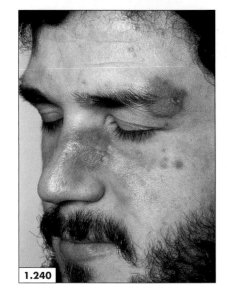

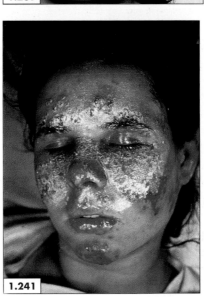

1.240
Sharply demarcated discoid plaques

1.241
Papular butterfly rash with erythema and scaling

Table 1.6 Some common drugs known to induce systemic lupus erythematosus

Dose–time-related drugs	Idiosyncratic drugs
Hydralazine	Aminosalicylic acid
Methyldopa	D-penicillamine
Procainamide	Griseofulvin
Isoniazid	Penicillin
Chlorpromazine	Ampicillin
Chlorthalidone	Streptomycin
Phenytoin	Tetracycline
Trimethadone	Methylthiouracil
Ethosuximide	Propylthiouracil
Carbamazepine	Phenylbutazone

as a smile), producing a mask-like appearance with a pinched-out nose (1.244). The mat-like telangiectasia (1.245) are present not only on the face (1.242–1.244) but also on the upper trunk, hands, neck, inside the mouth and in the gastrointestinal tract. This is a systemic disorder that involves many organs (e.g. gastrointestinal tract, heart, kidneys, lungs, joints and muscles) causing fibrosis and atrophy of the connective tissues and small vessel obliteration. The male to female ratio is 1:3 and the commonest presenting feature is *Raynaud's phenomenon* (p. **174**).

The heliotrope (reddish-purple) inflammatory rash over the eyelids, face, neck, upper chest (1.246) and dorsa of the knuckles (*Gottron's papules*) is the most arresting and characteristic feature of **dermatomyositis**. There is usually some degree of fine scaling and oedema of the affected

1.242
Systemic sclerosis. Note telangiectasia on the lip and stretched skin over the larynx

1.243
Rhagades (perioral furrowing) and nasal pitting

1.244
Rhagades, telangiectasia and stretched skin with nasal pitting

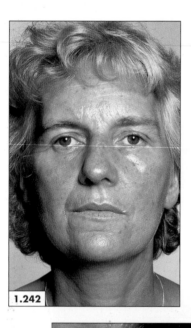

1.242

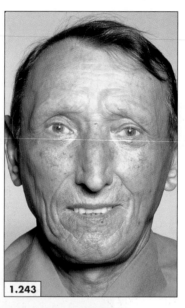

1.243

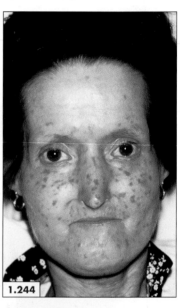

1.244

1.245
Systemic sclerosis: telangiectasia and pigmentation

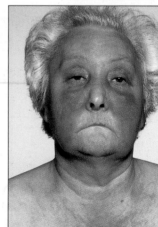

1.245

1.246
Dermatomyositis: heliotrope rash

1.246

areas. The oedema is particularly noticeable periorbitally when viewed from the side (1.247). The upper eyelids are almost invariably involved and there may be telangiectasia scattered on the erythematous rash (1.248). *Raynaud's phenomenon* occurs in approximately 20% of patients. *Fatiguability, muscle pains* and *proximal muscular weakness* occur in all patients. There is no agreement on the incidence of an associated malignancy (from 6 to 50%) but a search should be made, especially in patients over 40 years of age and in those who respond poorly to conventional treatment.

Genetic and metabolic disorders

Congenital erythropoietic porphyria (**Gunther's disease**) is a very rare disorder. Pink urine (stained nappies) and an acute cutaneous *photosensitivity* are two of its most characteristic features. The diagnosis is usually made in early childhood when the cutaneous manifestations of bullae, vesicles and ulcers occur on light-exposed areas. Patients surviving beyond childhood show the effects of recurrent exposure to the sun, and have diffuse and disfiguring scars on the face, with loss of portions of the fingers, nose, ears and eyelids (1.249). Erythrodontia, caused by the accumulation of porphyrins in the teeth, and splenomegaly associated with a compensated haemolytic anaemia occur in most cases.

In **variegate porphyria**, vesicles and bullae occur more frequently on the hands and feet; nevertheless inspection of the face may prove rewarding since there is usually a heliotrope hue on the eyelids and sometimes around the mouth (1.250). Acute neurological attacks (e.g. confusion, psychosis, generalized seizures, autonomic neuropathy, sensory and motor neuropathy sometimes leading to quadriplegia and respiratory paralysis) are its most important clinical features. Photosensitivity is not a presenting feature.

Mechanical fragility of the sun-exposed skin occurs in **porphyria cutanea tarda** and patients with this condition may present with *hypertrichosis* (1.251) especially in sunny climates. Papules and ruptured blisters may be seen on the sun-exposed face and ears (1.252). Tense bullae on normal-appearing skin occur on the dorsum of the hands

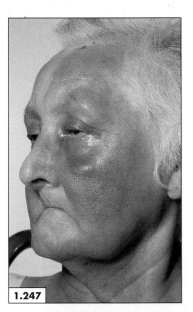

1.247

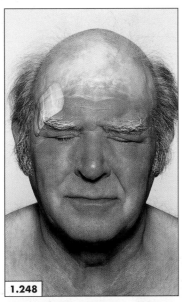

1.248

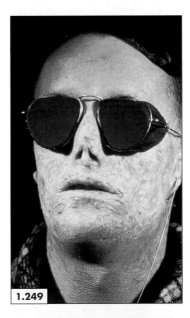

1.249

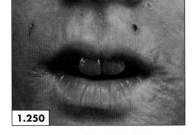

1.250

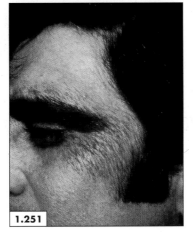

1.251

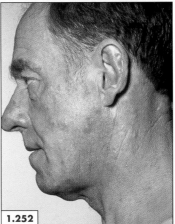

1.252

1.247
Heliotrope rash with fine scaling and oedema

1.248
Diffuse rash over the face and neck

1.249
Congenital erythropoietic porphyria: diffuse scarring with loss of nasal soft parts

1.250
Perioral heliotrope hue

1.251
Hypertrichosis

1.252
Papules and ruptured blisters

(**Chapter 9**). As in the variegate variety, a purple-red hue may be seen on the eyelids and around the mouth. Acute life-threatening attacks do not occur in this condition but it needs to be distinguished from variegate porphyria with which it shares cutaneous lesions. During acute attacks both conditions have increased levels of uroporphyrin in the urine, but the diagnostic hallmark in variegate porphyria is its markedly elevated *faecal protoporphyrin* level.

The diagnosis is confirmed by the presence of an *orange-red fluorescence* of the urine when examined with a Wood's lamp (1.253). It is always worth looking at a specimen of urine from a patient suspected of having porphyria cutanea tarda, since freshly passed urine may be orange-red or brown-red (1.254). In **congenital erythropoietic porphyria**, the colour of the urine ranges from pink to dark red (1.255) owing to the presence of uroporphyrins.

Neither xanthelasma nor the presence of an arcus is specific to **familial hypercholesterolaemia**; however, these signs point to the possibility that there may be an underlying lipid disorder that needs to be investigated. Xanthelasmata may be present in normolipaemic subjects, as in this patient with longitudinal, yellowish plaques just below the lower eyelids (1.256). The plaque has a brownish hue, it is slightly raised and there is a cluster of three yellowish papules medial to it (1.257).

An **arcus in a young adult** is highly significant and, together with xanthelasmata (1.258), suggests that there may be lesions elsewhere on the body, as in this patient with tuberous xanthomata (see also 9.177–9.179) and a positive family history for familial hypercholesterolaemia.

1.253
Fluorescence: viewed in Wood's lamp

1.254
Porphyria cutanea tarda: freshly voided urine

1.255
Congenital erythropoietic porphyria: darkish-red urine

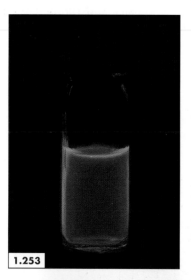
1.253

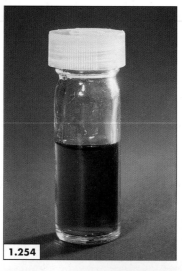
1.254

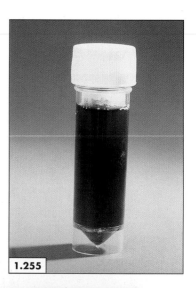
1.255

1.256
Bilateral xanthelasmata

1.257
Multiple, creamy xanthelasma papules

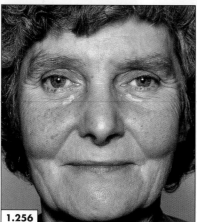
1.256

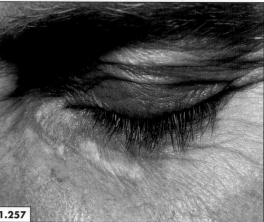
1.257

Tuberous sclerosis (epiloia), an autosomal dominant disease, is characterized by the presence of the red and white, firm and discrete papules of *angiofibromata* (1.259, 1.260) (sometimes mistakenly called adenoma sebaceum). These are pathognomonic of this condition but appear late in infancy. The lesions are reddish, telangiectatic papules with a yellowish tint, varying from 1 to 3mm in diameter, occurring mostly on the nasolabial folds and cheeks. Developmental and dysplastic lesions are found in other organs including the brain and kidney. The principal early manifestations are the triad of seizures, mental retardation and facial angiofibromata. The disease usually manifests in childhood but a mild form may present in adult life. Clusters of skin-coloured *fibromata* on the nasolabial folds are typical (1.261). The presence of *periungual fibromas* (see 10.92, 10.93) aid the diagnosis. Patients tend to have greasy skin; this is probably the reason why the angiofibromas were misnamed adenoma sebaceum.

Haemochromatosis is a common and easily overlooked autosomal recessive genetic disorder. This is because the cumulative iron deposition takes a long time (usually to the age of 40 years or over) to produce organ damage and there are very few early symptoms. As would be expected, clinical manifestations are more common in males and in postmenopausal women. Fatigue is a particularly distressing and common symptom and there may be arthralgias, abdominal discomfort, impotence and amenorrhoea. The *skin pigmentation* is often striking. With the increasing melanin and haemosiderin deposition, the skin has a slate-grey appearance (*bronzed diabetes*) in over-exposed areas such as the hands, neck and face (1.262, 1.263). Other manifestations include hepatomegaly, portal cirrhosis, hypogonadism and diabetes mellitus.

The hyperpigmentation of haemochromatosis should be distinguished from that caused by **transfusion haemosiderosis** (1.264), **chronic amiodarone therapy** (1.265, 1.266), and **alcoholic cirrhosis**, which causes both iron overload and pigmentation. Some patients on long-term amiodarone therapy develop a bluish or slate-grey pigmentation (1.265) caused by amiodarone deposition. A

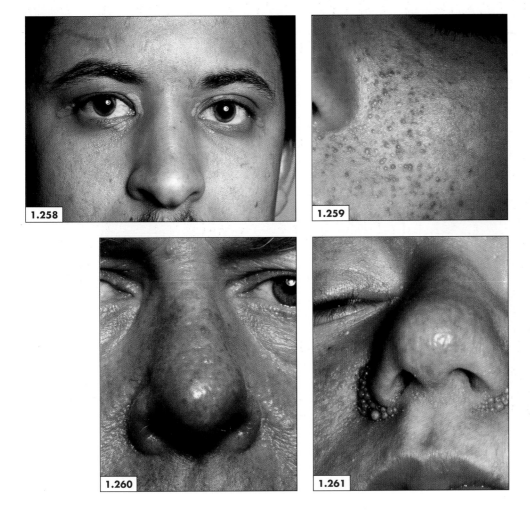

1.258
Arcus juvenilis and xanthelasmata

1.259
Tuberous sclerosis: confluent, small, angiomatous papules

1.260
Multiple reddish macules and papules on and around the nose

1.261
Clusters of skin-coloured and reddish papules in the nasolabial folds

spell of long exposure to the sun can cause intense bluish-grey pigmentation of the cheeks, nose and forehead (1.266). Corneal deposition of the drug, photosensitivity and an exfoliative dermatitis are some of its other manifestations. Patients with *increased saturation* of transferrin (more than 50%), and *elevated serum iron* and *ferritin levels* should have a **liver biopsy** for the definitive diagnosis of haemochromatosis. Once the diagnosis is made, other family members should be screened, since early treatment is quite effective in arresting the progression of the disease.

Mollusca fibrosa are soft, pink or skin-coloured, sessile (early) or pedunculated (late) tumours scattered over the face (1.267) and the rest of the body in **neurofibromatosis**. Small neuroma nodules develop along the course of cutaneous nerves and these may be numerous, tender and disfiguring. A malignant change to neurofibrosarcoma may occur in one of these, with a concomitant rapid increase

in size, as happened in a neuroma on the left side of the neck of this patient (1.267). Sharply defined, light-brown patches called *café-au-lait* spots appear in almost all patients. Freckling in the axillae (1.268) is pathognomonic.

Hereditary haemorrhagic telangiectasia is an autosomal dominant condition (also called **Osler–Weber–Rendu syndrome**) that affects blood vessels, especially on the face, in the mouth, the lungs and the gastrointestinal tract. Small, flat, violaceous telangiectatic lesions, approximately 1–3 mm in diameter occur on the face (1.269), lips, mouth and hands. The typical lesion is a punctate, purplish-red macule or papule with a tiny mesh of capillaries radiating from it (1.270). The telangiectasis results from dilatation, thinning and convolution of the venules and capillaries. These vascular meshes have neither contractile properties nor any anatomical support, and they bleed spontaneously or after minor trauma.

1.262
Haemochromatosis: generalized, slate-grey pigmentation

1.263
Haemochromatosis: intense, slate-grey pigmentation of sun-exposed face, neck and forearms

1.264
Haemosiderosis: cutaneous and mucosal pigmentation

1.265
Amiodarone pigmentation of the face, hands and nails

1.266
Chronic amiodarone therapy: dark, bluish-grey pigmentation of the face and forehead

1.267
Neurofibromatosis: multiple skin-coloured and pinkish papules and nodules. Note the larger swelling in the neck caused by a neurofibrosarcoma

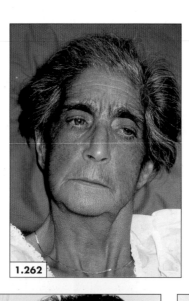
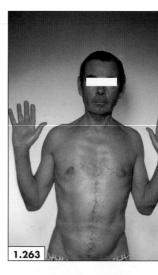
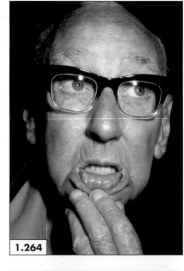
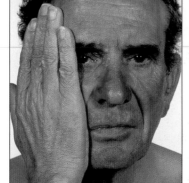
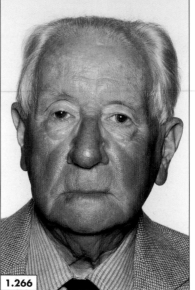
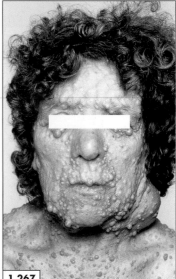

Vascular malformations in the lung result in pulmonary arteriovenous fistulas in approximately one-fifth of cases. These malformations increase in size and frequency with age and may cause recurrent haemoptysis, infections, hypoxaemia, clubbing and polycythaemia. The condition should be sought in patients with unexplained haemoptysis and anaemia.

Endocrine disorders

The endocrine disorders that cause major changes to the facial appearance have already been discussed (p. **3**). **Non-scarring alopecia** and **vitiligo**, possibly associated with some endocrine and autoimmune disorders, and a

hormone-secreting tumour with cutaneous manifestations (**glucagonoma**) will need to be considered here.

Alopecia areata is a localized, well-circumscribed, oval or circular loss of hair mostly affecting the scalp (1.271) but sometimes occurring on the beard, eyebrows or eyelashes. Erythema may be present in the early stages but in well-developed cases there are no inflammatory changes. Characteristically, the peripheral areas of hair loss are studded with the diagnostic broken-off hairs called '*exclamation mark hairs*'.

Occasionally the hair loss may spread to the entire scalp (*alopecia totalis*) (1.272). This may be difficult to recognize in a patient wearing a wig, although the profuseness of the hair on the wig, and the difference between the colour of the native hairs in front of the ears and those of the wig (1.273) may be obvious to the discerning clinician. Alo-

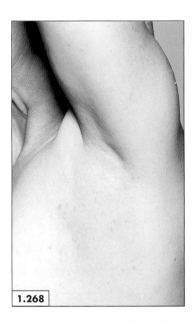

1.268

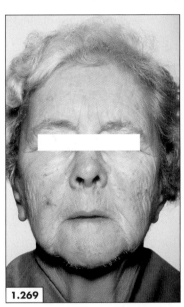

1.269

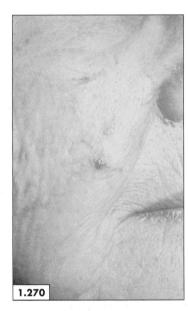

1.270

1.268
Neurofibromatosis: axillary freckling

1.269
Osler–Weber–Rendu syndrome: multiple, discrete, red macular and papular telangiectases

1.270
Telangiectasis: a mesh of capillaries radiates from the central punctum (arteriole)

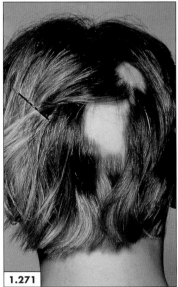

1.271

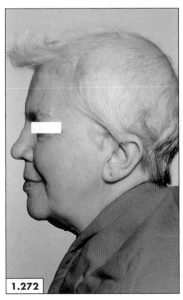

1.272

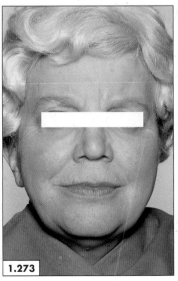

1.273

1.271
Alopecia areata

1.272
Alopecia totalis

1.273
Camouflaged alopecia totalis

pecia areata may be an autoimmune disease and is sometimes associated with Hashimoto's thyroiditis, pernicious anaemia and diabetes mellitus. Progressive hair loss may involve the entire body (*alopecia universalis*), as in this patient (1.274) who also had pernicious anaemia and diabetes mellitus. The hair loss was complete, affecting the scalp (1.275), eyelashes, eyebrows (1.276) and the rest of the body. The nails may show dystrophic changes, with the dorsal nail plate having multiple tiny depressions simulating 'hammered brass'.

Vitiligo may manifest as scattered, circumscribed areas of hypomelanosis of the skin and hair around body orifices such as the mouth and eyes (1.277). It also occurs over bony prominences, particularly of the hands, knees and elbows. In most cases, vitiligo is of idiopathic origin but there is an increasing association with certain autoimmune conditions such as thyroiditis, hyperthyroidism, diabetes mellitus, Addison's disease and pernicious anaemia.

Glucagonoma is a rare neoplastic condition with well-described cutaneous manifestations, caused by an over-production of glucagon in an alpha-cell tumour of the pancreas. The characteristic skin lesion is a superficial *migratory necrolytic erythema* with central blisters or erosions that crust together, a beefy red tongue and angular cheilitis (1.278). The clinical features include loss of weight, diabetes mellitus (without ketoacidosis), thromboembolic episodes, anaemia and psychiatric disorders.

Granulomatous and vasculitic disorders

This group includes all those conditions characterized by the presence of granulomata and associated cutaneous manifestations, such as **sarcoidosis**, which affects many organs and has distinctive cutaneous lesions.

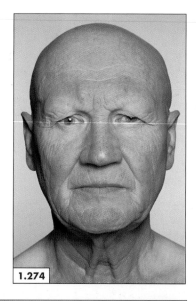

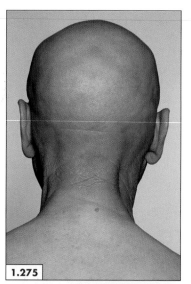

1.274 and 1.275
Alopecia universalis in a diabetic subject

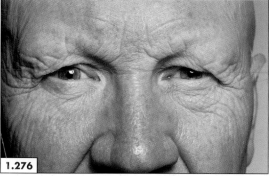

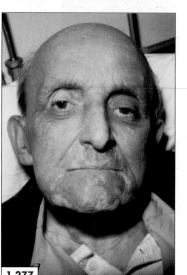

1.276
Alopecia universalis: loss of eyebrows and eyelashes

1.277
Vitiligo: sharply demarcated macules

Sarcoidosis is a chronic granulomatous disease of unknown aetiology that affects young adults and presents with skin lesions, pyrexia, ocular involvement, bilateral hilar adenopathy and pulmonary infiltrations. *Erythema nodosum* is the commonest cutaneous manifestation but multiple maculopapular lesions (1.279), lupus pernio and sarcoid infiltration of scars also occur. The maculopapular and nodular lesions spread peripherally in an annular fashion and some of the lesions coalesce into brownish-purple plaques on the face (1.280). On closer examination, papular invasion of the epidermis with a resulting purplish hue can be seen clearly (1.281). On diascopy, these lesions may look somewhat like the 'apple-jelly' (yellowish brown) of lupus vulgaris (see 1.207, 1.210 and 1.211) but there is no scarring in sarcoidosis. **Lupus pernio** (or chilblain) is a more homogeneous, dense, firm or soft, violaceous infiltration of the exposed parts such as the cheek, nose (1.282) and earlobes (1.283).

Wegener's granulomatosis is a distinct clinicopathological entity and consists of a triad of: (i) a necrotizing granulomatous vasculitis of the upper and lower respiratory tracts; (ii) a focal necrotizing glomerulitis; and (iii) a systemic small vessel vasculitis involving numerous organs. Cutaneous manifestations occur in approximately half the cases but in only approximately 10% of patients at initial presentation. In almost all patients a *history of symptoms referable to upper respiratory catarrh or infection* is obtainable. Common symptoms and signs include a persistent nasal discharge, fever, cough, haemoptysis and nasal granulomata.

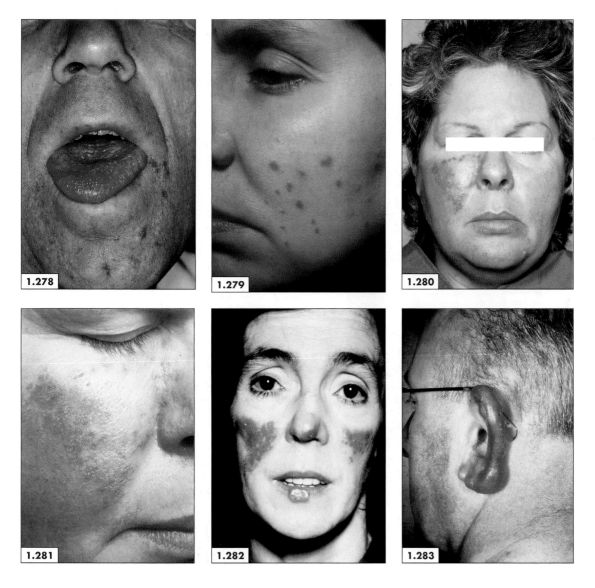

1.278 Migratory necrolytic erythema: inflammatory papules, angular cheilitis and beefy tongue

1.279 Sarcoidosis: maculopapular reddish pepules

1.280 Sarcoidosis: brownish-purple granulomatous plaque

1.281 Yellowish-brown granulomatous infiltration of the cheek and nose

1.282 Lupus pernio of the cheeks

1.283 Lupus pernio: swelling and congestion of the cold-exposed ear

Granulomatous involvement of the nasal mucosa may be betrayed by a reddish hue of the skin overlying the granulomata (1.284). The granulomata can be readily seen by looking up the patient's nostrils (1.285).

Renal disease is seen in approximately 80% of patients and virtually dictates the outcome. The diagnosis should be suspected strongly when an upper respiratory complaint is accompanied with haematuria and/or vasculitic lesions.

Vasculitides constitute a heterogeneous group of disorders that includes Wegener's granulomatosis and can be loosely classified under various subheadings:

- **Hypersensitivity angiitis** (e.g. Henoch–Schönlein purpura, cryoglobulinaemia, hypocomplementaemic vasculitis);
- **Allergic vasculitis** from drug reactions;
- **Underlying infections** (e.g. infective endocarditis, meningococcaemia);
- **Neoplastic diseases** (e.g. carcinoma, lymphoma, leukaemia);

- **Connective tissue diseases** (e.g. systemic lupus erythematosus, rheumatoid arthritis, polyarteritis nodosa);
- **Granulomatous vasculitis** (e.g. Wegener's, Churg–Straus disease);
- **Giant cell arteritis** (e.g. temporal arteritis, polymyalgia rheumatica, Takayasu's disease).

The hallmark of the group is the predominance of cutaneous involvement, which may appear as the classical palpable purpura on the face (1.286) and elsewhere on the body. In addition, there may be macules, papules, nodules, bullae, ulcers and recurrent urticaria. The crusted lesions represent cutaneous infarction associated with necrotizing vasculitis. The cutaneous manifestations, together with the involvement of one or more systems, suggest the possible presence of one of the vasculitides. For example, in meningococcaemia the tell-tale cutaneous vasculitic lesions may be red papules or petechiae (1.287), in association with fever, malaise, headache and meningism.

1.284
Wegener's granulomatosis: inflammatory granulomatous infiltration of the nose

1.285
Wegener's granulomata

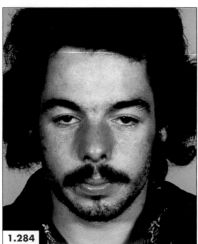

1.284

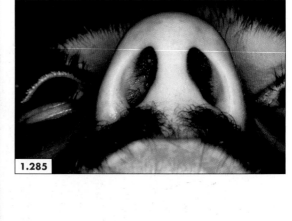

1.285

1.286
Vasculitis: multiple purpuric papules with same crusted (cutaneous infarction) lesions

1.287
Meningococcal meningitis: reddish papules

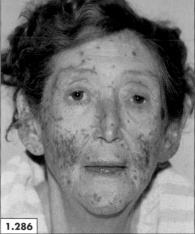

1.286

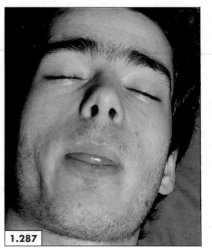

1.287

Vascular and haemovascular disorders

The **Sturge–Weber syndrome** is a nonfamilial congenital disorder of facial and cerebral blood vessels. It is characterized by an angiomatous malformation on the face (*port-wine stain*) (1.288), epilepsy and mental deficiency. The port-wine stain is an irregularly shaped red or violaceous haemangioma, and usually involves the area supplied by the first or second division of the trigeminal nerve (1.289). It does not cross the midline but the skin supplied by the corresponding branch of the opposite nerve may be similarly affected. In middle age it may darken and become studded with angiomatous nodules. There may be an angioma of the occipital and parietal leptomeninges on the side of the facial lesion. The underlying cerebral cortex is atrophic with deposits of iron and calcium, responsible for the characteristic *tramline* appearance on CT scan of the brain. The patient may have one of the other congenital abnormalities usually associated with this condition (e.g. glaucoma, strabismus, optic atrophy, etc.).

Haematological abnormalities causing changes in the constituents of blood (i.e. red and white blood cells, proteins, etc.) and cardiovascular disorders, individually as well as in combination, inevitably affect the colour of the skin (easily visible on the face) caused by alterations in the haematocrit and haemodynamics. *Facial flushing* and *facial pallor* are the two principal examples that are also two of the commonest findings encountered in the general population. A facial or *malar flush* may be seen in a healthy but sensitive young Caucasian female, particularly in a warm atmosphere, but it is also often found, irrespective of the weather, in association with **mitral stenosis** and is hence referred to as *mitral facies* (1.290). Chronic facial flushing causes permanent dilatation of the capillaries with telangiectasis (1.291).

In mitral stenosis, the malar flush is thought to be related to pulmonary hypertension and peripheral vasoconstriction, but the so-called mitral facies is not specific to mitral valve disease. It is also found in patients with **myxoedema** (1.291) and **aortic valve disease** (1.292).

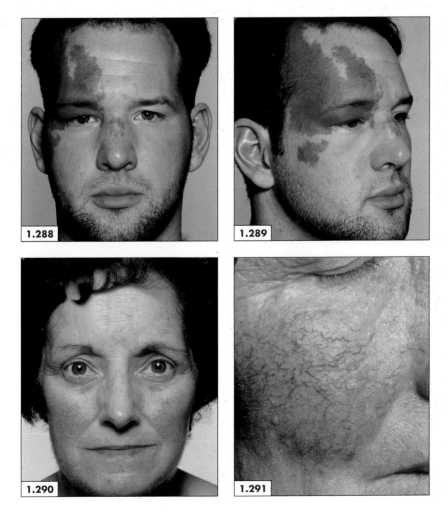

1.288
Port-wine stain. Note strabismus

1.289
Port-wine stain along the distribution of the first division of the trigeminal nerve

1.290
Malar flush in a patient with mitral stenosis

1.291
Long-standing malar flush with telangiectasis

A dusky red face (1.293) is often seen in patients with **polycythaemia rubra vera** although not all patients with facial plethora have polycythaemia. These patients may be asymptomatic or may complain of headaches, dizziness or visual symptoms. On questioning they may admit to having night sweats and generalized pruritus made worse by a warm bath. In addition to facial plethora, clinical examination may reveal retinal vein distension and a palpable spleen. At the other extreme, *pallor* is a dependable manifestation of either **a low volume**, **low perfusion state** or of **anaemia** (1.294). In either event, pallor as a clinical sign

should be confirmed by inspecting the mucous membranes, particularly by looking at the guttering between the palpebral and bulbar conjunctiva (see 3.24).

The signs associated with hyperlipidaemias and abnormal hyperproteinaemias are discussed elsewhere (pp. **50**, **110**, **192**).

Diagnostic considerations

The diagnosis of various skin lesions is dependent essentially on familiarity with their appearance which can be

1.292
Long-standing malar flush with telangiectasis in a butterfly distribution (aortic valve disease)

1.293
Polycythemia rubra vera: diffuse plethora

1.294
Pallor

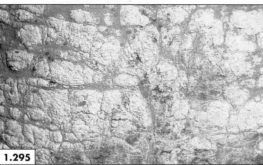

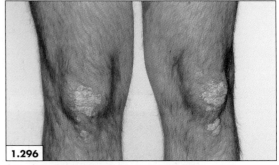

1.295
Psoriasis: well-defined plaques with silvery-white scales

1.296
Psoriasis: plaques on the knees

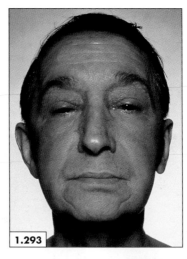

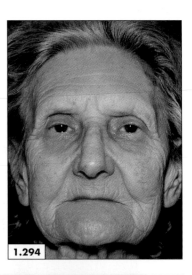

1.297
Familial hypercholesterolaemia: tuberous xanthomata

1.298
Psoriasis: pitting of the nails

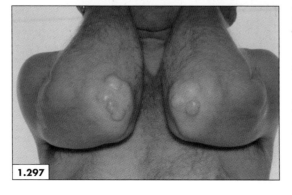

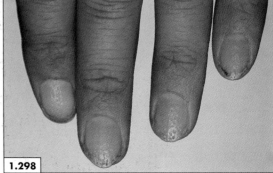

gained by looking at as many pictures and patients as possible. Any clinician who takes the trouble to study and understand the unique pattern of a lesion in an atlas will find it easier to identify it when it is seen on a patient. When studying a lesion, particular attention should be paid to its various components such as its size, shape, base, edges, surface, the state of the surrounding skin, and its areas of predilection. For example, even part of a lesion without its anatomical relationship can be recognized as psoriasis by the presence of sharply defined, keratotic, silvery-white plaques on erythematous skin (1.295). Its predilection for extensor surfaces (1.296, see also 9.61) is well known, as is that of tuberous xanthomata (1.297), yet the two can hardly be confused with each other since both lesions have strikingly different appearances. The knowledgeable clinician will also look for other familiar lesions known to be caused by the suspected disease such as the *pitting of the nails* in **psoriasis** (1.298).

Unfortunately, skin lesions of many diverse diseases can look the same, and even those known to have characteristic features do not always possess them. Thus, the lesions of **solar keratosis** (1.299) may not look much different from those caused by **dermatitis herpetiformis** (1.235), **discoid lupus erythematosus** (1.240) or **porphyria cutanea tarda** (1.252). Similarly, **lymphocytoma of the skin** over the nose (1.300) may not be easily distinguishable from **lupus pernio** (1.301) or **discoid lupus erythematosus** (1.240). Without a proper history and meticulous attention to the entire face and forehead, these lesions of **pellagra** with thickening, fissuring and scaling of the skin (1.302) may be accepted as simple facial plethora in a patient who subsists on alcohol for calories.

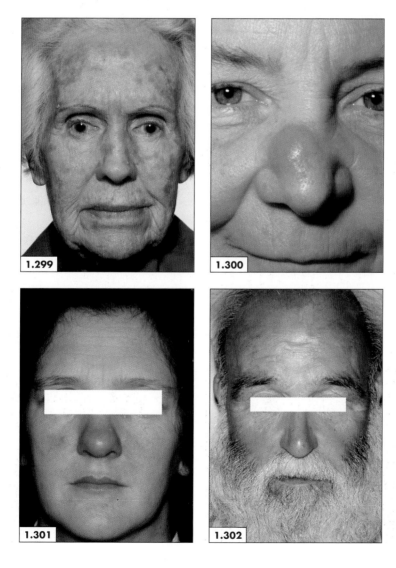

1.299
Solar keratosis: tanning, brownish-red macules and wrinkling (solar elastosis)

1.300
Cutaneous B-cell lymphoma: well-defined, bluish-red nodule

1.301
Lupus pernio: diffuse reddish-brown granulomatous infiltration of the nose and adjoining cheeks

1.302
Niacin deficiency: diffuse erythema with tanning of light-exposed areas

It is clear that many disorders of the skin, like those of any other system, cannot be diagnosed without a proper and comprehensive clinical assessment. Whenever the lesions look similar (e.g. pemphigus, pemphigoid and dermatitis herpetiformis), attention should be directed to the personal history of the patient, the mode of onset of the lesions, the pattern of their occurrence, their distribution, the state of the surrounding skin, and the associated symptoms. These points are well illustrated by considering the differential diagnosis of the various **blistering disorders** (Table 1.7). **Pemphigoid** blisters usually arise on erythematous skin (1.303) and, unlike those of **pemphigus** (1.304), intact ones are often seen because they are thick and rupture less easily. At first sight, the collapsed blisters of pemphigus (1.304) may look like those of dermatitis herpetiformis (1.305) but the lesions of the latter occur in groups whereas those of the former are more haphazardly distributed. In addition, *itching* is a major symptom of dermatitis herpetiformis and not of pemphigus.

As can be seen in Table 1.7, the age of onset, the presence or absence of constitutional symptoms, any associated symptoms, the uniqueness of lesions, the colour of the lesions and of their surrounding skin, their distribution and their sites of predilection all help to distinguish the various forms of blistering diseases. Similar logic can be applied in diagnosing other skin lesions, whether they reflect the primary skin or underlying systemic disorders.

Miscellaneous facial disorders

If there is no evidence of an endocrine or a neuromuscular disorder and there is no mucocutaneous abnormality, then the clinician should scan each part of the head sequentially. In practice, experienced clinicians usually scan the scalp and face in one glance, looking for the pres-

Table 1.7 The differential diagnosis of blistering diseases

Disease	History	Age of onset	Lesions	Distribution
Pemphigus	Weakness, wasting, no pruritus	40–60 years	Skin-coloured normal skin, thin/ruptured bullae	Mouth, face, scalp, chest, axillae
Pemphigoid	Prodromal urticaria/eczema, occasional pruritus	60–80 years, may occur in children	Tense bullae on erythematous skin	Generalized, rarely in oropharynx
Dermatitis herpetiformis	Intense itching and burning sensation	20–40 years	Erythematous papules, vesicles, urticarial weals	Scalp, face, extensor areas
Erythema multiforme	Exposure to drugs, fever, malaise	Usually below 30 years	Macules, papules, vesicles, bullae, target lesions	Hands, trunk
Porphyria cutanea tarda	May follow alcohol, oestrogens, etc.	30–40 years	Vesicles, bullae, hypertrichosis	Symmetrical, sun-exposed areas: hands, face, ears

1.303
Pemphigoid: intact blisters arising on erythematous skin

1.304
Pemphigus: ruptured blisters leaving non-healing red lesions

1.305
Dermatitis herpetiformis: groups of papulovesicular lesions

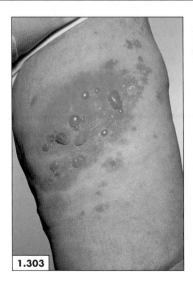

1.303

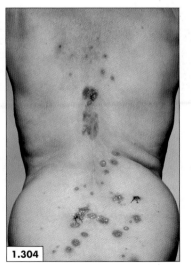

1.304

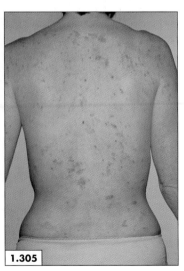

1.305

ence or absence of abnormalities in all the major groups. Since the objective is that nothing must be missed, the observer should follow a set pattern, taking into account all the groups without the need to exclude one group before looking for the lesions from the other group.

It is beyond any argument that a clinician familiar with the appearances of the typical facies of **Down syndrome** (previously known as mongolism) (1.306) will not wait to rule out the first three groups before making a diagnosis. He or she will use the same set routine on this face, since Down syndrome does not exclude the other possibilities.

The facial features are so characteristic that all Down patients look alike; their palpebral fissures are almond-shaped, and the eyes slant upwards with the outer canthi being higher than the inner ones. Most Down patients have epicanthic folds (a semicircular fold of skin crossing vertically over the inner canthus) (1.307). The mouth is often kept open with the tongue partially protruding through it.

The syndrome of mongolism is now named after J.H. Down (1828–1896) who suggested in an article ('*The Ethnic Classification of Idiots*') that the resemblance of many congenital idiots to mongolian and other allied races is related to their evolutionary status when intelligence had not reached its Caucasian apex. It is ironic that the term Down syndrome is used to avoid offending Chinese and Japanese investigators!

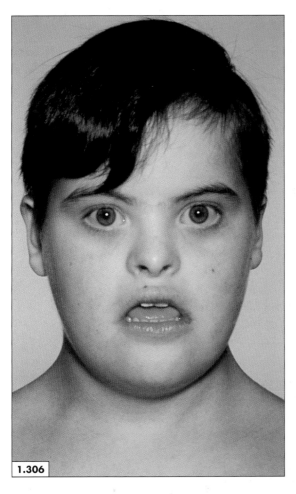

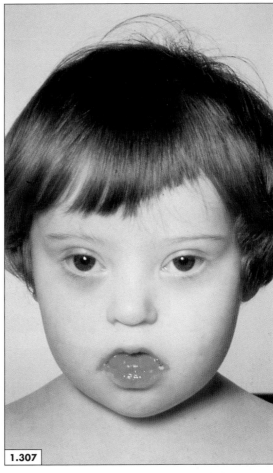

1.306
Down syndrome facies: upward slanting, almond-shaped eyes with open mouth

1.307
Down syndrome. Note the prominent epicanthic fold on the left side

In search of various abnormalities in this group, one should start by looking at the scalp to see whether there are any lesions on it, and whether the cranium looks enlarged (as in Paget's disease and hydrocephalus), paying particular attention to the frontal and occipital areas that look protuberant and irregular in **Paget's disease** (1.308). The enlargement of the frontal bones can be appreciated best by looking at the patient's frontal view (1.309). A simultaneous glance over the clavicles may reveal that these are also prominent and involved in the disease process. The cranium, the clavicles and the long bones of the legs are most commonly found to be abnormal. Occasionally, the diagnosis may be made on a chest X-ray, having been taken for some unrelated reason, where one or both clavicles may look enlarged with a fuzzy outline indicating a combination of *osteosclerosis* and *osteolysis*.

The *frontal bossing* of Paget's disease is sometimes difficult to detect – particularly in a patient with a large and square face. There is usually a sharp drop where the enlarged frontal bone curves laterally, the supraorbital ridges may be enlarged and prominent, and the clavicles may be abnormal (1.310). All these features can be seen clearly in the lateral view (1.311).

In some patients the base of the skull is involved as suggested by a bitemporal prominence in the frontal view (1.312). Severe enlargement of the base of the skull may lead to basilar impression and compression of the spinal cord, the brainstem, the vertebral and spinal arteries and the cerebellum producing a variety of symptoms (e.g. pain, syncope, dysarthria, visual disturbances, etc.).

While looking at a patient's face the clinician should not only search for a structural abnormality, important though that may be, but also examine facial expression, which will

1.308 and 1.309
Paget's disease: enlarged calvarium, lower jaw and clavicles

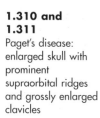

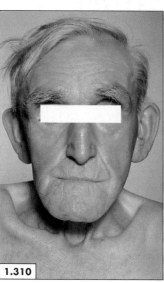

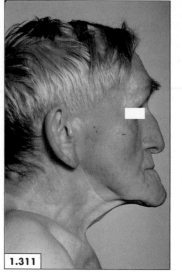

1.310 and 1.311
Paget's disease: enlarged skull with prominent supraorbital ridges and grossly enlarged clavicles

1.312
Paget's disease: bitemporal enlargement

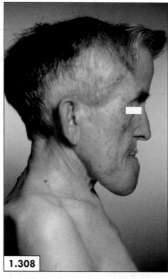

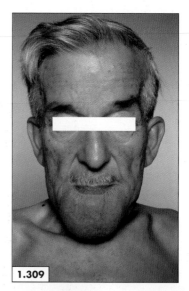

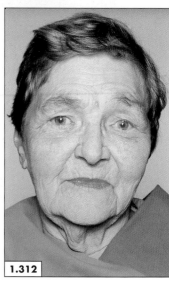

reflect inner emotion, and may suggest a psychological or an organic disorder. These signs are usually 'soft' and do not have a specific connection with any one particular disease, but emotional lability is an exception and suggests diffuse **cerebrovascular disease** or dementia. The patient appearing normal at first sight (1.313) may suddenly start crying (1.314) and equally abruptly erupt into a smile (1.315).

A history of pain in the temporal region of the scalp, headache, visual disturbances, or facial pain during chewing should direct the clinician's attention to the possibility of **temporal arteritis**. In such patients there may be a nonpulsatile, tender swelling of part of the temporal artery (1.316). It is a valuable sign of a medical emergency that if untreated may lead to loss of vision.

The inspection of the forehead may reveal some interesting features such as *coal-dust tattoos* as in this coal miner (1.317). Such coal-dust scars (1.318) present a relevant piece of *nonverbal history* in a patient with a respiratory complaint.

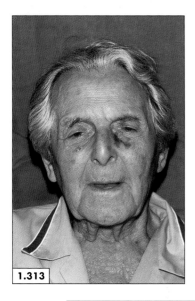

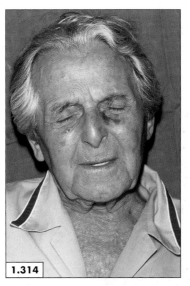

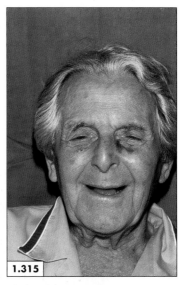

1.313
Cerebrovascular disease: recovering from a recent cerebrovascular accident

1.314
Starts crying in response to a 'hello'

1.315
Abrupt and unsolicited change into a smile!

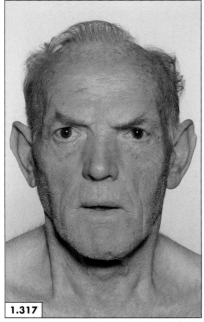

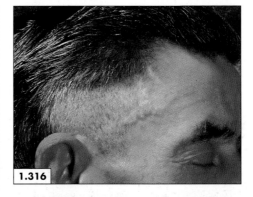

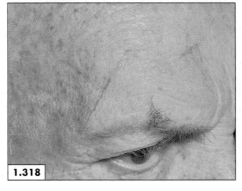

1.316
Temporal arteritis: enlarged superficial temporal artery

1.317
A coal miner with a chronic respiratory disorder and a tell-tale sign

1.318
Coal-dust tattoos

In the **Ehlers–Danlos syndrome** (1.319), *the bridge of the nose* tends to be *flat* and *wide* giving a characteristic appearance to the face. The skin, especially over the neck, axillae, groins and the trunk, is smooth and stretches like a piece of elastic when pulled out from the underlying structures (1.320). The syndrome consists of a group of more than 10 inherited connective tissue disorders characterized by soft, velvety and hyperextensible skin, marked joint laxity, easy bruising, hernias, kyphoscoliosis and 'cigarette-paper' scars in areas of trauma (1.321). In one variety there may be rupture of viscera and arteries. Many of these patients have varicose veins, abnormal joint mobility (1.322) and thin, translucent skin with visible veins.

A *depressed nasal bridge* (*saddle nose*) is classically associated with **congenital syphilis** (1.323, 1.324). This is a consequence of destruction of the nasal cartilage caused by

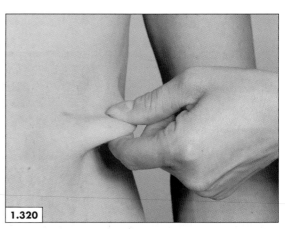

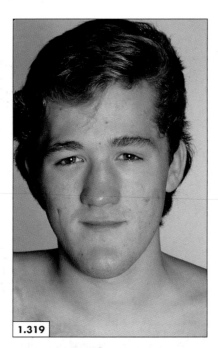

1.319
Ehlers–Danlos
syndrome: a flat,
wide nose

1.320
Ehlers–Danlos
syndrome: elastic
and mobile skin

1.319

1.320

1.321
'Papyraceous' scars

1.322
Hyperextensible
joints

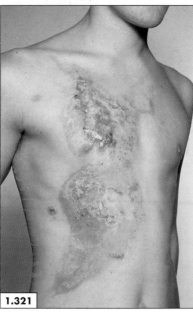

1.321

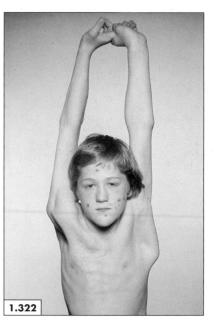

1.322

infection of the nasal mucosa (*snuffles*) soon after birth. These patients also have *periostitis* causing prominence of the frontal bones, poor development of the maxilla, and anterior convexity of the tibiae (*sabre shins*) (see 11.52).

A depressed nasal bridge is also a characteristic feature of the **mucopolysaccharidoses**, a group of inherited disorders caused by incomplete degradation and storage of acid mucopolysaccharides (glycosaminoglycans). **Hurler's syndrome** is the most severe form of these disorders. The facial features become progressively coarser after the first year

of life. The head is large and dolichocephalic with frontal bossing, the bridge of the nose is depressed and the nose is broad and flat (1.325). These patients also have hepatosplenomegaly, kyphosis, dysostosis multiplex and corneal opacities.

The soft parts of the nose may be enlarged either by multiple nasal polyps (1.326) or because of outgrowths of fibromata (1.327). In the latter condition (**hyaline fibromatosis**) there are recurrent outgrowths of fibromata on the nose, face, ears and joints.

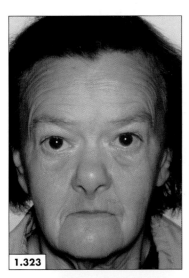

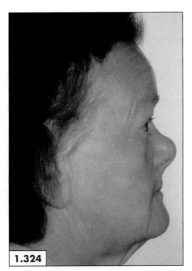

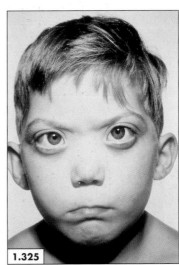

1.323 and 1.324
Congenital syphilis: flat, depressed nasal bridge

1.325
Hurler's syndrome: flat nasal bridge, wide-set eyes and frontal bossing

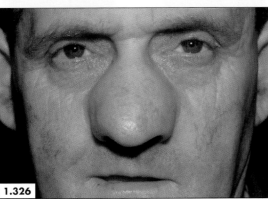

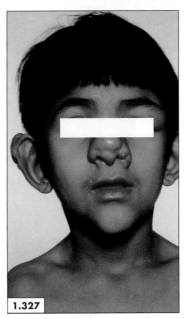

1.326
Multiple nasal polyps

1.327
Hyaline fibromatosis: fibromatous outgrowths

Alteration of the facial appearance can also be caused by underdevelopment, atrophy or enlargement of the various constituents of the face. An overall *thinning of the face*, particularly of the *temples*, may be a reflection of **generalized wasting**. Although the presenting complaints and the subsequent clinical assessment can lead to a correct diagnosis from the many possibilities that cause wasting (e.g. malignancy, malabsorption, gastrointestinal disorders, chronic infections, etc.), some cases may be seen initially with an unrelated complaint. Among these are **malnutrition caused by social deprivation** (1.328), **malabsorption** and **Crohn's disease** (1.329). Patients with **anorexia nervosa** often insist that they are eating well, many even believe that they are overweight, but their facial features suggest undernutrition (1.330).

Neuromuscular disorders including facial hemiatrophy have been discussed earlier in this chapter (p. **29**). Loss of facial fat may make the normal muscles look prominent in **lipodystrophy** (1.331; see also 1.15 and 1.16). *Asymmetry* of the face may be caused by **facial hemiatrophy** (see 1.145), or by a **cavernous haemangioma** (1.332). This lesion is not present at birth but appears during childhood. A cavernous haemangioma is a deep, vascular malformation characterized by a soft compressible deep-tissue swelling and surface varicosities.

The *maxillary hypoplasia* and other associated abnor-

1.328
Lonely and undernourished: smiles after a good hospital meal!

1.329
Crohn's disease: loss of weight and depression

1.330
Anorexia nervosa with marked loss of subcutaneous fat and muscle mass

1.331
Lipodystrophy with prominent musculature

1.332
Cavernous haemangioma: bluish swelling of the right face

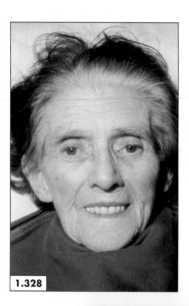
1.328

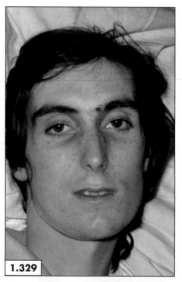
1.329

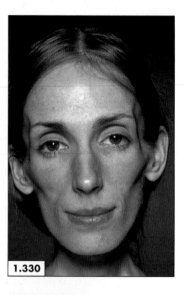
1.330

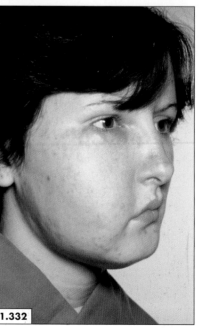
1.331

1.332

malities of the **Treacher Collins syndrome** (*mandibu-lofacial dysostosis*) can produce a characteristic facial appearance with sunken cheek bones, receding chin (mandibular hypoplasia), colobomas of the lower eyelids, downward pointing palpebral fissures, deformed pinnas and auditory canals (1.333). The condition can be diagnosed usually at birth, and certainly in early infancy, since there may be mandibular hypoplasia with a tapering chin, a blind fistula between the angle of the mouth and the ear (1.334), or a deformity of the eyelids and ears. Early diagnosis and the recognition of an associated conductive

hearing loss are important to prevent the possible delayed learning and retardation caused by deafness.

Even though the bulk of the muscles, fat and bones in the face may be normal, the rigidity of the muscles in **Parkinson's disease** may give the face an abnormal *mask-like* appearance (1.335). Evidence of poor muscular mobility, although often subtle in the early stages, can be seen when a patient tries to smile (1.336).

Enlargement of the parotid gland alters the facial appearance even though at times the change may not be very obvious, since the bulk of the gland lies below

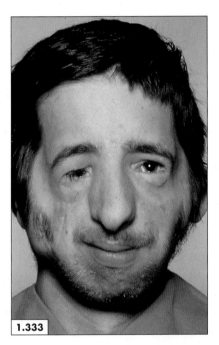

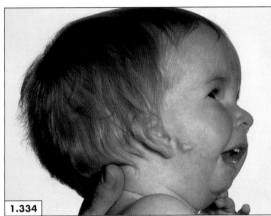

1.333
Treacher Collins syndrome: maxillary hypoplasia, downward-pointing palpebral fissures and colobomas of lower eyelids

1.334
Treacher Collins syndrome: mandibular hypoplasia, blind fistula and deformed ear

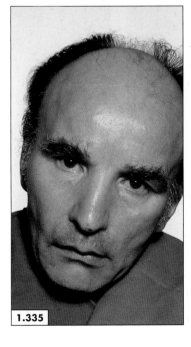

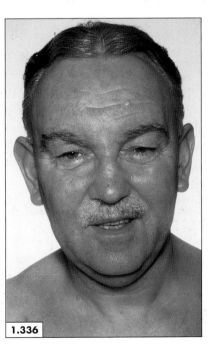

1.335
Parkinson's disease: mask-like facies

1.336
Poorly mobile facial musculature

and behind the ear, and the swelling may be only minimal (1.337). **Mumps** is the commonest cause of bilateral or unilateral enlargement of the parotid gland in children (1.338). Occasionally, it occurs in adults and may be complicated by oopheritis, epididymo-orchitis, meningitis and pancreatitis. Meningitis is a frequent complication in children but usually resolves without any sequelae.

The parotid glands are also enlarged in **portal cirrhosis** (especially of alcoholic origin), **Sjögren's syndrome** (1.339) and when involved in a neoplastic process. In **Sjögren's syndrome** the patient is usually female (with a female: male ratio of 10:1) and may have the *sicca complex* with dry eyes and dry mouth. The parotid glands are diffusely enlarged (1.340) and sometimes there may be swelling of the submandibular (1.341) and lacrimal glands. If only a part of the gland is enlarged then it is more likely to be neoplastic (1.342).

1.337
Parotid swelling

1.338
Mumps: unilateral parotid swelling

1.339
Sjögren's syndrome with bilateral parotid swelling

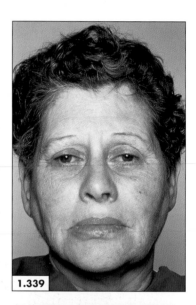

1.337

1.338

1.339

1.340
Diffuse parotid swelling causing a hollow anteriorly

1.341
Sjögren's syndrome with submandibular gland enlargement

1.342
Malignant tumour of the parotid gland

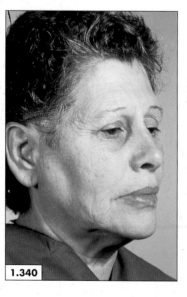

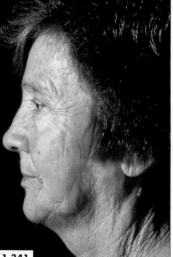

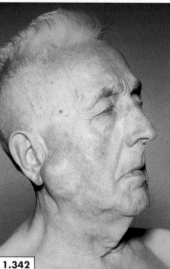

1.340

1.341

1.342

2 THE MOUTH

The mouth should be inspected with the patient facing a good natural source of light. This is particularly important when looking for cyanosis, pallor and excessive redness of the lips, gums, tongue and the buccal mucosa. The various individual components of the oropharynx should be examined sequentially.

The lips

An acute inflammation of the lips with painful fissuring and scaling (*cheilitis*) at the angles of the mouth (*angular cheilitis, angular stomatitis*) (2.1) is usually the result of physical damage to the lips by sunlight or cold wind. In patients with ill-fitting dentures, the skin and the mucosa at the corners of the mouth become macerated because of dribbling saliva, which causes fissuring of the angles of the mouth, or *cheilosis* (2.2). It is also a feature of *deficiency of the vitamin B complex, especially of riboflavin* (2.3). Angular cheilosis is sometimes complicated by monilial infection, particularly in immunocompromised states. Angular stomatitis may also be self-induced, as in this patient (2.4) who produced recurrent ulcers by digging his nails into the angles of his mouth.

By far the commonest infection of the lips is **herpes simplex**, which may start as a simple vesicle (2.5), later producing a cluster of vesicles and extending to the mucosa with ulceration (2.6). The infection may occur in healthy but susceptible subjects and it is often seen in association with the **common cold** and other acute febrile states such as **pneumococcal pneumonia**. The lips may also be

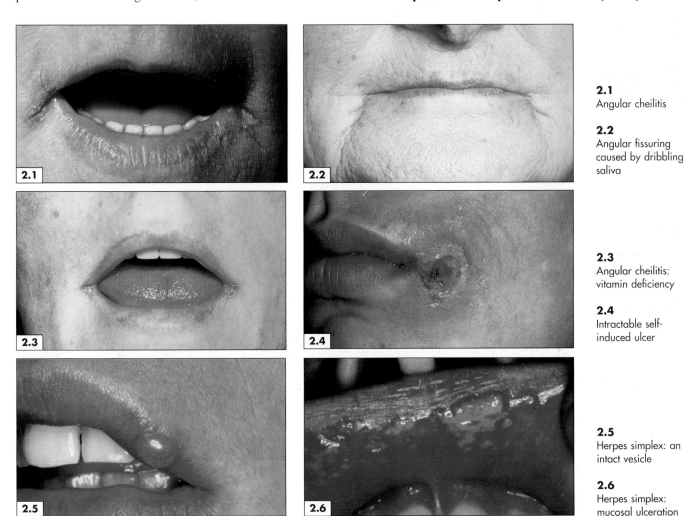

2.1
Angular cheilitis

2.2
Angular fissuring caused by dribbling saliva

2.3
Angular cheilitis: vitamin deficiency

2.4
Intractable self-induced ulcer

2.5
Herpes simplex: an intact vesicle

2.6
Herpes simplex: mucosal ulceration

involved in other cutaneous infections; for example in **tinea corporis** they have sharply marginated, red plaques (2.7).

A primary syphilitic **chancre** is a painless nodule that can ulcerate but it is rarely seen today. More commonly one may see a simple wart (2.8). A **cavernous haemangioma** is a bluish, compressible nodule that may occur on the lips (2.9). Both these lesions should be differentiated from a **squamous cell carcinoma**, which may start as a warty, crusted ulcer.

The granulomatous process of **Crohn's disease** may involve any part of the alimentary tract from the lips to

the anus. Oral lesions have been reported in 6–20% of patients; these occur more commonly in patients with colonic disease, and in those who have other extraintestinal manifestations such as joint and skin lesions. Oral lesions may precede the onset of intestinal disease, thus the condition should be suspected in any patient presenting with swollen lips (2.10, 2.11). Either of the lips may be involved with submucosal inflammation, oedema and fissuring, sometimes complicated by superadded cheilosis and ulceration (2.12). Aphthous ulcers and hyperplasia of the cheeks with fissuring of the buccal mucosa (2.13) may occur in some patients.

2.7
Tinea corporis: spreading erythematous ring

2.8
Simple wart

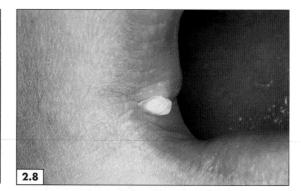

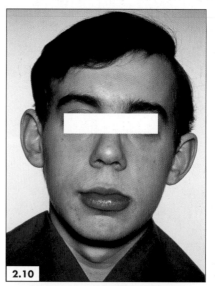

2.9
Cavernous haemangioma

2.10
Crohn's disease with granulomatous infiltration of the lower lip

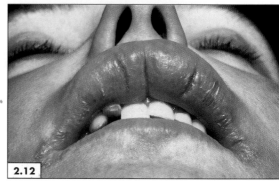

2.11
Crohn's disease lips

2.12
Crohn's disease: swollen lips with fissures and angular stomatitis

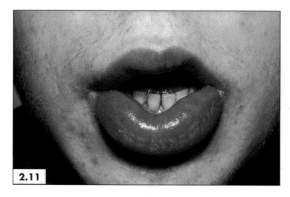

Multiple angiomas, varying from the size of a pinhead to 3 mm in diameter, occur on the mucous membranes in **hereditary haemorrhagic telangiectasia** (**Osler–Weber–Rendu syndrome**) (2.14) and in **systemic sclerosis** (2.15). Often the differential diagnosis is not difficult by the time the oropharynx is examined (see pp. **47, 52**). In general, the angiomata tend to be small, flat and discrete in systemic sclerosis, whereas those in hereditary haemorrhagic telangiectasia are larger, fleshy (2.16) and profuse involving the tongue and the buccal mucosa.

The brown, or brownish-black specks, of the **Peutz–Jeghers syndrome** should be looked for at the mucocutaneous junction of the lips and around the mouth (2.17).

Macules on the lips may disappear over time but oral pigmentation persists as an important diagnostic feature of this condition. As mentioned earlier (p. **46**), their clinical importance lies in their association with polyps in the small intestine which may cause intussusception and intestinal obstruction.

Sometimes a chance discovery of *pigmentation* in the mucous membrane of the lips (2.18) is the first clue of **Addison's disease**. More often the clinician has to look diligently for *buccal pigmentation* (see 1.95) in a patient suspected of having the disease. Although similar pigmentation may be seen in **haemosiderosis** (2.19) a history of multiple transfusions will resolve the issue.

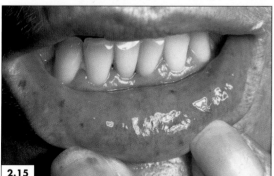

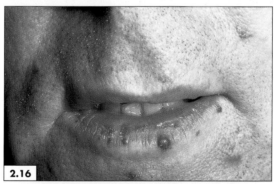

2.13
Crohn's disease: aphthous ulcer

2.14
Osler–Weber–Rendu syndrome: mucosal telangiectases

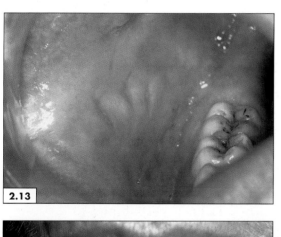

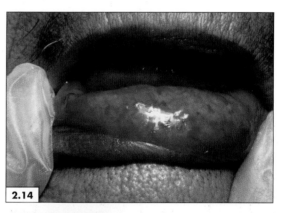

2.15
Systemic sclerosis: mucosal telangiectases

2.16
Osler–Weber–Rendu syndrome: large, fleshy angiomata

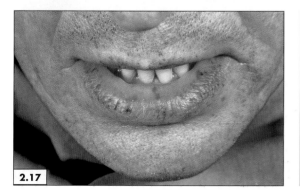

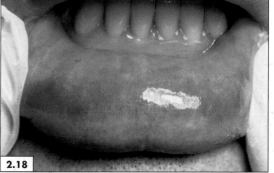

2.17
Peutz–Jeghers syndrome: mucocutaneous lentigines

2.18
Addison's disease: mucosal pigmentation

The gums and teeth

The gums, or gingivae, are part of the teeth-supporting apparatus and cover and protect the underlying tissues from the oral environment. Healthy gums are pinkish-red, firm, knife-edged and scalloped to conform with the contour of the teeth (2.20). The colour may vary with the melanin pigment in the epithelium, the vascularity and the amount of haemoglobin present in the blood. In Caucasian subjects, there is minimal pigmentation but some women may be left with marked gingival pigmentation after **multiple pregnancies** (2.21). A heavy and regular intake of coffee and prolonged smoking can cause staining of the teeth and gums (2.22). A high concentration of fluorine in the drinking water is also associated with marked staining of the teeth and gums (2.23). Chlorhexidine mouthwashes and red wines are also known to cause tooth stains.

Tetracycline staining of the teeth, often with *hypoplasia* (2.24), occurs when tetracycline is administered during the period of tooth formation, either to the pregnant mother or to a child up to the age of 12 years. This condition is rare today since there are safer alternative antibiotics available.

In **cystic fibrosis**, decreased saliva production associated with an inadequate attention to oral hygiene may cause discolouration, calculus formation (2.25) and *Pseudomonas aeruginosa* colonization of the mouth.

The gums, together with the alveolar bone, form the main components of the periodontium. **Periodontal**

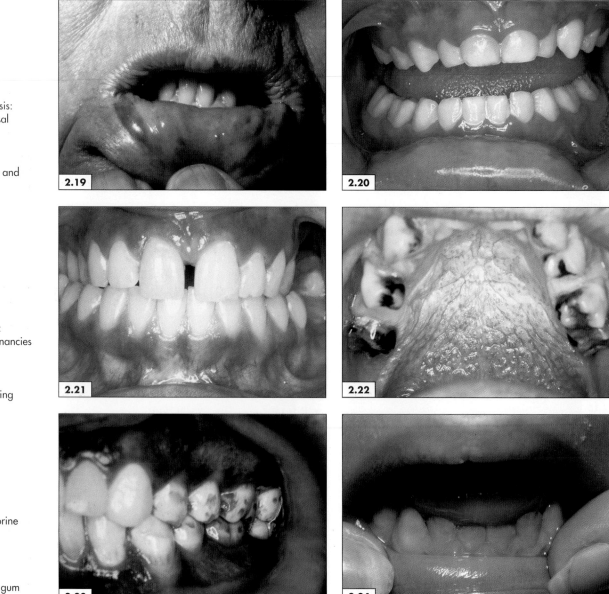

2.19
Haemosiderosis: diffuse mucosal pigmentation

2.20
Normal teeth and gums

2.21
Gingival pigmentation: multiple pregnancies

2.22
Tobacco and caffeine staining

2.23
Excessive fluorine staining

2.24
Tetracycline staining with gum hypoplasia

disease starts as gingivitis with red, swollen and friable gums (2.26) and leads to the loosening and loss of teeth (2.27). *Dental plaque* is a constant source of irritation, inflammation and pocketing of the gingival margin, which cuffs around the origin of the teeth. The plaque consists of numerous multiplying bacteria, which attach to the *salivary pellicle* (salivary glycoprotein forming a protective layer on the surface of the teeth) superadded with food residue. Although the dental plaques are invisible to the unaided eye, bad oral hygiene indicated by multiple plaques, food residues and inflamed gingival margin is easy to see (2.28), especially when compared with healthy gums free from plaques (2.29).

Some of the plaques become calcified and form a stony crust, or *tartar*, which deposits on the teeth and encroaches on to the undersurface of the gums (2.30, 2.31). **Supragingival calculus** is deposited first on the tooth surface opposite the salivary ducts, on the lingual surfaces of the lower incisors (2.30) and on the buccal surfaces of the upper molars. **Subgingival calculus** is attached to the root surface and its distribution is unrelated to the salivary ducts but related to the presence of gingival inflammation (2.31). It is dark green or black and tightly adherent to the tooth surface.

Plaque deposition, bacterial colonization, mineralization, gingivitis and pocket formation are the steps that lead to advanced periodontal disease and premature loss of teeth. Thus, plaque control and good oral hygiene form the cornerstone for prevention of periodontal disease and preservation of teeth, as illustrated by this sub-

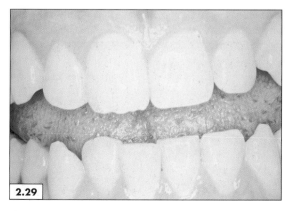

2.25

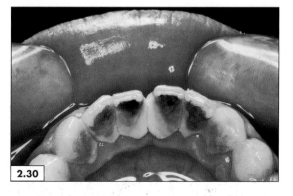

2.26

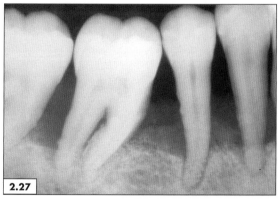

2.27

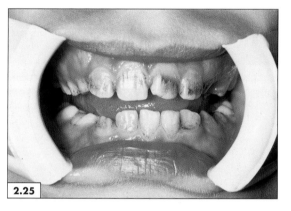

2.28

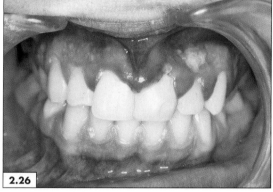

2.29

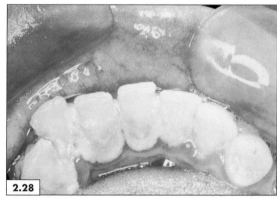

2.30

2.25
Cystic fibrosis: marked calculus formation

2.26
Gingivitis: inflamed and swollen gums

2.27
Advanced periodontal disease with loose teeth

2.28
Poor oral hygiene with food residue and plaque in between and around teeth

2.29
Good oral hygiene with clean gingival margins

2.30
Tartar on the teeth

ject (2.32) who had all his teeth intact at the age of 75 years.

Plaque is invisible and is often difficult to dislodge. Since plaques contain organic matter they can be stained with food-colouring agents such as **erythrosin**, which is the chief constituent of the so-called **disclosing tablets**, to make them visible (2.33). This method can be used to test the effectiveness of brushing of the teeth as illustrated in Figures 2.34 and 2.35, in which right-handed patients have missed more plaques on the right side than on the left side of the mouth.

Unchecked plaque formation leads to gingival inflammation (2.36). The gums become swollen, spongy, red, friable and bleed after minor trauma, such as eating an apple. The gums separate from the teeth giving rise to pockets, which may not be easy to detect unless exposed

2.31
Tartar eroding under the gums

2.32
Well-preserved teeth in a man aged 75 years

2.33
Disclosing agent revealing the widespread plaque formation

2.34 and 2.35
Disclosing agent after thorough brushing: residual plaques suggests inadequate brushing

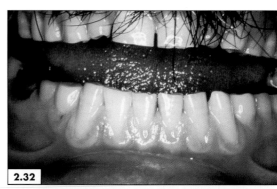

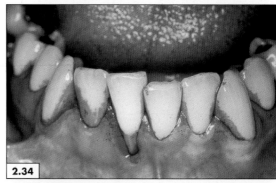

2.36
Gingival inflammation due to chronic plaque formation

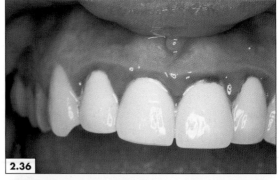

2.37
Gingival probe

2.38
Advanced periodontal disease with canine drifting

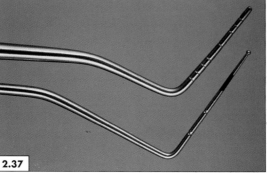

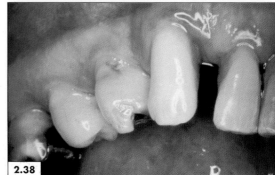

with a special probe (2.37). Advanced periodontal disease with *bone resorption* may cause drifting of canine teeth (2.38) and will eventually lead to tooth loss.

Periodontal disease, as described above, is very common in the general population but it is usually left to dental surgeons to diagnose and treat. In contrast, *swelling of the gums* (2.39), which is far less common than periodontal disease, attracts much more attention among physicians because of its connection with various drugs and medical disorders, for example:

- Puberty;
- Pregnancy;
- Drugs (e.g. phenytoin, nifedipine);
- Gingivitis (e.g. periodontal disease, Vincent's ulcerative gingivitis);
- Amyloidosis;
- Acute myeloid leukaemia;
- Scurvy.

Hyperplasia of the gums is frequently seen in association with long-term **phenytoin therapy for epilepsy** (2.40). Such a patient will give a history of seizures and may also have some of the other side-effects of the drug such as dizziness, nausea, hirsutism, diplopia, ataxia, lymphoma-like syndrome, lupus erythematosus, pulmonary fibrosis and megaloblastic anaemia caused by folate malabsorption. The differentiation from periodontal disease, with which it may coexist, may be difficult. In drug-induced hyperplasia (2.41) the dental margin of the gums is swollen and spongy but not inflamed and friable as in periodontal disease (2.36). Patients with gum hypertrophy need to take extra care to maintain good oral hygiene.

Prolonged vitamin C deficiency, or **scurvy**, characteristically leads to **gingivitis** with swollen, fragile and purplish gingival papillae (2.42, 2.43). The condition is uncommon today but is still found among socially deprived elderly patients.

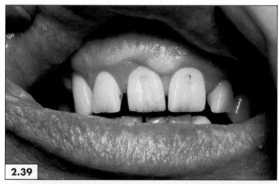

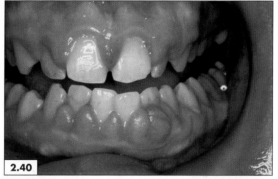

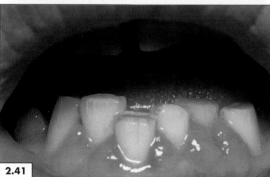

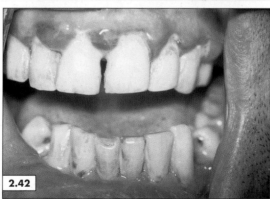

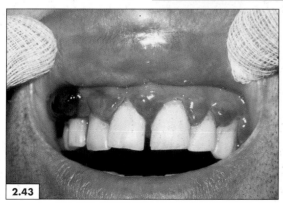

2.39
Swollen gums

2.40
Phenytoin gum hyperplasia: swollen, spongy gums

2.41
Drug-induced gum hyperplasia

2.42 and 2.43
Scurvy: gingival hypertrophy with purplish discolouration

One of the diseases with swollen gums that needs urgent attention is **acute leukaemia**, especially of the **myelomonocytic** variety (2.44). The dentist may be the first person to see such a patient and needs to be aware of the association. The absence of any of the other causes of gum hyperplasia, and a history of a haemorrhagic diathesis, should suggest the diagnosis of acute leukaemia.

The common conditions of dermatological interest that affect the oral mucous membrane are moniliasis, lichen planus, erythema multiforme, pemphigus, herpes and secondary syphilis. **Herpetic vesicles** appear on an erythematous base and then erode and form ulcers. These lesions are often seen in clusters (2.45). **Pemphigus** (2.46), and less often **pemphigoid**, also involve the oral mucous membrane. In the former the typical lesions are erosions, and

bullae are rarely seen, whereas in pemphigoid there may be erosions and bullae that are not easily ruptured.

Patients with acute lesions of the gums and lips usually present first to their general practitioners but they are also seen in hospital practice. **Self-induced injury** to the gums (2.47, 2.48) is often recurrent and erosions tend to occur in the same place. There are usually seen around the incisors which are easily accesible to the patient. **Self-biting ulcers** characteristically occur at the angles of the mouth (2.49) where the mucous membrane is easily trapped between the two sets of canine teeth.

Acute ulcerative gingivitis known as **Vincent's disease** or **acute necrotizing gingivitis** (2.50, 2.51) is caused by a variety of organisms, particularly *Borrelia vincentii* and *Fusobacterium nucleatum*. It is a disease of young adults,

2.44
Acute myelomonocytic leukaemia: gingival hypertrophy with haemorrhages

2.45
Herpes simplex: cluster of ulcers

2.46
Pemphigus: inflamed mucosa and ulceration

2.47
Self-induced erosion above the right incisor

2.48
Self-induced erosion above the incisors

2.49
Self-biting ulcer at the angle of the mouth

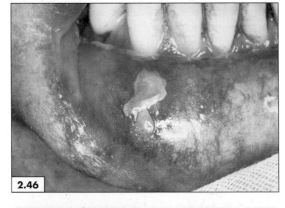
2.44

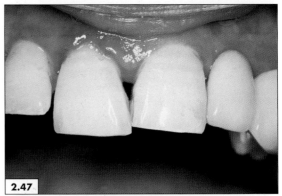
2.45

2.46

2.47

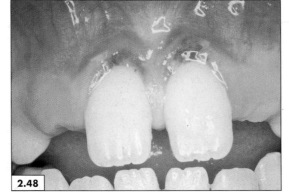
2.48

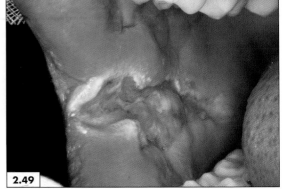
2.49

occurs equally in both sexes, and most cases are seen in spring and autumn. The presenting features are spontaneous bleeding, gingival soreness, alteration of taste and a disagreeable halitosis. Predisposing factors include malnutrition (*trench mouth* of soldiers in World War I), an extraoral malignancy, blood dyscrasias and heavy smoking.

Aphthous ulcers are the most common lesions of the oral mucosa. The ulcers may be small (**Mikulicz's aphthae**) and punched out with an inflamed margin (2.52). **Major aphthous ulcer (periadenitis mucosa necrotica recurrens)** starts as a submucosal nodule and soon breaks down to form a crater-like ulcer (2.53), which may last for over a month. The characteristic features of aphthous ulcers are that they are painful, recurrent, and may occur anywhere on the oropharynx. They are of unknown aetiology but are sometimes associated with a variety of conditions such as collagen disorders, gastrointestinal diseases and Behçet's syndrome.

Chronic desquamative gingivitis (gingivosis) occurs mostly in young females. In the moderately severe forms there is erythema of the marginal, interdental and attached gingiva, with desquamation of the epithelium of the intervening gingiva, revealing the underlying grey surface (2.54). Patients complain of a burning sensation and cannot tolerate tooth brushing, condiments and inhalation of air.

The gingiva may become swollen and red during puberty, pregnancy and in women taking the contraceptive pill, but frank gingivitis is uncommon in pregnant women who maintain good oral hygiene. Occasionally, a '**pregnancy tumour**', or **epulis** (2.55), develops from an inflamed gingival papilla. It is a form of pyogenic granuloma and

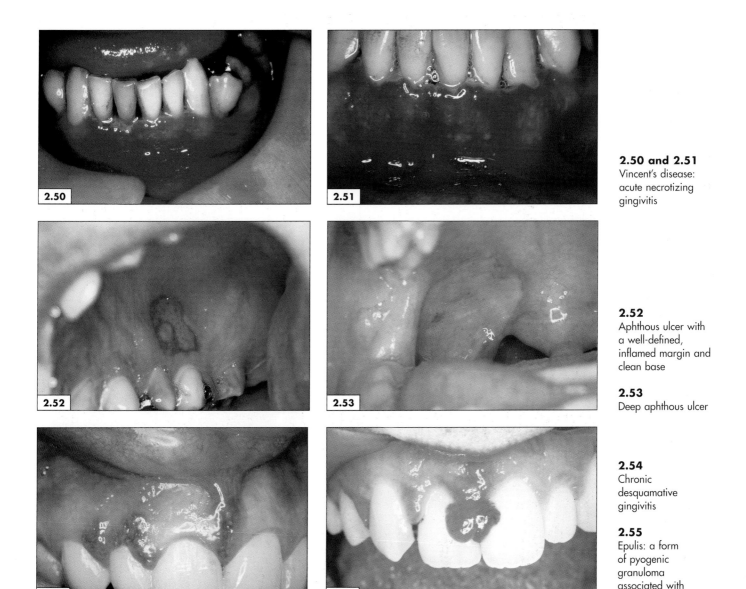

2.50 and 2.51
Vincent's disease: acute necrotizing gingivitis

2.52
Aphthous ulcer with a well-defined, inflamed margin and clean base

2.53
Deep aphthous ulcer

2.54
Chronic desquamative gingivitis

2.55
Epulis: a form of pyogenic granuloma associated with pregnancy

presents as a localized, red, pedunculated swelling (2.56), which may become large enough to displace a tooth (2.57, 2.58). The term **angiogranuloma** is often applied to avoid the implication of a neoplasm. Removal of the epulis should be associated with the removal of local irritants and with fastidious dental hygiene without which the swelling always recurs. Occasionally, an epulis may achieve gigantic proportions (2.59). They bleed easily and cause malocclusion of the teeth. Although spontaneous regression follows after delivery, the complete elimination of the residual inflammatory lesion requires the removal of all forms of local irritation.

Excessive sugar intake predisposes the teeth to **caries**. Even the *milk-teeth* can be affected, as seen in this infant who was habitually sucking a dummy covered with sugar (2.60.)

The tongue

The clinician should have a set of observations with definite questions and the possible answers as a litany when examining the tongue, since repeated requests to protrude the tongue become wearisome for the patient. It should be looked at for its **size** (e.g. macroglossia, hemiatrophy, global atrophy), **shape** (e.g. *triangular*, square or lobed), **colour** (e.g. *pink*, red, blue or pale), **state of hydration** (e.g. *moist*, dry, furred and coated), **papillae** (e.g. *normal*, enlarged or atrophied), **vessels** (e.g. prominent, angiomata), and for any **lesions** on it. At a single look the clinician should be able to obtain answers to several pre-set questions (Table 2.1). A prolonged or further inspection may be necessary only if an abnormality has been found.

The normal tongue is moist, red or pink-red, usually uncoated and triangular with the protruding tip being nar-

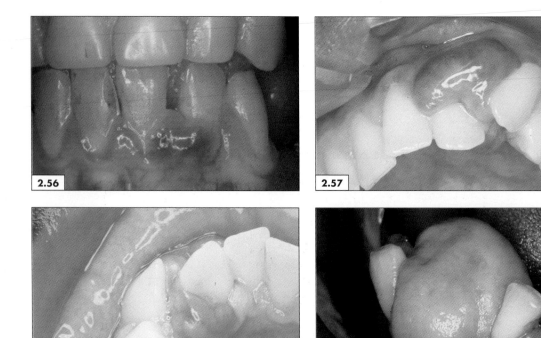

2.56
Large epulis

2.57
Large epulis displacing teeth

2.58
Large epulis encroaching on the canine tooth

2.59
Gigantic epulis

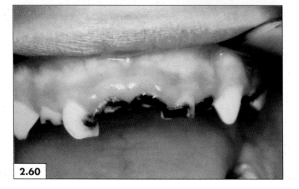

2.60
Caries in infantile teeth: the 'sugared dummy teeth'

rower than the base inside the mouth (2.61.) Sometimes the tongue of a healthy subject may be coated, in the absence of dehydration, pyrexia or mouth breathing. A **dry tongue** will impart little or no moisture to the examiner's finger tip touching it. Common causes of a dry tongue are mouth breathing, dehydration, and the ingestion of anti-depressants and atropine-like drugs. Sjögren's syndrome and local radiotherapy also cause a dry tongue but, in such cases, there will be other supportive signs and symptoms.

The **black hairy tongue** is a normal variant; the hair consists of elongated, filiform papillae on the dorsum. The colour varies from yellowish (2.62) to brown or black (2.63). The cause of a hairy tongue is often unknown but occasionally may follow antibiotic therapy.

Leucoplakia with thick, white, adherent patches or streaks on the tongue (2.64) is an important sign to recognize because of its significance as a *premalignant* condition. The patches have sharply defined edges, cannot be denuded from the mucous membrane of the tongue, and look like streaks of white paint (2.65).

Table 2.1 Examination of the tongue

Questions	Possible answers/observations
Normal variants	Coated, geographical, 'scrotal' tongue, black hairy, varicosities on the undersurface ('caviar' tongue)
Size	Macroglossia, hemiatrophy, global atrophy
Shape	Triangular, multilobed, square
Colour	Red, bright red, pale, blue
Papillae	Enlarged, absent (bald tongue)
Vessels	Prominent, angiomas
Hydration	Moist, dry, coated and furred
Movements	Immobility, deviation, fasciculation

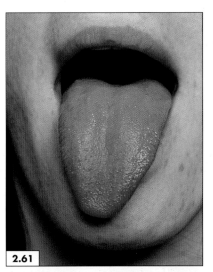

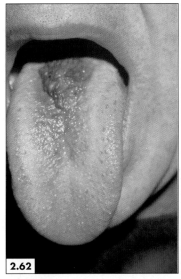

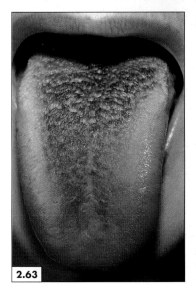

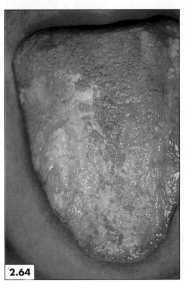

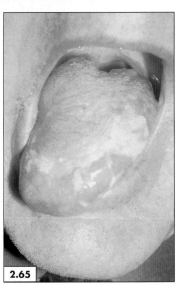

2.61
Normal tongue

2.62
Yellow, hairy tongue with elongated papillae

2.63
Black hairy tongue with filiform, elongated papillae

2.64
Sharply defined leucoplakia patches

2.65
Leucoplakia with well-defined white patches

Patients with **acromegaly** and **myxoedema** have fleshy, large tongues. In the former case, the protruded tongue may fill the entire oral orifice (2.66). **Primary amyloidosis** is a well-known cause of *macroglossia* and in some cases the tongue may be very large and multilobed owing to amyloid deposition (2.67). Similarly, other tumours can cause an irregular enlargement of the tongue.

A lower motor neurone lesion of the twelfth cranial nerve causes unilateral *wasting* of the tongue on the affected side, where the mucous membrane is raised into folds owing to the underlying muscular atrophy (2.68). The protruded tongue deviates to the side of the lesion (2.69) because of the unopposed action of the opposite genioglossus. The atrophied side is wrinkled and the median raphe curves with its concavity to the paralysed side. A unilateral lesion may be caused by **syringomyelia, motor neurone disease, tumours** and **fracture of the base of the skull**.

The most common cause of *bilateral wasting* of the tongue is **motor neurone disease**. The tongue is reduced in size and the mucous membrane of the dorsal surface is thrown into folds (2.70). The wasting may be asymmetrical and the protruded tongue will deviate to the worse affected side (2.71). *Fasciculations* are usually present and are often best seen if the tongue is in a relaxed position in the floor of the mouth.

Cyanosis, particularly a mild degree of blue discolouration of the mucous membranes, is one of the most difficult signs to recognize in clinical medicine. Nevertheless some clinicians can guess the arterial oxygen saturation to within 5%, simply by looking at the tongue and the buccal mucous membrane of a cyanosed patient, especially if it is a mildly hypoxaemic subject. Any careful observer can acquire this skill by comparing the abnormal with a normal tongue side by side (2.72, 2.73) for the first dozen or so observations.

An experienced clinician used to looking at the normal tongue should recognize easily the raw, beefy-red tongue associated with a **glucagonoma** (2.74), or the red and comparatively bald tongue of **iron deficiency anaemia** (2.75).

2.66
Acromegaly: large, square tongue fitting the oral cavity

2.67
Primary amyloidosis: multilobular, large tongue with amyloid deposits

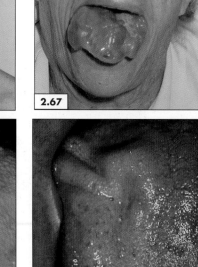

2.68
Right twelfth cranial nerve palsy with mucosal folds over an atrophied and shrunken tongue

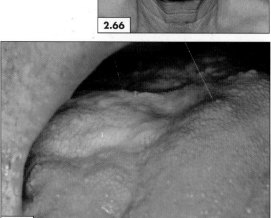

2.69
Right hypoglossal nerve palsy: the tongue deviates to the side of the atrophy

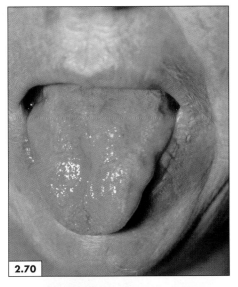

2.70

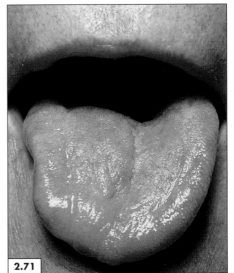

2.71

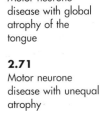

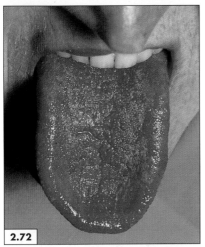

2.72

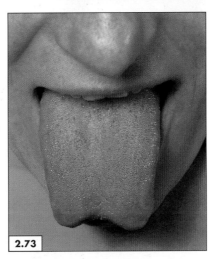

2.73

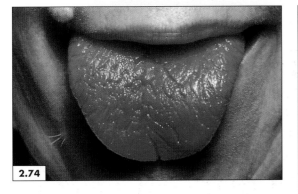

2.74

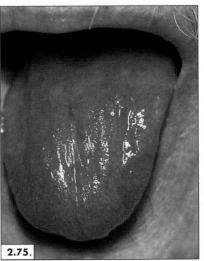

2.75,

2.70
Motor neurone disease with global atrophy of the tongue

2.71
Motor neurone disease with unequal atrophy

2.72
Bluish-red, cyanosed tongue

2.73
Normal tongue

2.74
Glucagonoma syndrome: beefy, red tongue

2.75
Iron deficiency anaemia: bald tongue with atrophied papillae and angular inflammation

Glossitis is not always very severe but there is usually some degree of atrophy of the lingual papillae, often associated with *angular stomatitis* and *facial pallor* (2.76). Although iron and vitamin B12 deficiency states (2.77) are comparatively commoner causes of a sore, red and smooth tongue, enquiry should also be extended to include a deficiency of riboflavin, niacin, folic acid and pyridoxine. Sometimes anticancer treatment may produce a similar appearance. A deficiency of more than one vitamin is much more likely to cause glossitis and loss of papillae, as may be seen in patients with **malabsorption, pellagra**, and **scurvy caused by malnutrition** in socially deprived patients (2.78).

In the **Peutz–Jeghers syndrome**, the freckle-like pigmentation not only involves the lips (see 2.17) but it also often extends to the tongue (2.79).

Although punched-out lesions resembling aphthous ulcers may be present on the tongue without any identifiable cause, these may suggest the possibility of **chronic inflammatory bowel disease** (2.80) as the two are frequently associated.

In one subgroup of **multiple endocrine neoplasia, MEN type IIb**, the tongue may have *mucosal neuromas* on its surface (2.81). These small mucosal outgrowths may also be present on the lips and eyelids. The syndrome consists of a

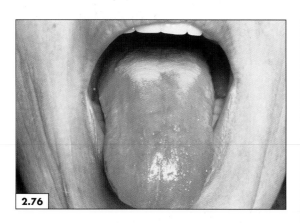

2.76
Iron deficiency anaemia with bald tongue and angular stomatitis

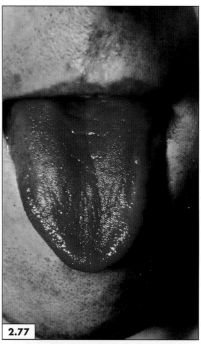

2.77
Iron and vitamin B12 deficiency: glossitis with angular stomatitis

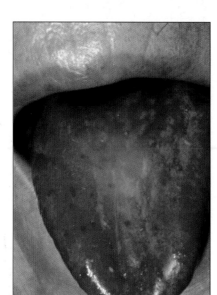

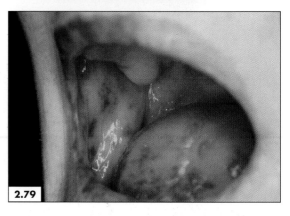

2.78
Undernutrition with multiple vitamin and iron deficiency: bald, fiery tongue

2.79
Peutz–Jeghers syndrome: mucosal lentigines and pigmentation

medullary carcinoma of the thyroid, mucosal neuromas, a Marfanoid habitus, and is sometimes associated with a phaeochromocytoma or a parathyroid adenoma. Apart from the mucosal lesions there may be a swelling in the neck or an operation scar of previous thyroidectomy for the medullary carcinoma (2.82). Some patients also have a proximal myopathy and ganglioneuromatosis of the bowel.

Both the dorsal and ventral surfaces of the tongue should be inspected carefully to look for the small *telangiectasia* (2.83, 2.84) associated with the **Osler–Weber–Rendu syndrome**. Such a finding can help considerably in investigating a patient with an iron-deficiency anaemia of undetermined cause.

In patients with **superior vena caval obstruction**, the undersurface of the tongue may show the presence of multiple angiomata and distension of the venules (2.85),

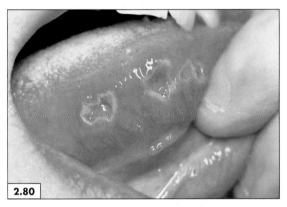

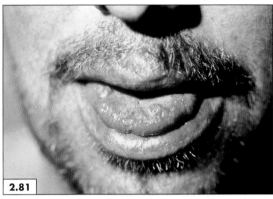

2.80
Ulcerative colitis: punched out aphthous ulcers

2.81
Multiple endocrine neoplasia type IIb: mucosal neuromas

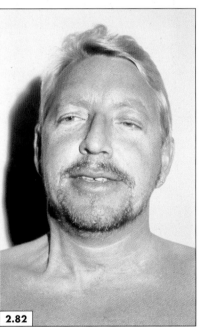

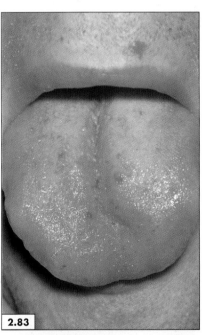

2.82
Multiple endocrine neoplasia type IIb. Note scar of previous thyroidectomy

2.83
Osler–Weber–Rendu syndrome: glossal telangiectases

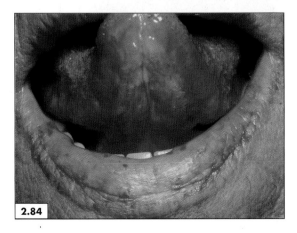

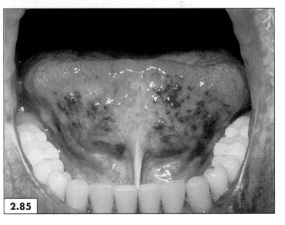

2.84
Osler–Weber–Rendu syndrome: telangiectasia on the undersurface of the tongue

2.85
Superior vena caval obstruction: multiple angiomata due to prolonged, venous stasis

which resembles the 'caviar tongue' of some elderly patients with varicosities on the undersurface. An isolated, single haemangioma may be seen on the dorsal surface of the tongue (2.86). Such swellings are bluish in colour and often compressible.

Mucosal eruptions of the oropharynx occur in a variety of mucocutaneous disorders and the mouth should always be examined whenever a skin lesion is seen. In some cases the mucosal lesions may be the first to appear, as for example in measles, pemphigus, Behçet's syndrome, and purpura.

Koplik's spots (see also p. **44**) are not always easy to find. In a febrile child, the buccal mucosa should be inspected carefully with the help of a good light. During the prodromal stage of **measles**, these spots can be seen as small, 'salt-grain' white dots (2.87) or patches on the inside of the cheeks (see also 1.223).

Mucosal ulcers associated with severe erythema and haemorrhagic exudation occur in the **Stevens–Johnson syndrome** (2.88, 2.89). There is usually a positive drug history (of, for example, sulphonamides, antibiotics, etc.) and erythematous and *target lesions* may be seen on the skin (see 1.189).

Viral infections such as herpes and Coxsackie may cause eruptions on the tongue (2.90).

The oral mucous membrane is often affected early in the course of **lichen planus** with slightly raised, white lesions usually in a characteristic lacy-pattern distribution (2.91). A similar trabecular appearance is also seen on the inner surfaces of the cheeks (2.92). These lesions are asymptomatic and easily missed but are nonetheless very important for confirming the diagnosis, since the cutaneous lesions may sometimes resemble psoriasis.

Recurrent, painful aphthous ulcers of the tongue (2.93) and buccal mucosa (2.94) are the hallmark of **Behçet's syndrome**. The pharynx and palate are rarely involved. Apart from the recurrent oral and genital ulcers, the syndrome

2.86
Haemangioma

2.87
Measles: Koplik's spots

2.88 and 2.89
Stevens–Johnson syndrome: multiple mucosal ulcers with erythema

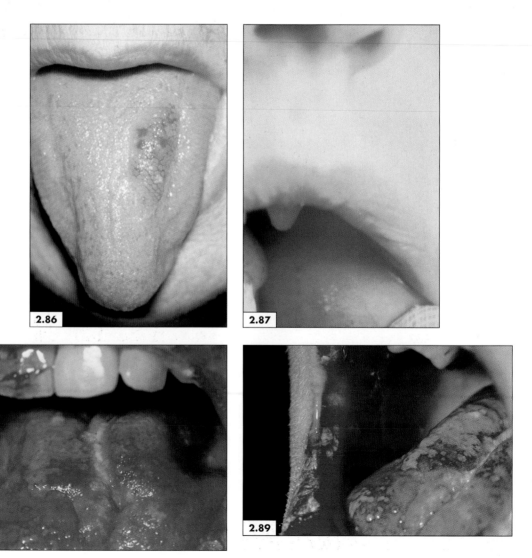

frequently involves the eyes (e.g. recurrent hypopyon, iritis, iridocyclitis, chorioretinitis), the skin (e.g. erythema nodosum, thrombophlebitis), the joints, gastrointestinal tract, and the central nervous system (e.g. brainstem syndromes, confusional states).

Oral candidiasis, or **thrush**, is caused by *Candida albicans*, which is a normal commensal of the gastrointestinal tract. The organism becomes invasive at the extremes of age, in immunocompromised patients, and in those whose microbial flora has been altered by disease or by antibiotic therapy. The typical lesions are adherent white patches on the tongue (2.95, 2.96) and buccal mucosa, and there is often associated angular stomatitis (2.97). The infection may also involve the urogenital area, the

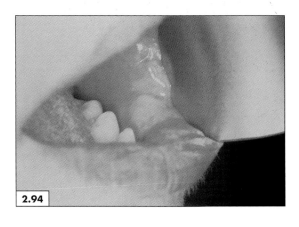

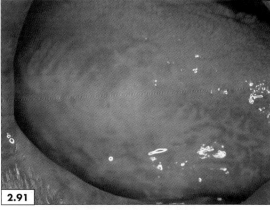

2.90
Coxsackie eruption: ulcers with inflamed margins

2.91
Oral lichen planus: confluent, white papules coalesced in a lacy pattern

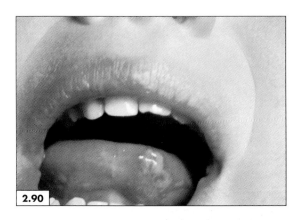

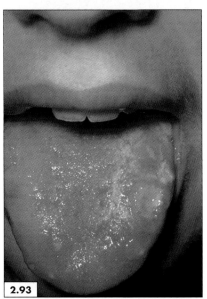

2.92
Buccal lichen planus with a lacy pattern

2.93
Behçet's syndrome: aphthous ulcers

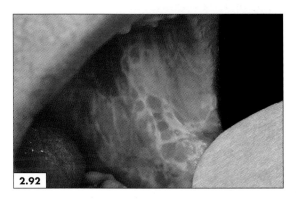

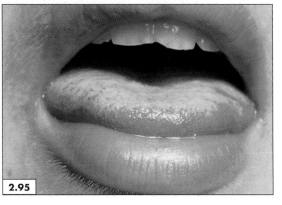

2.94
Behçet's syndrome: aphthous ulcers of the buccal mucosa

2.95
Pseudomembranous candidiasis (thrush)

oesophagus causing dysphagia, and the alimentary tract producing intractable, and sometimes 'unexplained', diarrhoea.

Carcinoma of the tongue (2.98) may be easily missed because it is painless in the initial stages and usually occurs on the edges or the undersurface of the tongue. **Tertiary syphilis** may occasionally involve the tongue causing a *gumma* (2.99). This may prove very helpful when there are unexplained symptoms referable to the liver or bones.

The palate and pharynx

The fauces and pharynx must be examined with the aid of a good light. A tongue depressor should be used to get

2.96
Widespread colonies of *Candida* with erythematous (atrophic) patches

2.97
Candidiasis with angular cheilitis

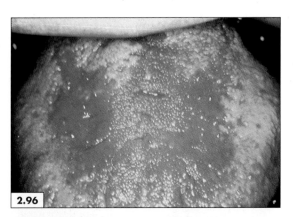
2.96

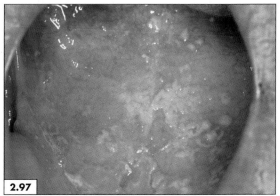
2.97

2.98
Painless ulcer (carcinoma) of the tongue

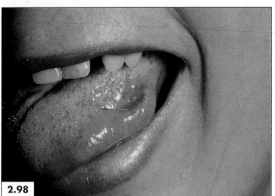
2.98

2.99
A well-defined gummatous nodule

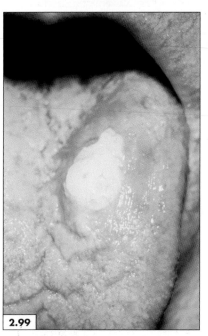
2.99

2.100
Palatal purpura

2.101
Aplastic anaemia: a blood blister with surrounding haemorrhagic spots

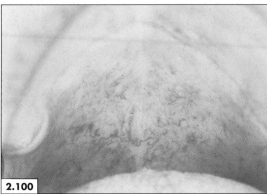
2.100

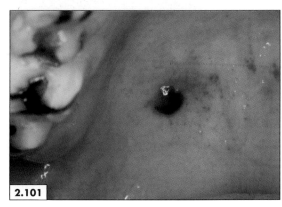
2.101

an adequate view of the uvula, posterior wall of the pharynx and the tonsils. Some of the mucosal lesions mentioned already also involve the palate and should be looked for.

Purpuric spots may be seen scattered on the mucous membrane of the palate in any condition causing **thrombocytopenia**. In some systemic disorders, such as **rheumatoid arthritis**, the association may spring to mind if these spots are seen, as in this patient with **Felty's syndrome** (2.100). *Blood blisters* with a few purpuric spots on the palate (2.101) may be caused by heat burn or by trauma from a fork or fishbone but their presence may also be an important clue to an unsuspected **acute leukaemia** or **aplastic anaemia**. The two conditions are frequently asso-ciated with small haematomas on the buccal mucosa (2.102) from trauma caused by the neighbouring teeth.

Streptococcal pharyngitis and **diphtheria** (rare today) cause an exudative pharyngitis with yellowish-white patches covering the tonsils and fauces. Sometimes the former may herald **infectious mononucleosis** (2.103).

Nodular involvement of the pharynx (2.104) is suggestive of **Wegener's granulomatosis**, particularly when it is associated with *haematuria, vasculitis* and/or *pulmonary infiltrations*.

Perforation of the palate is one of the legacies of **congenital syphilis** and it may be seen in an adult (2.105) who may have some of the other features of the disease (see 1.323, 1.324, 3.52, 3.53 and 11.52).

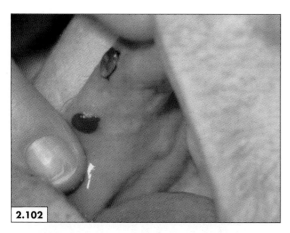

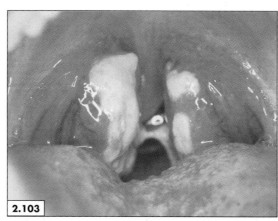

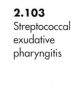

2.102
A buccal haematoma in a patient with acute leukaemia

2.103
Streptococcal exudative pharyngitis

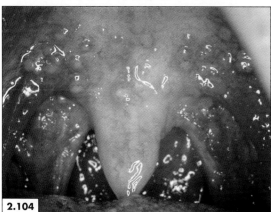

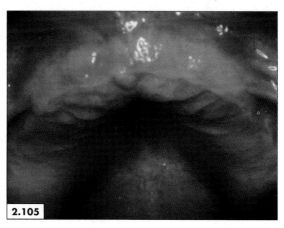

2.104
Wegener's granulomatosis: granulomatous nodules in the fauces and pharynx

2.105
Perforation of the soft palate

During the examination of the oropharynx (with the patient saying 'Aah'), note should be taken of the shape of the palate and arch which may be narrow and high as in **Marfan's syndrome** (2.106). The teeth may be crowded and maloccluded and there may be other associated skeletal stigmata (see 11.48, 11.49; p. **225**).

The usual central position of the uvula may be altered by an injury to the tenth cranial nerve, which supplies the muscles of the palate. The tenth nerve, together with the ninth and the eleventh cranial nerves which accompany it, may be injured as they exit through the jugular foramen. The uvula is drawn to the opposite side as in this patient with a left-sided **jugular foramen syndrome** (2.107). There is an *absent gag reflex* on the affected side, impaired taste over the posterior third of the tongue (ninth cranial nerve), and a *weak and wasted sternomastoid muscle* (eleventh cranial nerve).

The deviation of the uvula may not be obvious in its resting position but it can be highlighted if the patient is asked to open the mouth as widely as possible and say 'Aah', as in this patient with a **left lateral medullary syndrome** (2.108). This patient also had an ipsilateral Horner's syndrome and diminished pain and temperature sensation on the face, signs of cerebellar dysfunction, and contralateral decreased pain and temperature sensation on the trunk and limbs.

A neoplasm of the pharynx is easy to detect in an advanced stage when it also involves and distorts the soft palate (2.109).

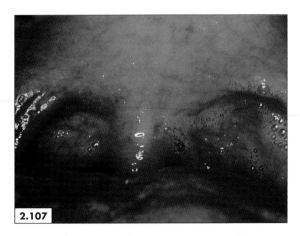

2.106
Marfan's syndrome: gothic arch

2.107
Left tenth cranial nerve palsy. Note deviation of the uvula to the right

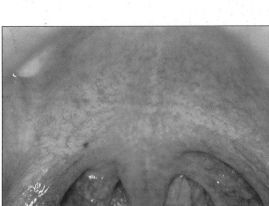
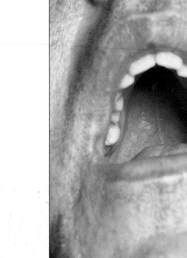

2.108
Left lateral medullary syndrome: on saying 'Aah' the palate contracts on the healthy (right) side

2.109
A marauding carcinoma of the pharynx

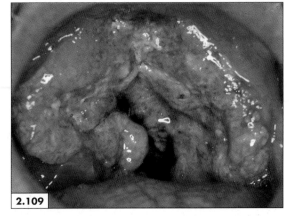
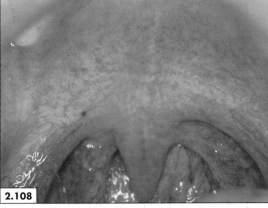

3 THE EXTERNAL EYE

A generalist needs to have some knowledge and understanding both of the conditions that cause local ocular diseases and of the ocular manifestations of various systemic disorders. The initial inspection should focus on each subsection of the external eye (3.1, 3.2) namely: the orbit, the eyebrows, the eyelashes, the eyelids; the two canthi where the lower and upper eyelids meet; the caruncle; the conjunctiva; the cornea; the iris; and the lens. A sequential inspection of these areas completes a full assessment of the eyes.

The eyelids and orbit

Herpes simplex and **herpes zoster** can both involve the eyes in susceptible subjects. In **herpes simplex 1 infection** clusters of vesicles usually appear on the lower eyelids which, after rupture, leave erythematous spots (3.3). In patients with **atopic eczema**, the infection can take a more aggressive form, **eczema herpeticum**, affecting both lids and conjunctiva (3.4). The infection rapidly becomes widespread involving the lips and face (3.5), the extremities, the

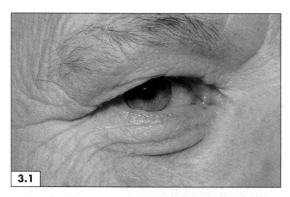

3.1

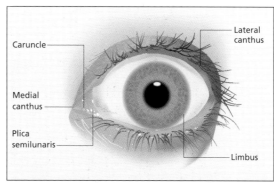

3.1
Normal eye

3.2
Structures of the eye

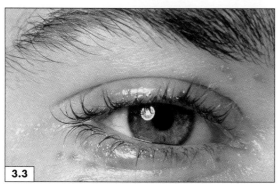

3.3

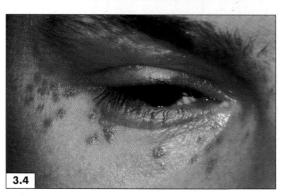

3.4

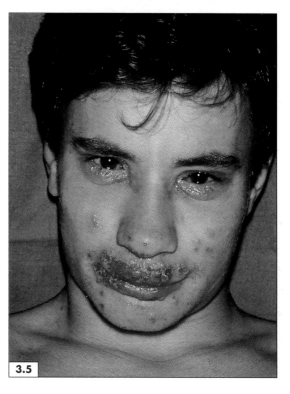

3.5

3.3
Herpes simplex: ruptured vesicles

3.4
Eczema herpeticum: clusters of ruptured vesicles

3.5
Herpes of the eyes, face and lips: confluent, ruptured, crusted vesicles

trunk and, in some cases, the central nervous system. The cornea develops a **superficial punctate keratitis** with tiny, whitish plaques (3.6) that desquamate, form erosions and usually heal without scarring. The keratitis is associated with irritation, lacrimation and blepharospasm. *Dendritic ulceration* is the hallmark of epithelial involvement. The opaque cells of the initial lesion become arranged in a dendritic, coarse punctate or stellate pattern (3.7). Healing is usually complete.

After the initial episode, the infected person becomes a carrier and periodic attacks may erupt on the lips, nose, eyelids, cornea and genitalia, particularly in association with intercurrent febrile illnesses. Sometimes infection with **herpes simplex 2** may be acquired by sexual contact, resulting in a herpetic eruption on the genitalia and eyelids with associated **keratoconjunctivitis** (3.8). The appearances are indistinguishable from herpes simplex 1 and the diagnosis can be made by obtaining an appropriate history.

In **herpes zoster ophthalmicus** rows of vesicles, or crusted small ulcers and residual scabs, are scattered along the course of one or more branches of the ophthalmic division of the fifth cranial nerve (3.9; see also 1.214, 1.215; p. **42**). The surrounding skin becomes red and oedematous. The pain can be excruciating but sometimes ceases after the outbreak of the eruption. Unfortunately, in many patients the pain persists for months and even years.

The eyelids may be affected like the rest of the body in **neurofibromatosis** and sometimes there may be a single neuroma on one of the lids (3.10) with no other visible tumours. Such a nodule (3.11) has a firm feel unlike a haemangioma. The nerves may be hypertrophied and felt as hard strings through the skin, and there may be *café-au-lait* spots on the trunk (see 7.37; p. **148**). In some cases, the ciliary nerves are affected and sometimes there may be a glioma of the optic nerve.

Erysipelas of the face may involve the corresponding orbit (3.12) when both eyelids are red, shiny and swollen. The patient is unable to open fully the affected eyelids and often there is associated fever and leucocytosis.

3.6
Keratoconjunctivitis: well-defined, whitish plaques of punctate keratitis

3.7
Ulceration of the cornea with greyish discolouration and irregular margins

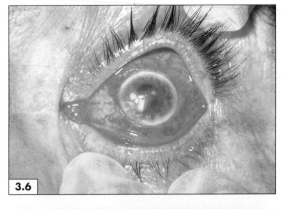
3.6

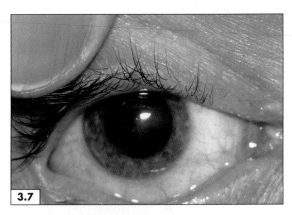
3.7

3.8
Herpetic keratoconjunctivitis

3.9
Herpes zoster, involving the eye, along the distribution of the ophthalmic branch of the fifth cranial nerve

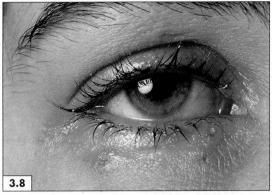
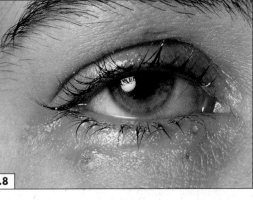
3.8

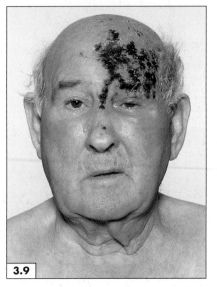
3.9

The redness and swelling seen only on the eyelids is the result of **orbital cellulitis** (3.13). The infection spreads most frequently from a nasal sinus but occasionally it may be caused by a retained foreign body or a staphylococcal septicaemia. There is usually severe pain aggravated by movement of the proptosed eye, the latter often obscured by the swollen and chemosed eyelids. In some patients there is a retrobulbar neuritis, which may progress to optic atrophy. Panophthalmitis may develop, with the danger of extension to the meninges and brain. **Proptosis** has been discussed earlier (p. **27**) and the exophthalmos of Graves' disease has been discussed in Chapter 1 (p. **14**).

The exophthalmos and reddish induration of the upper eyelids of **histiocytosis X (Langerhans' cell granulomato-** sis) (3.14) may mimic orbital cellulitis but the former is of long-standing duration, predominantly affects male children and there are no local or systemic signs of infection. In its *multifocal form*, there may be involvement of the bones (destructive lesions), hypothalamus (diabetes insipidus), lungs (interstitial infiltrates leading to a honeycomb appearance) and lymphoid and other tissues (hepatosplenomegaly, lymphadenopathy). A painless, nodular swelling within the orbit, without any signs of inflammation, should alert the clinician to the possibility of a tumour. Although the majority of **neuroblastomas** arise in the adrenal gland, presentation as proptosis or bruising around the eyelids (3.15) is sometimes seen.

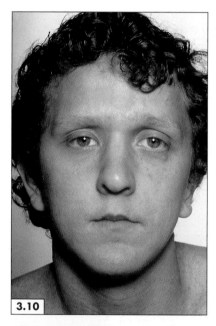

3.10

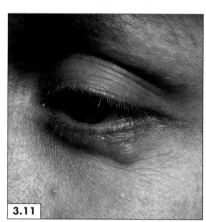

3.11

3.10
Neurofibromatosis: a neuroma in the lower eyelid

3.11
A single neuroma of the lower eyelid: greyish-pink, firm nodule

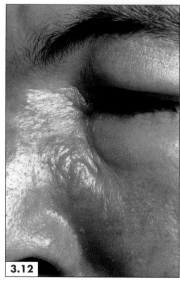

3.12

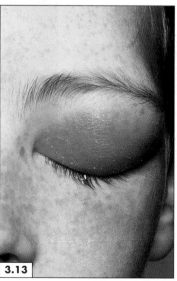

3.13

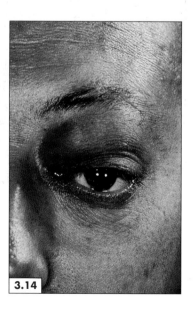

3.14

3.12
Erysipelas of the face and orbit: inflamed, oedematous skin

3.13
Orbital cellulitis

3.14
Langerhans' cell granulomatosis

Orbital pigmentation, or *raccoon eyes* (3.16), caused by the discolouration of extravasated blood is an important sign of a fracture of the base of the skull. This is particularly significant in an unconscious patient when no history may be available. There may also be subconjunctival haemorrhage but the movement of the eyeballs may not be affected if the upper cranial nerves are spared (3.17).

A painless, bluish-red induration of the lower eyelid and face (3.18) can be caused by the granulomatous infiltration of **sarcoidosis** and is referred to as *lupus pernio*. This process may involve the face, nose and ears (see also 1.280–1.283).

The yellowish plaques on the lower eyelid of this patient (3.19) are caused by lipid deposition in the periorbital skin called *xanthelasmata*. In just under one-half of the patients there is an associated **hypercholesterolaemia**.

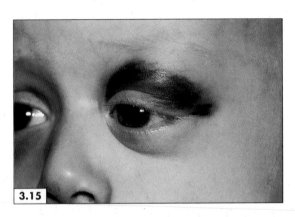

3.15
Neuroblastoma: bruised proptosis

3.16
Raccoon eyes: bluish discolouration of the extravasated blood after a fracture of the anterior cranial fossa

3.17
Intact eye movements

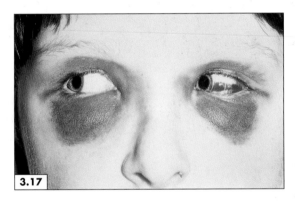

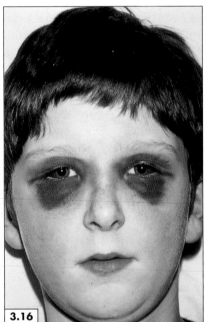

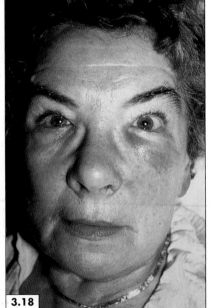

3.18
Lupus pernio: sarcoid granulomatous infiltration

3.19
Xanthelasma

A **stye** is a localized abscess in an eyelash follicle caused by a staphylococcal infection (3.20). Recurrent infection should raise the suspicion of an underlying disorder such as diabetes mellitus.

Retention of the secretion from a meibomian gland (modified sebaceous glands in the lids) together with a concomitant infection results in a reddish swelling (**chalazion**), which, unlike a stye, points away from the lid margin (3.21).

Lateral to the outer canthus of the eye, the *hypertrichosis* of **porphyria cutanea tarda** (3.22) is easily missed. It is usually only noticed when a clinician is specifically looking for it, having first noticed some lesions on the hands (see 9.196–9.201; p. **195**).

Blepharitis is a chronic inflammation of the lid margins and may occur in two forms. In **squamous blepharitis**, small white scales accumulate among the lashes, which fall out but are replaced without distortion. This condition is often associated with **seborrhoeic dermatitis of the scalp. Ulcerative blepharitis** is an infective condition and, in its chronic form, may lead to conjunctivitis and permanent loss of lashes (3.23).

The conjunctiva

The most common observations about the conjunctiva are regarding its *pallor* or excessive *redness*. The latter observation is often first made by patients or their relatives. The certainty about the presence of pallor, however, is compromised by the transparency of the conjunctiva, which imparts extra shine to the blood vessels even when they contain less than the normal level of haemoglobin. The best area to look for pallor is in the conjunctival fornix, which is the guttering between the palpebral and bulbar parts. Here a fold of conjunctiva can be raised by pulling

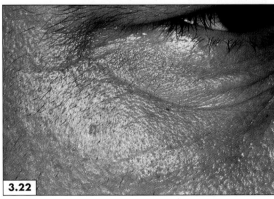

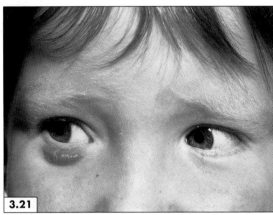

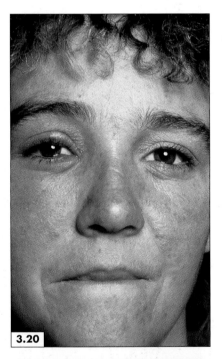

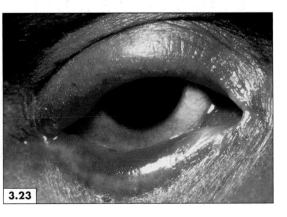

3.20
Stye in the upper lid

3.21
Chalazion: swollen and inflamed meibomian gland

3.22
Porphyria cutanea tarda: increased hairiness at the outer canthus

3.23
Chronic blepharitis with loss of eyelashes

down the lower lid (3.24). The guttering looks unambiguously pale compared with the vascular tarsal rim of the conjunctiva.

Often the pallor is first suspected by looking at the face, as can be seen in this patient with an **iron deficiency anaemia** and an unrelated goitre (3.25). However, facial appearances are influenced by the ambient temperature, the normal colour of the patient, and by the associated cutaneous and systemic disorders. Many elderly patients look paler than can be justified by their haemoglobin levels. The conjunctival fornix is a more reliable place as it is almost always pale in patients with anaemia (3.26) and low-output states.

The red eye is caused by chronic or recurrent congestion of the conjunctiva and may be the result of either constant exposure to a dusty environment or of heat, smoke, toxic fumes and other allergens. Often the conjunctiva looks normal until the lower fornix is exposed but, in some cases,

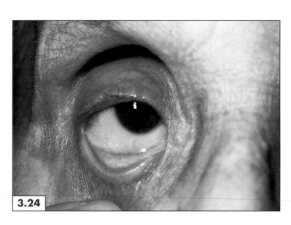

3.24
Clinical anaemia. Note the pallor of the fornix against the reddish tarsal rim

3.25
Facial pallor

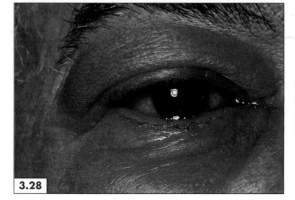

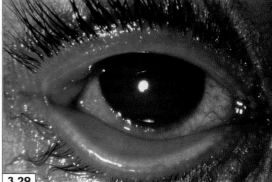

3.26
Pallor of the face and conjunctival fornix

3.27
Congested conjunctiva

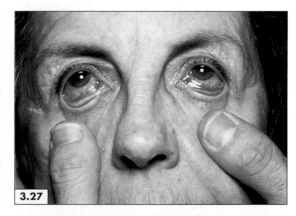

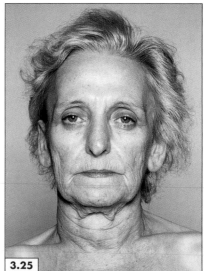

3.28
Allergic conjunctivitis and contact dermatitis

3.29
Vernal conjunctivitis

the bulbar conjunctiva also looks congested (3.27). Some allergic conditions such as hay fever are always associated with congestion of the conjunctiva and increased watery secretions. Contact with allergens, such as plant products at home or chemical irritants at work, can produce a florid reaction involving the conjunctiva as well as the lids (3.28).

Spring catarrh (**vernal conjunctivitis**) is a recurrent bilateral conjunctivitis (3.29) occurring with the onset of hot weather in summer time and affects mainly young people, usually boys. The patients experience burning, itching, lacrimation and some degree of photophobia.

Mucopurulent conjunctivitis can be caused by several organisms producing an intense reaction with photophobia and a purulent discharge. It is usually associated with an infection of the cornea and eyelids with chemosis. A particularly severe form of purulent conjunctivitis can occur in infants during the first few days of their life (**ophthalmia neonatorum**) (3.30) after having contracted the infection (usually gonococcal) during birth. However, this condition is not so common these days.

The commonest cause worldwide of conjunctivitis leading to blindness is **trachoma.** It is endemic in central and eastern Europe, Asia, north and central Africa, central and many areas of South America. In western countries, infection of the eyes and genital tract by *Chlamydia trachomatis* is spread mostly by sexual transmission.

The disease usually starts insidiously, first affecting the upper palpebral conjunctiva, which appears congested, red and velvety and then the characteristic *trachoma follicles* develop (3.31). The follicles have a diameter of up to 5 mm and characteristically appear in rows on the upper fornix, although they are also found on the lower conjunctiva and on the caruncle. As the disease advances, *trachomatous pannus* develops as a lymphoid infiltration (3.32) with vascularization towards the upper margin of the cornea (3.33). Gradually both the haziness and vascularization at the upper half of the cornea spread downwards and indolent corneal ulcers develop, starting at the advancing edge of the pannus.

In the absence of secondary infection, trachoma may remain a very mild disease causing few symptoms. However, the recurrent follicular process causes cicatrization of the lids, corneal vascularization and ulcera-

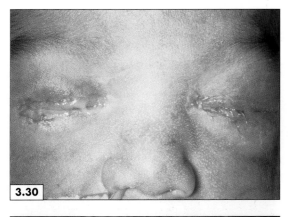

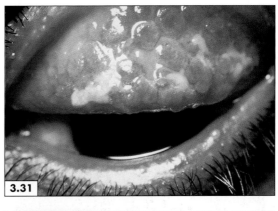

3.30
Ophthalmia neonatorum with purulent discharge

3.31
Trachoma follicles in the inverted upper lid

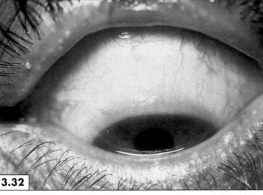

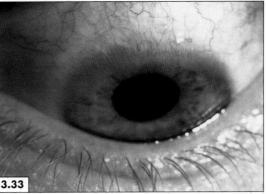

3.32
Trachomatous pannus

3.33
Trachoma: vascularization of the conjunctiva encroaching on the upper margin of the cornea

tion leading to opacification of the cornea and blindness (3.34).

A **pterygium** appears as a triangular, vascularized growth advancing from the conjunctiva to the cornea and usually arising from the inner canthus but may also encroach from the outer canthus (3.35). It extends gradually across the cornea but does not cross the midline. The condition is commoner in hot, sunny and dusty climates.

A **pinguecula** is a yellowish-white deposit on the bulbar conjunctiva adjacent to the limbus but it does not encroach onto the cornea. It is commoner than pterygium and not confined to hot countries. In **Gaucher's disease**, yellowish deposits may be present on either side of the cornea (3.36) in both eyes.

Vitamin A is an integral component of light-sensitive proteins in retinal rod and cone cells. Its deficiency causes follicular hyperkeratosis and night blindness. **Severe vitamin A deficiency**, as a result of chronic, uncorrected malabsorption or prolonged undernutrition, causes conjunctival xerosis, indicated by the presence of *Bitot's spots* (3.37), degeneration of the cornea (*keratomalacia*), retinal dysfunction and permanent blindness.

The inspection of the conjunctiva may yield critical and pathognomonic signs in some cases of septicaemia. For example, the discovery of *petechial haemorrhages* on the bulbar conjunctiva in this febrile patient (3.38) with a

*This sign was detected by a medical student on a ward round. The patient had inexorable malabsorption from an ileojejunal bypass, which had been performed for her gross obesity.

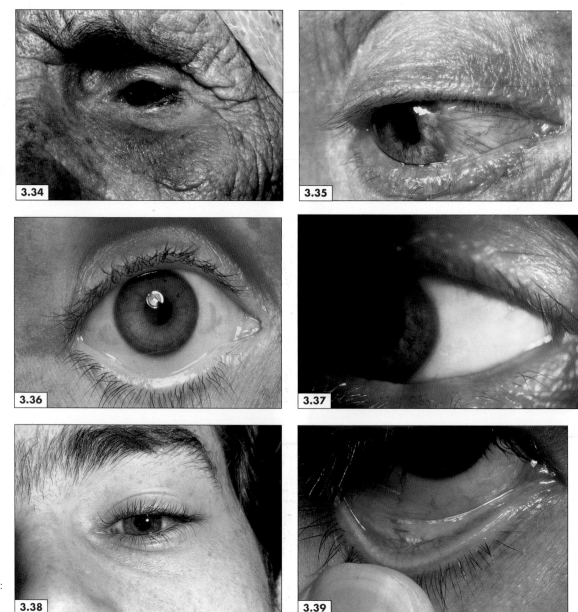

3.34
'Burnt out' trachoma

3.35
Pterygium

3.36
Gaucher's disease with yellowish glycolipid deposits

3.37
Bitot spot: focal area of conjunctival xerosis with a foamy appearance*

3.38
Petechial haemorrhage on the bulbar conjunctiva

3.39
Infective endocarditis: petechial haemorrhage

headache reinforced the clinical impression of a **meningococcal meningitis**. Similarly, the presence of *petechiae* on the conjunctival fornix in this patient (3.39) with a pyrexia of undetermined cause suggested the diagnosis of **infective endocarditis**. Both these patients were treated appropriately before the confirmatory evidence had become available.

Spontaneous subconjunctival haemorrhages (3.40) are the result of the rupture of small vessels from increased intravascular pressure, during the explosive and repetitive bouts of coughing associated with **whooping cough** and in patients with hypertension. These haemorrhages also occur in patients with a blood dyscrasia such as **aplastic anaemia** and **thrombocytopenia**. The appearance of subconjunctival haemorrhages in a patient with metastatic carcinoma (3.41) may suggest medullary infiltration by neoplastic cells (**leucoerythroblastic anaemia**).

The cornea

In addition to a general look at the conjunctiva and cornea for any obvious abnormality, the cornea should be examined specifically through the plus lenses of an ophthalmoscope for the structural detail of an inflammatory process, or if a specific lesion such as band keratopathy or Kayser–Fleischer rings is suspected. Sometimes a slit-lamp examination may be required; this is often undertaken by an ophthalmologist.

Injuries and acute infections of the cornea (exogenous or secondary to conjunctival infections) lie in the domain of the ophthalmologist, since prompt treatment is necessary to relieve distress and to prevent serious sequelae. However, any doctor in the emergency room of a hospital, or a general practitioner, may be the first to see a patient with a corneal injury or infection. Doctors who have not specialized in eye diseases should familiarize themselves with the appearance of some of the common corneal diseases. Furthermore, some abnormal corneal signs are characteristic of some systemic disorders (e.g. band keratopathy, arcus juvenilis, etc.).

Good history-taking is the single most helpful step towards making a sensible assessment of a corneal disease. This is illustrated by the story of this patient who presented to his doctor with a painful, red right eye (3.42). He used contact lenses and took care to wash them regularly in the saline solution used for this purpose. He complained of pain and could not fully open the right eye. A close look at the cornea showed an ulcer on the upper half with a whitish appearance (3.43) caused by the ensuing lymphoid cell infiltration. As in this case, the washing solution can be the source of the ubiquitous *Acanthamoeba*, which can cause keratitis with devastating results unless diagnosed and treated early.

Corneal ulcers are *exquisitely painful* and not difficult to diagnose so long as the accompanying *blepharospasm* is gently overcome, and the lids are separated to reveal the

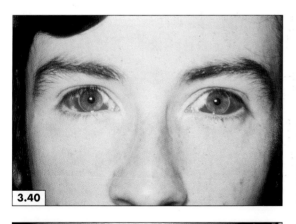

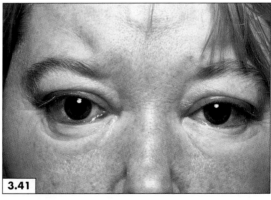

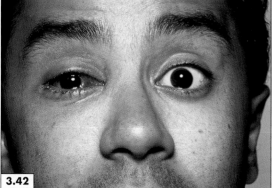

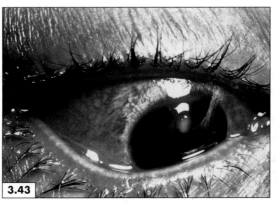

3.40
Subconjunctival haemorrhage

3.41
Unilateral proptosis and subconjunctival haemorrhage

3.42
Acanthamoeba keratoconjunctivitis

3.43
Corneal ulcer

ulcerated cornea (3.44, 3.45). Such patients should be referred urgently to an ophthalmologist, since untreated or inadequately treated ulcers can lead to abscess formation (3.46) and loss of vision. Superficial ulcers heal without permanent damage but deeper ones tend to leave a scar (3.47).

Band keratopathy (3.48) starts as a grey patch spreading from the pupillary margin towards the periphery but often remains sharply marginated from the limbus. It is caused by a deposition of calcium salts in the subepithelial space and anterior part of the Bowman's layer. The appearance is characteristically associated with **hypercalcaemia** but may be the result of **chronic iridocyclitis** in children; it can also occur spontaneously in the elderly.

Kayser–Fleischer ring may be seen as a yellowish-brown deposit, due to copper overload, on the limbus at the upper and lower poles of the eye (3.49) in Wilson's disease. The rings are always present in association with the neurological involvement but may be difficult to see in the early stages except with slit-lamp examination. This is the reason why Wilson, astute clinician though he was, did not see them when he first described the disease.

The cornea may be involved secondary to inflammation in the neighbouring sclera – known as **sclerosing keratitis**. An opacity develops at the margin of the cornea near the affected sclera (3.50). The opacity is caused by lipid deposition and lymphoid cell infiltration. It is tongue-shaped with the rounded apex towards the centre of the cornea (3.51). It can become intractable, causing discomfort in the eyes, but there is usually no ulceration, unlike an infective

3.44
Corneal ulcer with early abscess formation

3.45
Corneal ulcer with associated conjunctivitis

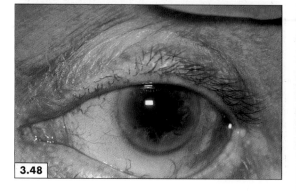

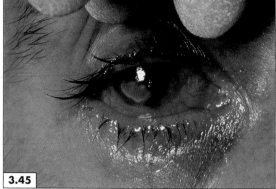

3.46
Corneal abscess

3.47
Corneal scar

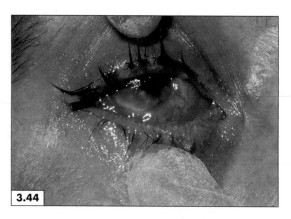

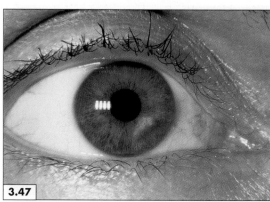

3.48
Band keratopathy: grey discolouration spreading radially towards the limbus

3.49
Kayser–Fleischer ring: a yellowish-brown thin band of copper deposit at the upper and lower limbus

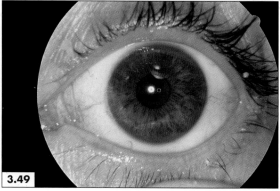

process which, if unchecked, can cause opacification of the entire cornea.

Interstitial keratitis from inherited syphilis most commonly affects children in their first two decades although delayed infection may occur over the age of 30 years. The inflammation tends to be unilateral and may be precipitated by an injury to the eye. The patient complains of irritation in the affected eye and there is usually some *ciliary congestion*, with one or more hazy patches appearing in the deep layers of the cornea near the margin (3.52). Gradually the haziness spreads and the whole cornea looks lustreless and dull, giving a ground-glass appearance (3.53). A closer look shows the underlying vascularization with radiating, brush-like vessels likened to a *salmon-patch* appearance.

Arcus senilis is an annular infiltration of lipid in the peripheral rim of the cornea (3.54). It is an ageing process and usually occurs in the sixth or seventh decade. It starts as a crescentic grey-white line at the upper (3.55) or lower margin of the cornea. It gradually spreads around the whole cornea as an annular ring (3.56), leaving a line of clear cornea between it and the limbus. Its importance lies in its association with **hypercholesterolaemia** and **diabetes mellitus** when it appears under the age of 40 years. Even in younger subjects an arcus may be present without any cause but the serum cholesterol should always be measured. Some of these patients may have **familial hypercholesterolaemia**, in which case other family members will also need to be screened.

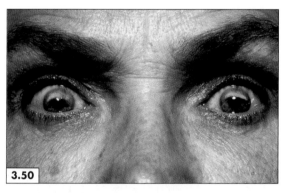

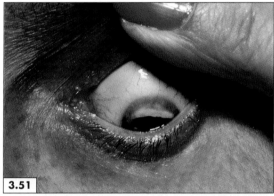

3.50
Sclerosing keratitis: tongue-shaped lipid–lymphoid cell deposit advancing from the limbus

3.51
Sclerosing keratitis: a yellowish-white lipid and lymphoid cell deposit

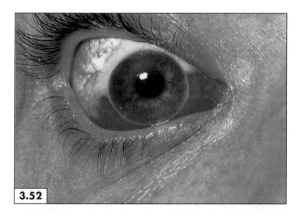

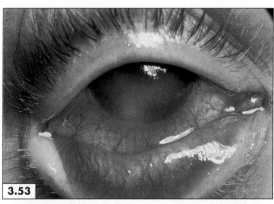

3.52
Interstitial (early) keratitis: hazy nasal cornea with associated ciliary injection

3.53
Late interstitial keratitis. Note the underlying 'salmon-patch' appearance

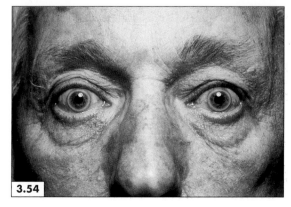

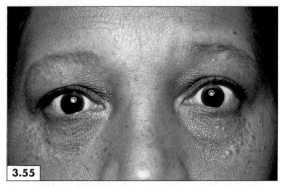

3.54
Arcus senilis

3.55
Start of the arcus in a younger subject with diabetes mellitus

The uveal tract

The uveal tract comprises the iris, ciliary body and the choroid. The choroid forms the posterior part of the tract and will be considered in the following section. **Iritis** or **iridocyclitis** is the term applied to inflammation affecting the anterior portion of the uveal tract resulting in a characteristic clinical picture.

The causes are as follows:

- **Exogenous infection** from perforating injuries;
- **Secondary infection** from the cornea, sclera or retina;
- **Endogenous infection** (e.g. tuberculosis, gonorrhoea, syphilis, brucellosis, viral, mycotic and protozoal infections);
- **Systemic diseases** (e.g. rheumatoid disease, Still's disease, systemic lupus erythematosus, Wegener's, sarcoidosis, ankylosing spondylitis, Reiter's disease, Behçet's syndrome, relapsing polychondritis, etc.).

Although there are many causes of iritis, the gross appearance of the eye does not differ very much from one condition to another. Severe pain, photophobia and *circumcorneal congestion* (*ciliary injection*) (3.57) with numerous white cells, aggregating into white dots, often inferiorly, on the cornea (*keratic precipitates*) (3.58) are the principal features of iritis. The iris becomes blurred and loses its distinctive radial appearance ('*muddy iris*').

Leakage of protein from the dilated vessels in the iris may cause it to adhere to the cornea (anterior synechiae) or to the lens (posterior synechiae). Excessive accumulation of the white blood cells may form a *hypopyon*, which is seen as a collection of pus in the anterior chamber (3.59). In **chronic anterior uveitis**, neovascularization of the iris (*rubeosis iridis*) may develop, together with posterior

3.56
Complete annular arcus juvenilis. Note its separation from the limbus

3.57
Iritis with ciliary injection

3.58
Keratic precipitates: white dots on the inferior pupillary cornea

3.59
Hypopyon: a collection of pus at the bottom of the anterior chamber

3.60
Rubeosis iridis: a reddish ring around the pupillary margins of the iris with ciliary injection of chronic anterior uveitis

3.61
Chronic anterior uveitis with lustreless lens (treated with atropine)

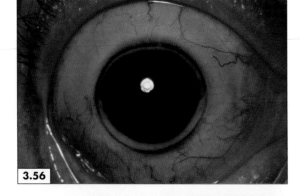
3.56

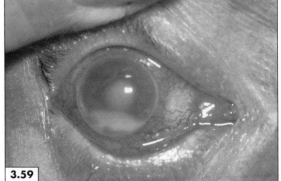
3.57

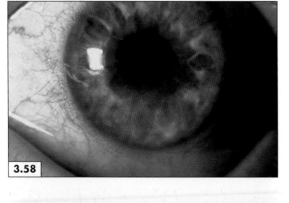
3.58

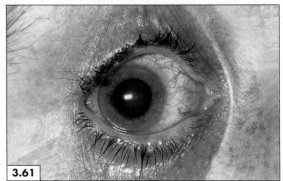
3.59

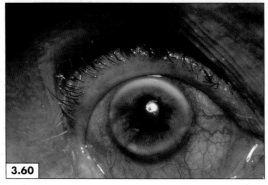
3.60

3.61

synechiae (3.60). In untreated cases, the pupil is constricted and the lens becomes less clear, as in this patient with **ankylosing spondylitis** (3.61). Sometimes it may progress to cataract formation (3.62).

Glaucoma is a well-known complication of iridocyclitis. It should be distinguished from iritis as the treatment of the latter (with atropine) is contraindicated in the former. In acute glaucoma, the onset is often sudden with severe pain, the pupil is large and either circular (3.63) or oval (3.64), there is corneal oedema and the intraocular pressure is high. Ciliary injection is common to both and the tension may be high in iritis, particularly in the presence of synechiae.

The diagnosis of iritis is not complete unless the underlying condition has been uncovered. This may be straightforward when a patient known to have a disorder such as ankylosing spondylitis develops iritis (3.65, see 3.61); however, in many cases an aetiological diagnosis remains unclear even after exhaustive investigation. In both the examples shown, the pupil is dilated because of treatment with atropine since iritis is often associated with a constricted pupil.

The neurological pupillary abnormalities have already been discussed in Chapter 1 (p. **28**).

A **congenital coloboma** is caused by a defective closure of the embryonic cleft. It occurs in the lower part of the iris (*typical coloboma*) extending from the pupil outwards (3.66). This can offer useful circumstantial evidence in support of a coexisting congenital disease. Figure 3.66 was obtained from a patient with **Klinefelter's syndrome**.

Melanoma of the iris (3.67) usually presents as a solitary nodule. It may, however, be difficult to distinguish from a benign naevus. The features that should arouse suspicion are an associated distortion of the iris, neovascularization, pupillary abnormalities, localized lens opacification and a high intraocular pressure.

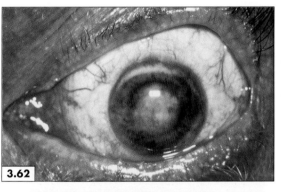
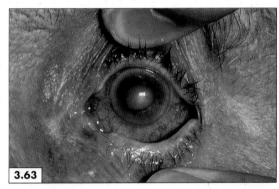

3.62 'Burnt out' chronic anterior uveitis with cataract formation

3.63 Acute congestive glaucoma with ciliary injection

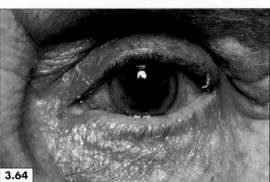
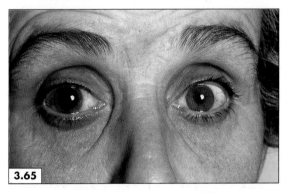

3.64 Acute glaucoma: large, somewhat oval pupil

3.65 Iritis on the right side (treated with atropine)

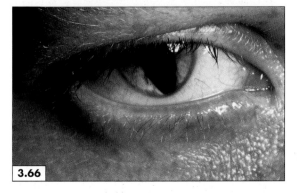
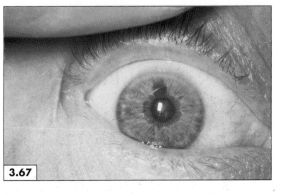

3.66 Congenital coloboma. Note the triangular shaped gap in the iris

3.67 Melanoma of the iris

The sclera

The sclera should be examined specifically for its colour and for the presence of **episcleritis** or **scleritis**.

The normal colour of the sclera is white, which aids the detection of any discolouration to a yellowish or bluish tinge. It is preferable to examine the sclera in natural light for the presence of jaundice (3.68).

The sclera is bluish in babies but a more pronounced blue colour is seen in **osteogenesis imperfecta** (3.69). This may be seen in several members of the same family, as the mode of transmission in most forms is recessive. The sclerotics retain their blue colour throughout life, although in adults it is less pronounced than in children (3.70). In osteogenesis imperfecta, the sclera and cornea are very thin and the uveal pigment shines through to produce the blue colouration.

Episcleritis is a common, self-limiting and frequently recurring disorder that typically affects young adults. It is sometimes associated with a systemic disease (e.g. rheumatoid arthritis, Crohn's disease, etc.). It may be either simple or nodular when there is usually a circumscribed nodule, 1–4 mm in diameter and approximately 2–4 mm from the limbus. The lesion is traversed by the deeper episcleral vessels giving it a purplish hue (3.71). It is *painless* and frequently involves both eyes (3.72).

Scleritis is less common, affects the older age groups and favours women over men. It is often *painful* and occurs in association with connective tissue diseases and herpes

3.68
Deep yellow discolouration of sclera

3.69
Blue sclerae

3.70
Marked blue-tinged sclerae

3.71
Episcleritis: a reddish nodule, 2 mm in diameter

3.72
Bilateral episcleritis with increased vascularity

3.73
Scleromalacia perforans: the necrotic patch reveals the underlying dark uvea

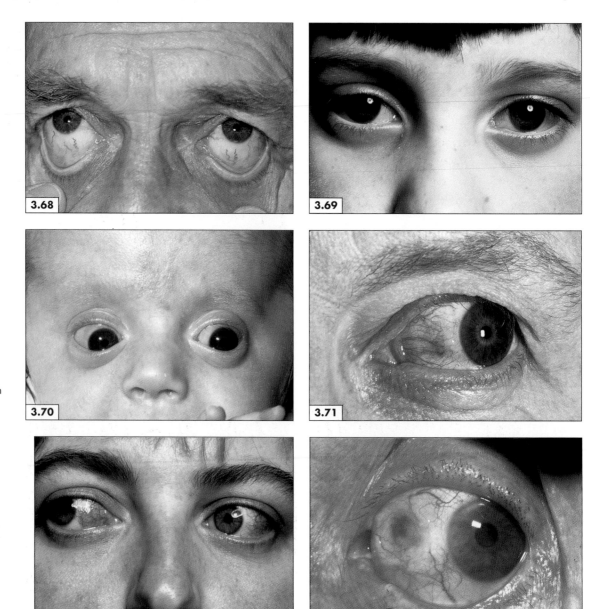

zoster. One or more nodules appear and the area is less circumscribed than episcleritis. It may even extend around the cornea to form an *annular scleritis*. The essential difference between episcleritis and scleritis is that the latter is painful and also involves the cornea and the uveal tract. The involvement of the cornea may persist and become a **chronic sclerosing keratitis** (p. **98**).

Scleromalacia perforans (3.73) typically occurs in females with long-standing seropositive **rheumatoid arthritis**. The condition is asymptomatic and starts as a yellowish necrotic patch gradually exposing the underlying uvea.

The lens

Opacification of the lens (cataract) with a steady decline in vision may bring a patient to their doctor. **Senile cataracts** develop in people over the age of 60 years, but the process may appear under the age of 50 years because of a systemic disorder. The causes of acquired cataracts in the young are as follows:

- **Ocular diseases** (e.g. iridocyclitis, choroiditis, high myopia, retinal dystrophy or detachment);

- **Genetic/inborn causes** (e.g. mongolism, galactosaemia, cretinism, myotonic dystrophy);
- **Metabolic disorders** (e.g. diabetes mellitus, hypoparathyroidism);
- **Skin diseases** (e.g. atopic eczema, scleroderma, poikiloderma vasculare atrophicus, keratosis follicularis, etc.);
- **Trauma** (e.g. concussion, perforating wounds);
- **Miscellaneous causes** (e.g. heat (infrared), irradiation, electric discharge).

A mature cataract is usually easy to see (3.74) and all that is required is a good source of light. However, if the cataract is *immature* and the opacity does not fill the entire pupil, or if the opacities lie in the centre or in the posterior capsule, the cataract may not be easily visible to the unaided eye.

All forms of cataract can be seen with the help of an ophthalmoscope. With its light on the eye, the observer should approach from a distance of approximately 30 cm (12 inches) and gradually move nearer the eye. A *red reflex* of the vascular retina will be seen at the pupil (3.75) if the path of the light to the retina is not obstructed by an opaque lens. The red reflex is absent if the lens is cataractous (3.76, 3.77).

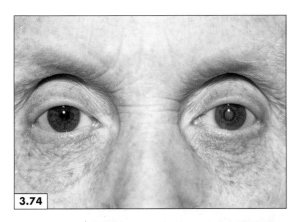

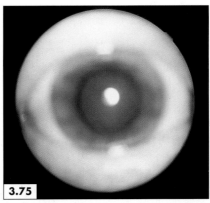

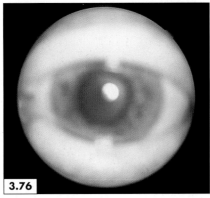

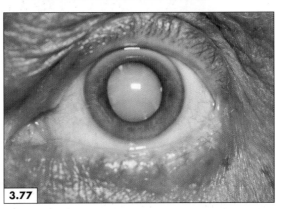

3.74
Cataract

3.75
Red retinal reflex visible through the clear lens

3.76
Absent red reflex: cataractous lens

3.77
Cataractous lens

4 THE OPTIC FUNDUS

The examination of the optic fundus with the aid of a suitable ophthalmoscope is important for three main reasons. First, the fundus is an extension of the brain that can be seen directly and, therefore, provides information about many of the disorders of the central nervous system. Second, the fundus is the only area where the blood vessels can be *seen*, and one can get some idea about the state of the vasculature in other organs in conditions such as atherosclerosis and hypertension. Third, the optic fundus may be involved in a systemic disorder (e.g. bacterial endocarditis, AIDS, sarcoidosis, etc.) and may provide critical diagnostic clues. For all these reasons it is important to take care to obtain fundal views under optimal conditions.

Since access to the optic fundus is through the pupillary aperture, it is self-evident that this path should be widened as much as possible. This can be achieved by placing the patient in a dark room for a few minutes, or by dilating the pupils with a mydriatic such as the short-acting (approximately 3h) tropicamide. Patients known or suspected of having glaucoma, and those who have had eye surgery in the past, should not be exposed to a mydriatic. Before the instillation of these drops, the patient should be warned about the immediate sting and of photophobia in the sunshine, both of which are caused by the tropicamide. Care should be taken to instil only one or two drops on the *lower* eyelid (4.1) and not directly on the cornea, since this causes pain and blepharospasm.

Any of the conventional ophthalmoscopes (4.2) with a range of lenses from +20 (4.3) to −20 dioptres (4.4) is satisfactory for viewing the fundus and the structures leading to it. In a severely myopic patient, the fundus is best viewed with the patient *wearing* their glasses. The fundus should be examined methodically, starting from the optic disc, tracing the vessels emerging from it into the four quad-

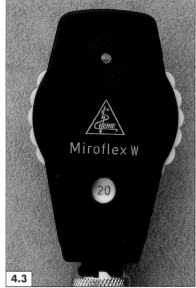

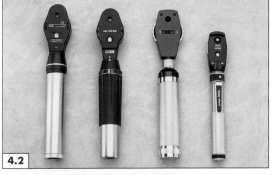

4.1
Instilling a drop of tropicamide on the everted lower eyelid

4.2
A series of available ophthalmoscopes

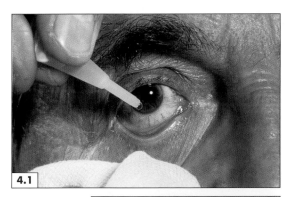

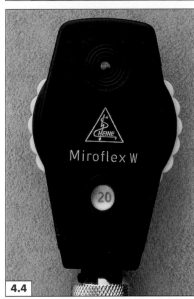

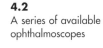

4.3
Set at +20 dioptre lens

4.4
Set at −20 dioptre lens

rants, followed by the macula, which will come into view when the patient looks at the light of the ophthalmoscope.

The normal fundus

The colour of a normal Caucasian fundus varies from orange to vermilion (4.5), that of a dark Asian person may be yellowish-grey (4.6) or coffee-brown, and that of an African subject tends to be chocolate-brown, owing to the combined colour of the pigmented epithelium and the underlying vessels.

The optic disc is pale red with a yellowish tint. It is usually circular (4.7) or vertically oval. The relative pallor

of the disc is largely the result of the reflection of light from the myelin sheaths of the optic nerve. In most normal fundi the disc has a funnel-shaped depression (known as *physiological cupping*) at its centre from which the retinal vessels seem to emerge. In **chronic glaucoma** this funnel is deep (*glaucomatous cupping*) and the emerging vessels appear to bend sharply at its edge (4.8).

The **retinal vessels** form four groups to supply the four quadrants of the fundus (4.9). These four principal divisions of the retinal vessels follow a sinuous course and divide dichotomously as they proceed to their respective quadrants (4.10). From the superior and inferior temporal vessels, small branches pass towards the **macula** where they terminate in fine twigs around the margin of the macular

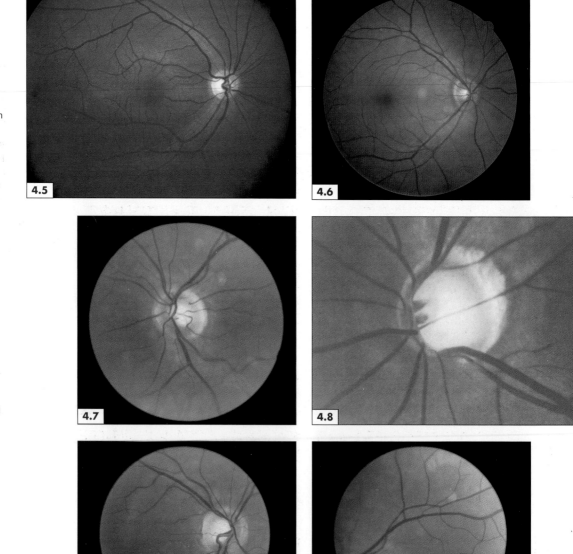

4.5
A normal Caucasian fundus

4.6
A yellowish-brown fundus of an Asian subject

4.7
Yellowish-pale optic disc

4.8
Glaucomatous cupping: sharply angulated emerging vessels

4.9
Retinal vessels distributed to four quadrants

4.10
Branching vessels

depression. They stop short of the *avascular* fovea (4.11), which gets its red colour, and oxygen, from the underlying choroidal vessels. The ophthalmoscopic white *axial reflex*, which runs along the centre of each vessel, is caused by the surface of the blood column and the vessel wall.

The **macula** lies at approximately 1–1.5 disc widths from the temporal border of the optic disc. It is a horizontally oval depression recognizable by the contrast of its red colour with that of the paler surrounding fundus (4.11, 4.12). At the centre of the macula lies a smaller depression called the fovea (4.13); this is a very thin part of the retina and allows the brighter red colour of the underlying choroidal circulation to shine through. This is the normal *foveal reflex*.

The abnormal fundus

The optic disc

The shape, width and depth of the physiological cup, the margin and the colour of the disc, together with the state of the vessels, should all be scrutinized carefully for evidence of disease. In simple, or primary, **optic atrophy** (from injury, ischaemia or toxic damage to the optic nerve) the disc is pale with sharply defined borders and a shallow physiological cup (4.14). Sometimes the pallor is not very striking unless a comparison is made with a normal fundus (4.15). In advanced cases, there is marked narrowing of the

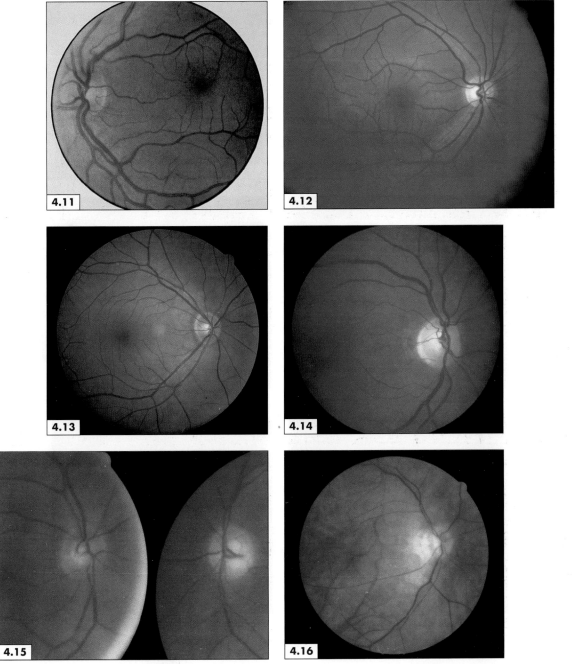

4.11
Vascular branches terminating around the darker avascular macula

4.12
The bright-red macula lateral to the yellowish-pale disc

4.13
The red foveal reflex: the thin avascular fovea reflects underlying choroidal vascularity

4.14
Optic atrophy with a pale, shallow physiological cup

4.15
Normal and pale optic discs

4.16
Optic atrophy with pale disc and thin vessels

retinal vessels as in this patient with bilateral optic atrophy (4.16, 4.17), who was found to have a large pituitary tumour compressing the optic chiasma. In **glaucomatous optic atrophy**, the cup is enlarged and occupies a larger part of the disc. Its margin shows an abrupt step down from the retinal level and the emerging vessels appear to bend sharply outwards (4.18).

Papilloedema, or a noninflammatory oedema of the optic nerve head, is an important diagnostic sign of many systemic, intracranial and orbital disorders. The earliest changes are a blurring of the disc margin, hyperaemia and swelling of the papilla (4.19). These changes start at the periphery of the disc leaving the central cup well-preserved until late on in the disease (4.20). As the intracranial pressure remains elevated the cup fills up, the disc becomes hyperaemic with dilated capillaries and the margin becomes completely obliterated (4.21). There is venous dilatation and the surrounding retina becomes involved with the appearance of soft, white patches. At this stage, clinical examination often reveals *enlargement of the blind spot*.

4.17
Optic atrophy with pale disc and attenuated vessels

4.18
Glaucomatous optic atrophy: sharply angulated vessels and pale disc

4.19
Papilloedema: swollen, hyperaemic disc with blurred margins

4.20
The pale central core of the disc surrounded by hyperaemia

4.21
Advanced papilloedema with congestion and oedema of the disc

4.22
Advanced papilloedema: tortuous and congested veins with oedema

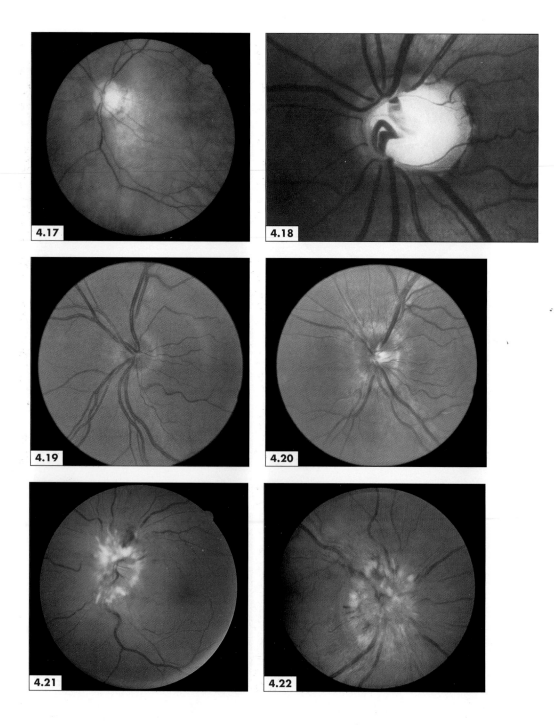

In many of these well-established cases there are several fine wrinkles in the retina just adjacent to the disc (4.20, 4.21). The veins become tortuous with a darker blood column near the disc and circumferential folds, caused by spacing of the nerve fibres and overfilling of the capillaries, that radiate from the optic head (4.22, 4.23). Cotton wool spots and haemorrhages appear in most cases (4.24).

Flame-shaped retinal haemorrhages may extend for several millimetres around the disc (4.25) and deeply placed linear exudates radiate from the macula, the so-called *macular fan* (4.26). These changes and the association of papilloedema with multiple exudates and haemorrhages (4.27) are often, but not always, suggestive of **accelerated hypertension**. An additional distinguishing feature of papilloedema caused by accelerated hypertension is that the papilla, and the surrounding retinal vessels, are obscured by the widespread presence of the oedema fluid. This ophthalmoscopic appearance contrasts well with that of an intracranial tumour (4.21–4.23) in which the swollen optic head, as well as the retinal vessels, can be seen clearly.

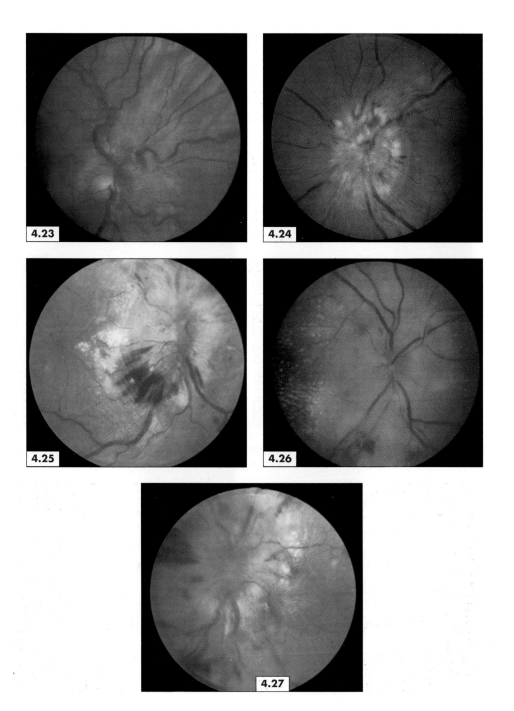

4.23
Papilloedema with completely obscured disc. Note tortuous veins with dark blood columns

4.24
Papilloedema with exudates and haemorrhages

4.25
Papilloedema with linear, flame-shaped haemorrhages and soft exudates

4.26
Papilloedema with the macular fan caused by multiple, confluent exudates

4.27
Papilloedema with haemorrhages and exudates (accelerated hypertension)

Myelinated nerve fibres are seen as a white patch spreading from the disc (4.28). The patch has a feathered margin reflecting the course of the nerve fibres in the retina. The condition is present at birth, does not change and causes no visual impairment.

A **subhyaloid haemorrhage** is often seen near the disc (4.29). It has a characteristic, sharply defined, rounded appearance and, in the presence of an appropriate clinical picture, is pathognomonic of a subarachnoid haemorrhage.

The retinal vessels

The blood vessels of the retina are involved in many disorders that also affect other parts of the fundus, such as diabetes mellitus, hypertension and optic atrophy. However, there are certain conditions that affect predominantly (the hyperviscosity syndrome), or primarily (vascular occlusion), the retinal vessels; some of these will be considered here.

In the **hyperviscosity syndrome** (caused by an excess of one or more constituents of blood, e.g. para-proteinaemias, macroglobulinaemias, polycythaemia, leukaemias, etc.), the outstanding fundal appearance is of an increased tortuosity and fullness of the retinal veins. These vessels have a marked axial light reflex facilitated by a large column of blood within, and there are also engorged capillaries in the retina (4.30). The venous engorgement is often associated with prominence of the underlying capillary network, micro-aneurysms and blot haemorrhages, as seen in this patient with multiple myeloma (4.30, 4.31).

Occlusive disorders of the retinal circulation are dramatic events and often bring together a physician and an ophthalmologist. In **central retinal artery occlusion** (usually caused by an embolus from the heart or a large vessel), there is sudden loss of vision in one eye and, within minutes, the retina looks pale with thin arteries and a cherry-red spot at the macula (4.32). An interesting variation of the ophthalmoscopic picture, seen in some cases, is the presence of the *cilioretinal artery*. This does not spring from the central retinal vessels and usually supplies a small area at the temporal edge of the disc (4.33). The cherry-red spot reflects the underlying choroidal

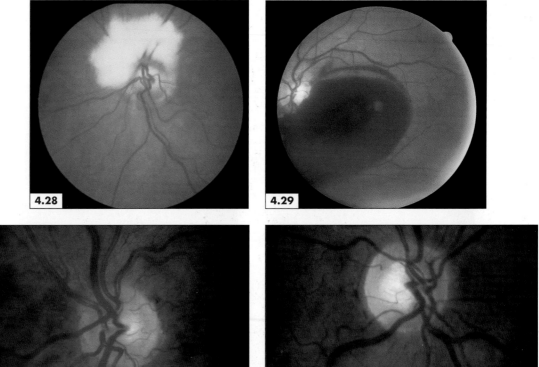

4.28
Myelinated nerve fibres. Note the irregular, finely feathered margin

4.29
Subhyaloid haemorrhage with a clearly delineated margin

4.30
The hyperviscosity syndrome with dilated, congested veins

4.31
Multiple myeloma: engorged veins and capillaries

circulation, which looks brighter in contrast with the neighbouring pale retina (4.32, 4.33). The occlusion may be confined to a branch retinal vessel where the area supplied will be pale in comparison to the rest of the retina, as illustrated by Figure 4.34 where the inferior temporal artery is occluded. Sometimes, the offending obstructive lesion, such as a cholesterol embolus, may be concomitant with an occluded arterial branch and a pale area distal to it (4.35).

Occlusion of the central retinal vein is much commoner than that of the corresponding artery and is a major cause of blindness in the elderly.

Among the associated conditions are hypertension, chronic simple glaucoma (often undetected), diabetes mellitus and a hyperviscosity state. In complete occlusion of the central vein, the fundus shows haemorrhages scattered prodigiously, resembling wallpaper splashed with blood (4.36, 4.37). The haemorrhages tend to congregate around the course of the venules and look like berries on a twig when the occlusion is incomplete (4.38) or when only a branch is involved (4.39).

The condition affects both males aged between 70 and 80 years and females (usually younger). Patients complain of blurring of the vision in one eye on awakening. In most

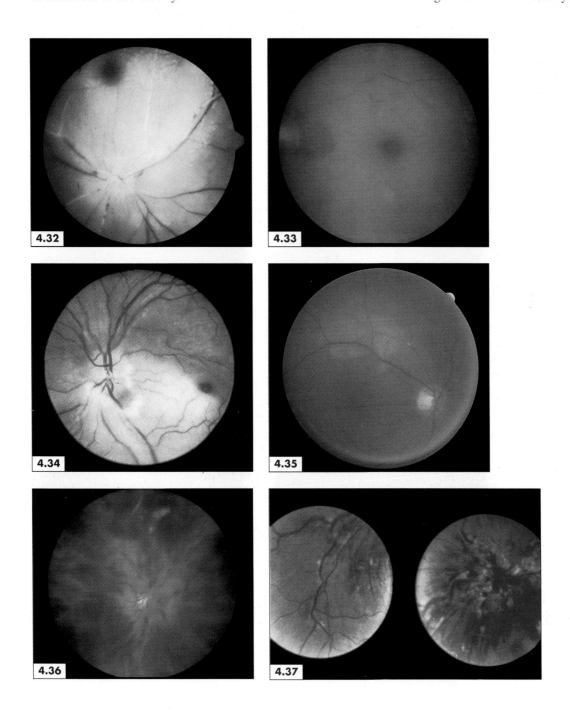

4.32
Central retinal artery occlusion: pale retina with attenuated vessels and a circular, cherry-red macula at the upper pole

4.33
Central retinal artery occlusion. Note the intact tongue-shaped vascular area, supplied by the cilioretinal artery, lateral to the optic disc

4.34
Inferior temporal artery occlusion. Note the cherry-red macula

4.35
A refractile cholesterol embolus occluding the inferior branch of the superior temporal artery

4.36
Central retinal vein occlusion with scattered haemorrhages

4.37
Central retinal vein occlusion: multiple haemorrhages along the course of veins

cases, the vision shows progressive deterioration and the disc becomes pale (4.40). In patients with a partial occlusion, the prognosis is good.

Hypertensive retinopathy affects the vessels of the retina through a dual process of *involutionary* (or senile) *sclerosis* and *reactive sclerosis* caused by the increased peripheral resistance. The ophthalmoscopic view of the vessels in elderly subjects (aged 60 years and over) shows that the arteries are narrower, straighter, paler with a reduced axial reflex, and that they branch more acutely

(4.41; cf. normal vessels in 4.10, 4.11). The veins are proportionately narrower with a less distinct axial reflex. The fundus generally shows signs of ageing with colloid bodies, peripheral choroidal degeneration and loss of the normal colour. The perifoveal arterioles become thin, straight and scanty. All these changes associated with advancing years are also seen in younger patients with sustained hypertension (4.42) and show a striking contrast with the fundal picture of a normotensive subject (4.43).

Traditionally, these changes described above are classi-

4.38
Haemorrhages along the course of the occluded vein

4.39
Occlusion of a branch of the central retinal vein

4.40
End-stage central retinal vein occlusion with optic atrophy

4.41
Involutional sclerosis of the retinal vessels: thinner vessels with reduced axial reflex

4.42
Hypertensive fundus (grade I)

4.43
Normotensive fundus

fied as **grade I** hypertensive retinopathy. With persistent hypertension a phase of hyperplasia follows with calibre variation, particularly at the arteriovenous crossings (**grade II**), where veins show tapering before and after the crossing. This is known as *Gunn's sign* (4.44).

This so-called *arteriovenous 'nipping'* is not caused by the pressure of a rigid and hyperplastic artery on the vein; rather, it can be explained by masking of the vein as it buries into the retina at the crossing, a loss of transparency in the retina, and by the associated hyperplasia in the arterial wall. Sometimes, this concealment of the vein, as it passes underneath the artery, is so complete that the vein looks as though it is 'cut in two' (4.45). In this form of Gunn's sign the venous blood column terminates abruptly on both sides of the crossing; here the concealment is probably caused mainly by the loss of transparency in the hyperplastic arterial wall. At this stage there may also be associated flame-shaped haemorrhages and hard exudates (**grade III**) (4.45). There are several variations at the arteriovenous crossings; it may be the vein that crosses the artery and the vein may rise at this level and form a 'hump' over the artery (4.44 and 4.46).

Focal ischaemia, seen as soft exudates, and vascular leakage, showing as hard exudates and haemorrhages (**grade III**), are both ominous signs suggesting an **accelerated phase** of hypertension (4.45–4.48). Some degree of oedema of the disc may be seen at this stage; however,

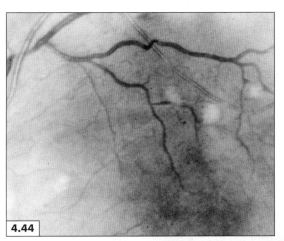

4.44

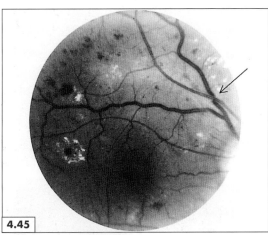

4.45

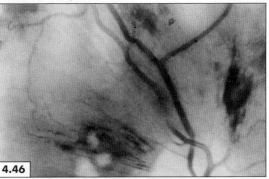

4.46

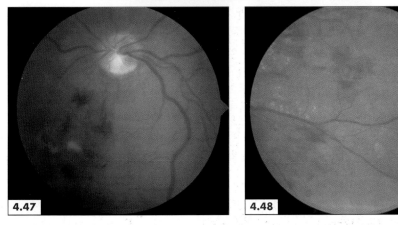

4.47

4.48

4.44
Arteriovenous nipping (Gunn's sign) where the main branches cross each other

4.45
Grade III hypertensive retinopathy. The venous shadow is lost where the artery crosses it (arrow). Note the haemorrhages and the circinate exudate around a blot haemorrhage

4.46
Arteriovenous crossings with the vein arching over the artery in the superior region

4.47 and 4.48
Grade III hypertensive retinopathy with haemorrhages

frank **papilloedema** (4.49, 4.50) may occur with or without any of the other changes (**grade IV**).

Diabetes mellitus is by far the commonest disease that can affect any part of the eye and produces vascular changes in the fundi of most patients within a few years of diagnosis. *Venous dilatation* is the earliest change (4.51), which may persist while *microaneurysms* (dots) and *retinal haemorrhages* (blots) develop. These changes of dot and blot haemorrhages are collectively called *background*

retinopathy (4.52–4.56), which does not cause any visual impairment unless a haemorrhage involves the macula. Patients with only background changes should have their visual acuity and fundi checked at least once a year.

Soft exudates are seen as fluffy, white spots with indistinct margins (4.57, 4.58) reflecting infarcted areas caused by the occlusion of arteriolar precapillaries. These occur early in the course of the disease, particularly if the patient also has hypertension. Patients with soft exudates should

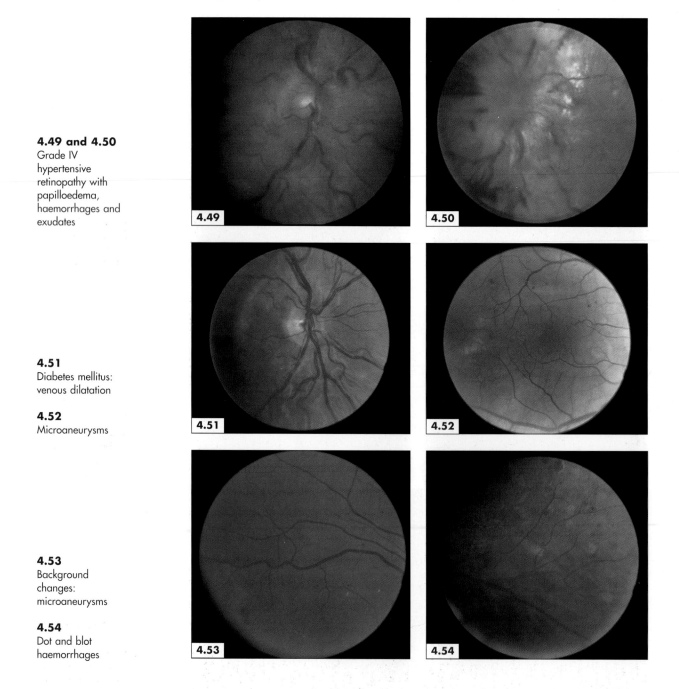

4.49 and 4.50
Grade IV hypertensive retinopathy with papilloedema, haemorrhages and exudates

4.49

4.50

4.51
Diabetes mellitus: venous dilatation

4.52
Microaneurysms

4.51

4.52

4.53
Background changes: microaneurysms

4.54
Dot and blot haemorrhages

4.53

4.54

be examined more frequently than once a year. If the exudate is near the macula, or if more than two exudates appear, or if there is any visual deterioration, the patient should be referred to an ophthalmologist.

Hard (serous) exudates are small, white or yellowish-white dots with well-defined margins scattered singly, in clusters (4.59), or in circinate rings (4.60). These remnants of vascular leakage comprise glycoproteins, lipoprotcins and phospholipids, and are located within the outer molecular layer. The concentrated material initially fills the individual cystic spaces in that layer but gradually breaks down

the barriers between these spaces and forms compact, hard, waxy masses (4.61). Preretinal haemorrhages with flat surfaces, which lie in a subhyaloid position in front of the retina, can also be seen in this figure. These haemorrhages are from new vessels, which lie hidden behind them.

Patients with hard exudates should be monitored regularly for their visual acuity and the location and number of the exudates should be charted. They should be referred to an ophthalmologist if there is a deterioration in their vision, if the exudates increase in number, if they form a

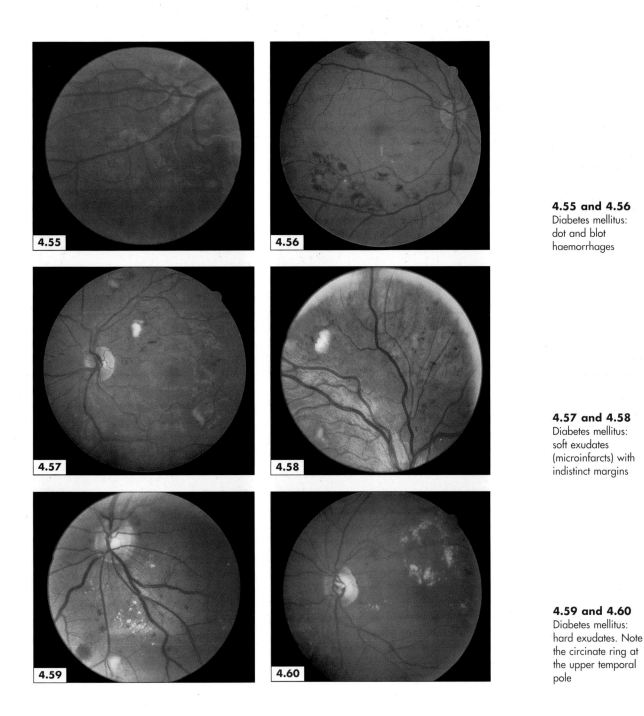

4.55 and 4.56
Diabetes mellitus: dot and blot haemorrhages

4.57 and 4.58
Diabetes mellitus: soft exudates (microinfarcts) with indistinct margins

4.59 and 4.60
Diabetes mellitus: hard exudates. Note the circinate ring at the upper temporal pole

4.61
Proliferative retinopathy: confluent hard exudates and preretinal haemorrhages with sharply defined margins

4.62
Microaneurysms and hard exudates coalescing in circinate rings

4.63 and 4.64
Diabetes mellitus: hard exudates forming circinate rings

4.65
Confluent hard exudates in a circinate ring around the macula

4.66
Maculopathy with exudates encroaching on to the macula

4.67 and 4.68
Maculopathy: exudates on and around the macula

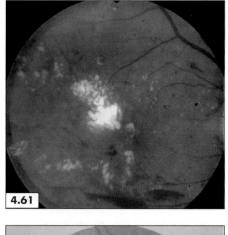
4.61

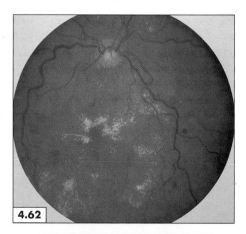
4.62

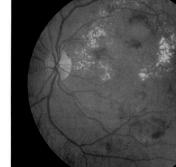
4.63

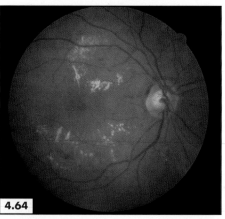
4.64

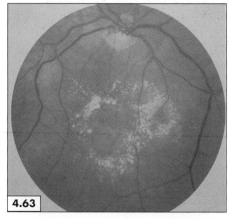
4.65

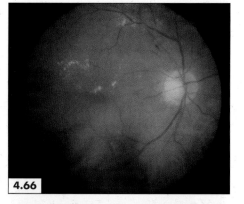
4.66

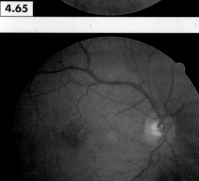
4.67

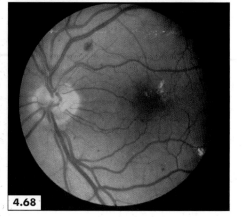
4.68

circinate ring around the fovea (4.62–4.65), or if they encroach on to the macula (**maculopathy**) (4.66). The circinate exudate represents both the capillaropathy (i.e. increase in permeability, damage and leakage) and the reactive stage of the retinopathy in which macrophages invade to clear the exudate. The number of exudates is less important than their location; even a small number of exudates on the macula (4.67, 4.68) can cause marked visual deterioration.

Maculopathy is best treated prophylactically by referring for laser therapy those patients in whom the exudates are near the macula and threatening to invade it (4.69).

Neovascularization is a common and dangerous mani-

festation of **diabetic retinopathy** and usually occurs after the reactive stage when there are hard and soft exudates, haemorrhages and venous dilatation (4.70). Serous exudates and haemorrhages precede new vessel formation in most cases.

Hypoxia is the critical factor that stimulates new vessel growth. Arteriolar capillaropathy, as indicated by chronic leakage of plasma or blood, is often the initiating phenomenon of new vessel formation. A **preproliferative stage** can be recognized when there are haemorrhages and venous dilatation (4.70, 4.71), often with a beaded outline (4.72). In addition there may be soft exudates, arterial sheathing and venous reduplication.

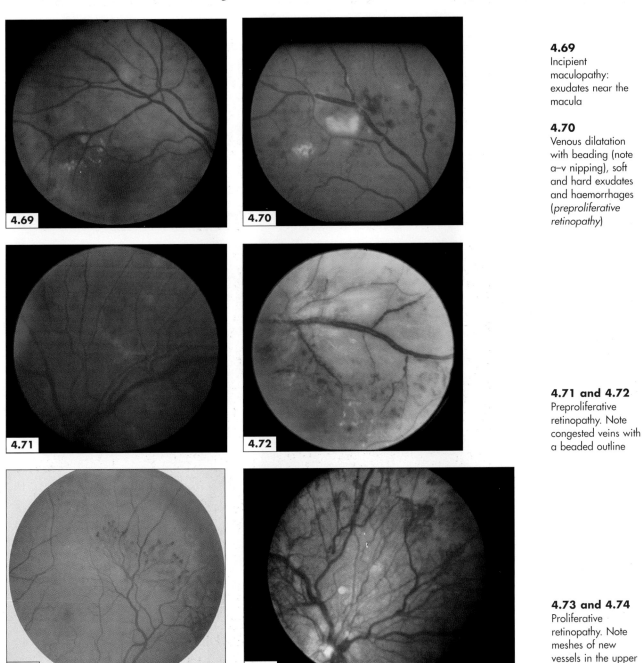

4.69
Incipient maculopathy: exudates near the macula

4.70
Venous dilatation with beading (note a–v nipping), soft and hard exudates and haemorrhages (*preproliferative retinopathy*)

4.71 and 4.72
Preproliferative retinopathy. Note congested veins with a beaded outline

4.73 and 4.74
Proliferative retinopathy. Note meshes of new vessels in the upper regions

Patients with preproliferative changes should be referred to an ophthalmologist. Venous dilatation, even without the presence of massive exudates, should be regarded with suspicion. Venous stasis from a diminished arteriolar blood flow and capillaropathy can stimulate neovascularization, usually in the superior temporal quadrant (4.73). Once begun, the proliferative stage is usually progressive and new vessels appear in various parts of the retina in an unpredictable manner (4.74, 4.75). Important information regarding the microcirculation and new vessel formation can be obtained using fluorescein angiography (4.76). Retinal photocoagulation can arrest the rapid progression of neovascularization and subsequent loss of vision. It leaves the fundus with laser scars and some remnants of the new vessels (4.77).

Retinitis proliferans (4.78) is a serious complication of progressive neovascularization. Leashes of vessels protrude into the vitreous followed by fibrosis (4.79), cicatricial contraction (4.80), retinal detachment and blindness.

4.75
Proliferative retinopathy with masses of new vessels

4.76
Fluorescein angiogram revealing a mesh of new vessels medial to the disc

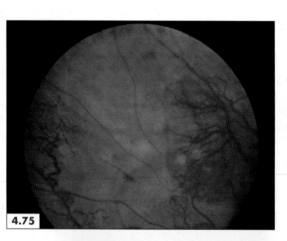

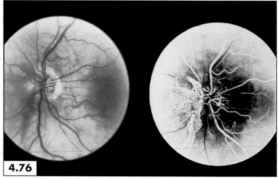

4.77
Neovascularization with laser scars

4.78
Retinitis proliferans: leashes of new vessels bleeding into the vitreous

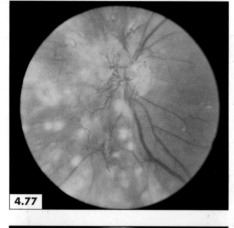

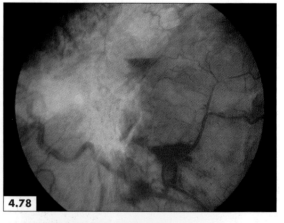

4.79
Fibrosing new vessels

4.80
Cicatricial contraction of fibrosed new vessels and retinal detachment

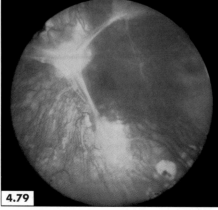

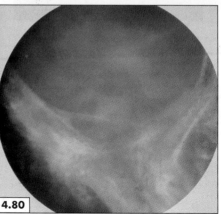

The retina and macula

The retina and the choroid are involved in a variety of systemic infections and, although the usual processes of inflammation, reaction and atrophy may not vary much from one condition to another, some appearances are quite distinctive and helpful when making a specific diagnosis.

Most inflammatory changes in the choroid are of endogenous origin (Table 4.1) but exogenous infection may be imported through a perforating injury or surgery.

Table 4.1 Causes of choroiditis/choroidoretinitis	
Bacterial	Tuberculosis, syphilis, leprosy, leptospirosis
Rickettsial	Q fever
Viral	Variola, measles, vaccinia
Granulomatous	Sarcoidosis
Mycotic	Histoplasmosis, aspergillus, candida, cryptococcosis, coccidioidomycosis
Protozoal	Toxoplasmosis, toxocara
Nematodal	Onchocerciasis
Malignant	Retinoblastoma

Choroiditis may also occur from an infection in the sclera and retina.

In diffuse **choroiditis** from any cause the choroid shows yellowish plaques of exudate with ill-defined margins and crossed by the vessels of the retina, which is frequently oedematous (4.81). In acute cases, there may be blurring of vision resulting from the vitreous haze. Loss of vision will result if the macula is involved. In chronic or 'burnt-out' forms there is clumping of pigment around the lesions, which themselves look white because of the presence of scar tissue (4.82).

The pigmentation is not specific to any particular form and merely surrounds any lesion where the entire choroid and the retina may have been destroyed, exposing the white sclera (4.83). Scattered patches of pigmentation with whitish lesions can be seen in old, diffuse choroidoretinitis. A patch of complete destruction of the choroid and retina will show the sclera and its vessels, as seen in the figure showing a case of **sun choroiditis** (4.84).

Toxoplasma and **cytomegalovirus** infection of the retina occur frequently in immunosuppressed patients (e.g. in AIDS, cytotoxic therapy, acute leukaemia, etc.). A single lesion may be seen in the centre of the fundus, both in the congenital and acquired forms of toxoplasmosis, and often involves the macula (4.85). As this heals, clumps of pigmentation appear within and around it.

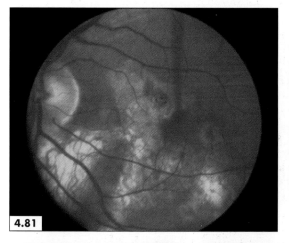

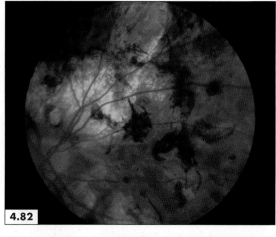

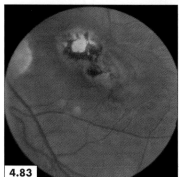

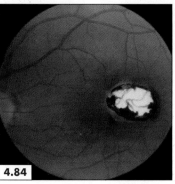

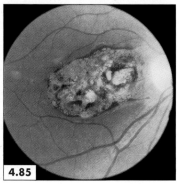

4.81
Choroiditis: yellowish plaques of exudates in the choroid underlying the retinal vessels

4.82
Chronic choroiditis with pigmentation

4.83 and 4.84
Choroidoretinitis: the destruction of retina and choroids exposing sclera and its vessels

4.85
Toxoplasma choroidoretinitis involving the macula

Retinal infection with **cytomegalovirus** usually spares the choroid.

The initial white granular dots on the retina soon become confluent, forming yellowish-white necrotic lesions. This is in close association with intraretinal haemorrhages, simulating the distinctive 'scrambled egg and tomato-sauce' appearance (4.86).

Scattered whitish patches with retinal haemorrhages are highly suggestive of cytomegalovirus infection (4.87), particularly in patients with underlying AIDS. Figure 4.87 also shows the involvement of the macula with oedema and streaks of exudates. The progression to complete loss of vision is often disastrously rapid.

In the presumed *ocular histoplasmosis* syndrome there are small pale foci of choroidoretinitis associated with pigmentation and surrounded by a rim of haemorrhage (4.88). These lesions are thought to be related to a hypersensitivity response to the products of *Histoplasma capsulatum*.

In **retinitis pigmentosa**, large pigmented spots looking like bone corpuscles start in the periphery and gradually encroach towards the centre of the fundus (4.89). The choroid becomes atrophied and tesselled. The visual deterioration progresses inexorably, starting with loss of temporal fields, leading to tunnel vision and eventually to complete blindness.

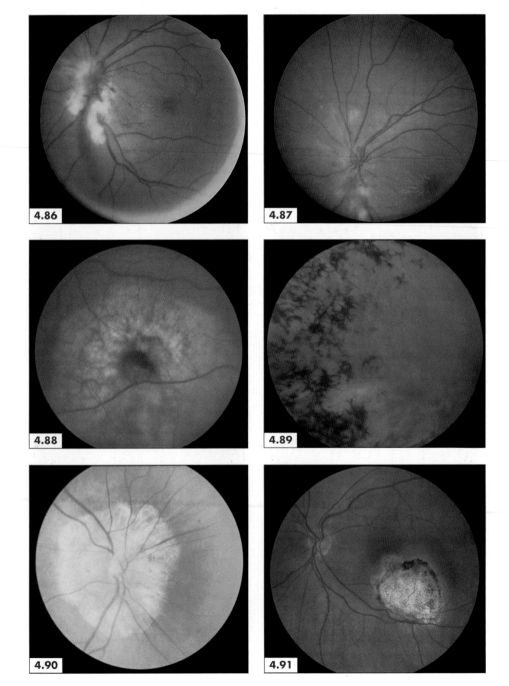

4.86 and 4.87
Cytomegalovirus retinitis with necrosis of the retina and haemorrhages

4.88
Histoplasma choroidoretinitis with confluent exudates and haemorrhages around a clump of choroidal pigment

4.89
Retinitis pigmentosa

4.90
Malignant melanoma: a yellowish mass under the retinal vessels

4.91
Malignant melanoma after laser therapy

The commonest tumour arising from the choroid is a **malignant melanoma**. The ophthalmoscopic picture is variable but a rounded, yellowish, somewhat elevated, patch under the retinal vessels should arouse suspicion of a tumour (4.90). Figure 4.91 shows a melanoma that has been subjected to laser therapy.

Angioid streaks, like the retinal vessels, radiate outwards from the disc but they do not arise from the vessels. They are more deeply situated, may be dark grey or red in colour and are sometimes outlined on either side by a thin white line. Figure 4.92 is from a patient with the **Ehlers–Danlos syndrome**; it shows a greyish streak lying superiorly round the disc and another one radiating outwards at 1 o'clock, crossing under two superior temporal vessels. Figure 4.93 is from a patient with **pseudoxanthoma elasticum** and it

shows a reddish angioid streak radiating at 1 o'clock outwards to the periphery under the superior temporal vein. The *triad* of skin changes (p. **64**), angioid streaks and vascular abnormalities is called the **Gröenblad–Strandberg syndrome**. In most cases the macula is affected and this may seriously impair the visual acuity.

The fundus in patients with **septicaemia** may have characteristic round, oval or elliptical haemorrhages, with a pale centre (caused by a collection of lymphocytes) called *Roth spots* (4.94). In a patient with suspected subacute infective endocarditis the fundus should be examined daily, since the discovery of a Roth spot could be very helpful. Roth spots may also be found in patients with haemolytic anaemias and in collagen diseases.

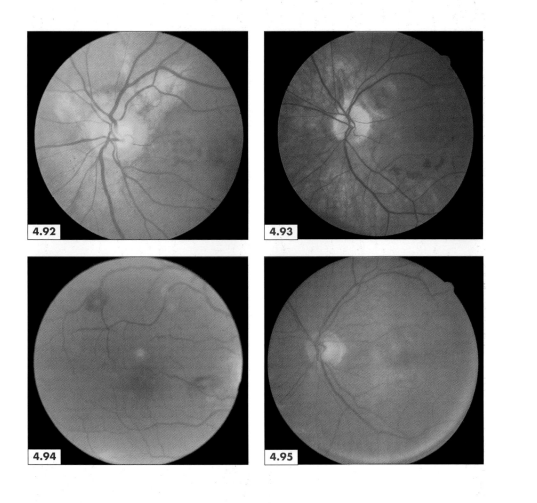

4.92
Angioid streaks: a greyish, ill-defined streak round the disc superiorly and one radiating outwards at 1 o'clock

4.93
Angioid streak radiating at 1 o'clock, running under the superior temporal vein

4.94
Roth spots

4.95
Senile macular degeneration

Senile macular degeneration is a common cause of deteriorating vision in the elderly. In the early stages there may be pigmented stippling at the macula (4.95) with the later appearance of faint, yellowish-white spots known as colloid bodies (4.96). In most cases the condition is slowly progressive and haemorrhages followed by scars appear at the macula.

Retinal detachment is usually heralded by complaints of flashes of light, snowstorm vision, dark spots or clouded vision. In the acute state, the fundal view may be obscured by a vitreous haze. In established cases, the detached area may show whitish folds (4.97) and the overlying vessels may look dark and *devoid of their axial reflex*. The choroidal detail is obscured by the detachment and the lenses of the ophthalmoscope may have to be changed to bring different parts of the fundus into focus. The folds of the detached portion may look like crests and valleys and the vessels are greatly attenuated (4.98, 4.99).

4.96
Senile macular degeneration: rounded, colloid bodies in the macula

4.97
Retinal detachment with whitish folds in the detached retina

4.98 and 4.99
Retinal detachment: obscured choroidal features, attenuated vessels and prominent, yellowish retinal folds

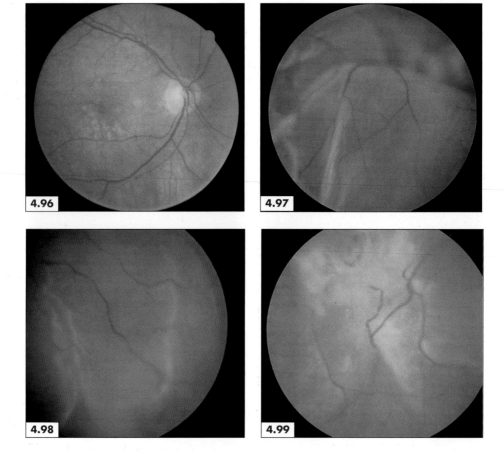

5 THE EARS

A complete and thorough examination of the ears is rarely performed by the average doctor, usually being left to the specialist ENT surgeon. This is unfortunate as the ear may often reveal useful clinical information about systemic disorders (e.g. sarcoidosis, gout, porphyria, etc.) and infections, and occasionally evidence of an early neoplasm may be found.

The external ear (5.1, 5.2) consists of the expanded **pinna (auricle)**, and the **external auditory meatus** leading to the **tympanic membrane**. The lateral surface of the pinna is irregular with numerous depressions and ridges to which various names have been assigned (5.2).

A diagonal crease may be seen in the ear lobe (5.3). This is referred to as *Frank's sign* and is associated with **ischaemic heart disease**. This crease may not fully traverse the ear lobe or may only be superficial. There is a statistical association between ear lobe creases and coronary artery disease in various populations studied.

Congenital malformation or absence of all or part of the ear is rare but clinically significant because of its association with deafness and facial asymmetry. A grossly abnormal external ear with an *absent* external auditory meatus (5.4) may be associated with some degree of *hypognathism* (5.5) resulting from the underdevelopment of the

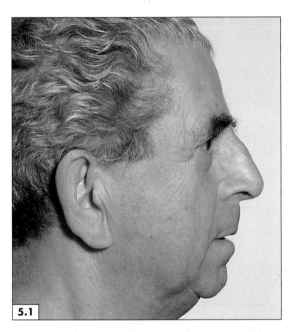
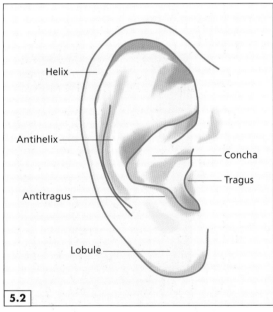

5.1
Normal external ear

5.2
Structure of the external ear

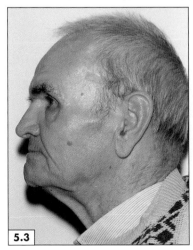
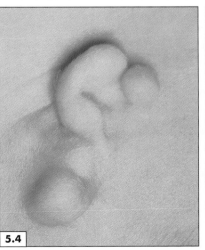
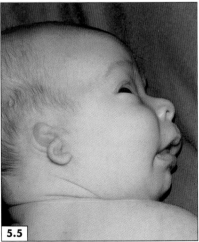

5.3
Frank's sign: a diagonal ear lobe crease (This sign was incidentally identified by a postgraduate student in a patient on a neighbouring bed, during a teaching session.)

5.4 and 5.5
Treacher Collins syndrome: deformed external ear and mandibular hypoplasia

mandible, as in the **Treacher Collins syndrome** (see also 1.334). The pinna may be almost completely absent and represented by a rudimentary bud (5.6) with major implications for hearing (absent external auditory canal) and facial appearance (5.7). This patient with severe *conductive deafness* also had hypoplasia of the left mandible and maxilla.

The ears are often exposed and therefore vulnerable to the extremes of temperature. Patients living in cold climates may get chilblains, while those exposed to the hot sun may develop **solar keratosis**, which can manifest as a small papule (5.8) or as a hyperkeratotic warty nodule (5.9). Some of these can develop into **squamous cell carcinomata**.

The ears should not be overlooked in patients with **porphyria cutanea tarda** (5.10). The helix of the pinna is a common site for *gouty tophi* (5.11), although these may also occur on the antihelix and on the medial surface of the pinna. The entire pinna should be palpated for the presence of swellings. The reddish, papulonodular lesions

of **sarcoidosis** can also occur on the ears (5.12) and on the face, nose and forehead (5.13). Granulomatous induration may involve the entire pinna in this condition (**lupus pernio**) (5.14).

In **fulminant meningococcaemia** (associated with septicaemic shock, hypotension and disseminated intravascular coagulation), peripheral vasoconstriction and acral cyanosis may involve the extremities and the ears (5.15). With such overwhelming meningococcaemia this process is often irreversible, leading to gangrene of the ear (5.16).

Nodular infiltration of the skin with an erythematous hue may occur on the face and ears in **leprosy** (5.17). Similar lesions are also found on the elbows, buttocks and knees.

Otitis externa (5.18) is the most frequent disorder involving the external auditory meatus and often, as in this case, extends to the pinna. Many such patients have an atopic or eczematous background with accompanying bacterial or even fungal superinfection. Figure 5.18 is an example of herpes zoster recognizable by the vesicular

5.6 and 5.7
Congenital absence of ears

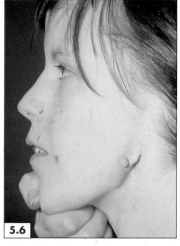

5.6

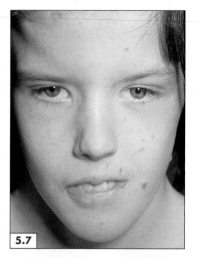

5.7

5.8
Solar papule: pigmented papule arising on a sun-exposed area

5.9
Hyperkeratotic, warty solar nodule

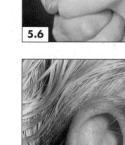

5.8

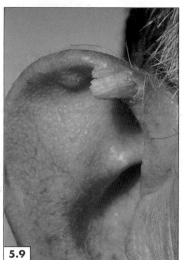

5.9

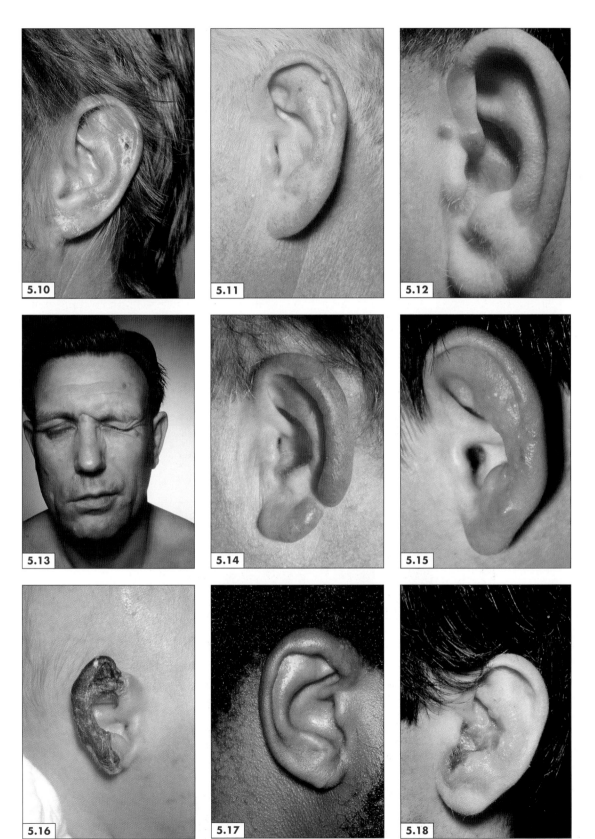

5.10
Porphyria cutanea tarda: atrophic scars

5.11
Gouty tophi

5.12
Sarcoidosis: granulomatous papules

5.13
Sarcoid papules

5.14
Lupus pernio

5.15 and 5.16
Fulminant meningococcaemia with vasoconstriction of the ear leading to necrosis

5.17
Leprosy: erythematous infiltration in the helix

5.18
Otitis externa: herpes zoster

eruption. This patient also had an ipsilateral seventh cranial nerve palsy (**Ramsay Hunt syndrome**). Recurrent bacterial infections occur frequently in atopic individuals and in those who have impaired immunity, causing scarring and deformity of the pinna (5.19).

Various skin tumours such as **keratoacanthoma (molluscum sebaceum)** and **squamous cell carcinoma** sometimes arise on the pinna. The former is less common, occurs earlier (50–60 years of age), and characteristically arises abruptly from the surface of the skin (5.20, 5.21). It

5.19
Recurrent infections with atrophic deformity of the ear

5.20
Keratoacanthoma: erythematous, dome-shaped tumour with a central necrotic scab

5.21
Keratoacanthoma: a glistening nodule with a central ulcer

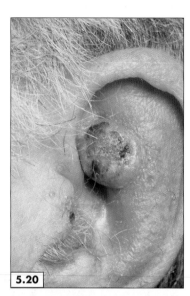

5.19

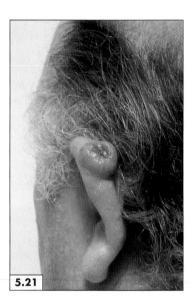

5.20

5.21

5.22
Squamous cell carcinoma: an erythematous plaque with haemorrhagic scabs

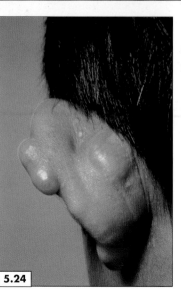

5.22

5.23
A large, transparent cyst

5.24
Hyaline fibromatosis with fibromatous outgrowths

5.25
Auriscope/otoscope

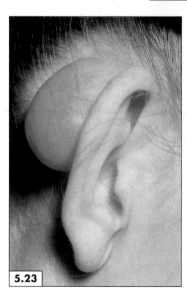

5.23

5.24

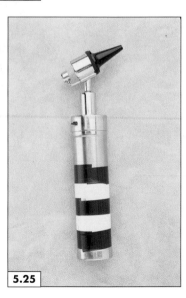

5.25

enlarges rapidly and then separates gradually, leaving a puckered scar. In contrast a **squamous cell carcinoma** (5.22) usually appears between the ages of 60 and 80 years, is commoner in males, and often arises on pre-existing **solar keratosis**.

Cysts (5.23) and **fibromata** (5.24) may be found on the pinna as elsewhere on the body but, because of their disfiguring appearance, the patient seeks help earlier than if the lesions were on the abdomen. In **hyaline fibromatosis**, outgrowths of fibrous tissue occur on the ears, face, hands and feet. They recur incessantly after excision and grow to enormous proportions (see also 1.327.)

After the external examination of the ear, the inner end of the external auditory canal and the **tympanic membrane** should be inspected with the aid of an otoscope (5.25). To obtain an adequate view of the tympanic membrane, the pinna is stretched gently and the otoscope is angled slightly downwards and anteriorly to follow the curve of the canal (5.26).

The **tympanic membrane** (5.27, 5.28) lies obliquely across the end of the external canal, separating the external from the middle ear. The healthy eardrum has a cone-shaped light reflex with its apex near the handle of the **malleus**. The light is not usually reflected by a diseased membrane, although in some cases of **otitis media** with effusion the reflex may not be totally lost. The most useful feature is the **malleus**, as the demarcation of its various parts is lost in various disorders such as **cholesteatoma**. The superior lateral process of the malleus appears rather like a knuckle in the top right-hand corner. The blushed seam is a normal feature as it does not extend onto the drum. In contrast, Figure 5.29 is an example of early **otitis media;** the entire drum is bulging and hyperaemic, with dilated vessels and an absent light reflex.

Figure 5.30 shows 'burnt-out' chronic otitis media with a posterior central *perforation* and dense sclerotic change within the rest of the pars tensa. As would be expected, there is no light reflex.

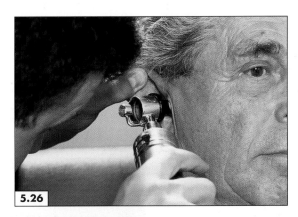

5.26
Examining the external auditory canal and tympanic membrane

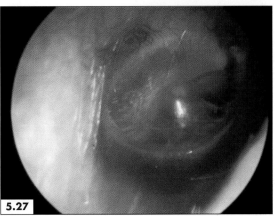

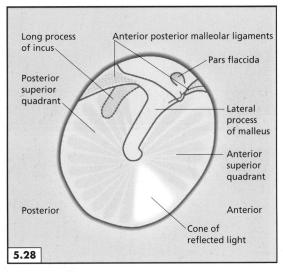

5.27
The tympanic membrane as viewed through an otoscope

5.28
The detail of the tympanic membrane

Chronic middle-ear disease often involves the surrounding bone (the tympanic ring, ossicles, mastoid air cells) and the walls of the attic, aditus and antrum. Erosion of these bony areas, together with the chronic inflammatory process, leads to the formation of a sac or **cholesteatoma** (5.31). In this particular case, there is keratinization over the attic, and the white mass visible over the posterosuperior quadrant is the fundus of the cholesteatoma sac descending into the mesotympanium.

One important feature of a cholesteatoma is that it contains constituents of the skin; in other words there is 'skin in the wrong place'. A cholesteatoma may be **congenital, primary** (without antecedent infection) or **secondary** to middle-ear infection. Figure 5.32 is another example of a cholesteatoma showing the presence of pus in the attic. The drum is also abnormal and bulging, with a whitish colour betraying the massive cholesteatoma, originating in the attic. Its sac is occupying, and almost obliterating, the entire middle ear.

One of the characteristics of a cholesteatoma is an attic granuloma (5.33). The pars tensa is intact and looks normal but the fundus of the cholesteatoma sac can be seen extending down from the posterosuperior region, occupying approximately two-thirds of the space behind the drum. Figure 5.34 shows an atelectic, but intact, tympanic membrane. There is evidence of previous infection but the eardrum has healed with some atrophic replacement of the drum. There is an attic retraction pocket but this is of no clinical significance.

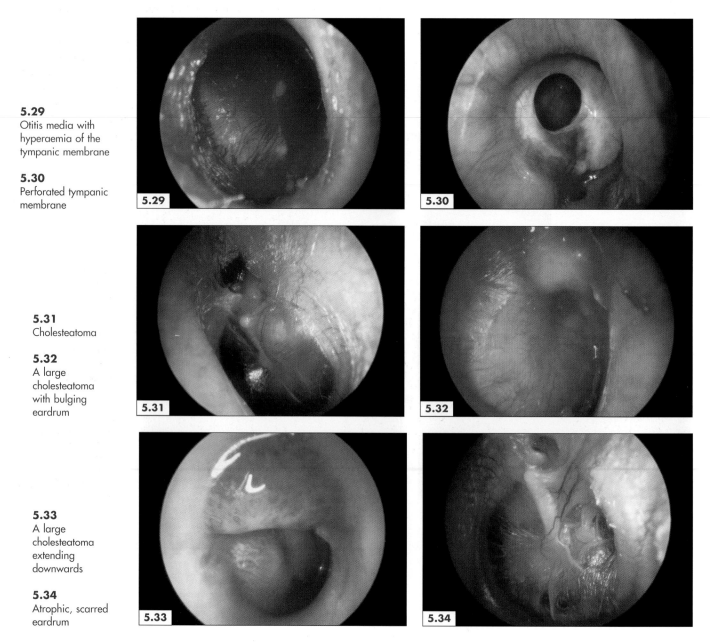

5.29
Otitis media with hyperaemia of the tympanic membrane

5.30
Perforated tympanic membrane

5.31
Cholesteatoma

5.32
A large cholesteatoma with bulging eardrum

5.33
A large cholesteatoma extending downwards

5.34
Atrophic, scarred eardrum

6 THE NECK

The diagnostic problems and signs usually encountered in the neck are as follows:

- **Congenital** (e.g. webbing, craniovertebral anomalies, thyroglossal cyst, sublingual dermoid, branchial cyst, cystic hygroma, cervical rib, laryngocoele, etc.);
- **Lymph glands** (e.g. lymphomas, infections, secondaries);
- **Salivary glands** (e.g. submandibular gland swelling, Mikulicz's syndrome);
- **Thyroid gland** (e.g. goitre, neoplasia);
- **Jugular veins** (e.g. congestive cardiac failure, superior vena caval obstruction, tricuspid incompetence);
- **Carotids** (e.g. Corrigan's sign, de Musset's sign, kinked carotid, absent/unequal pulses);
- **Cutaneous** (e.g. herpes zoster, scleroderma, scars, etc.);
- **Muscular** (e.g. muscular dystrophy/palsy).

Although any structure in the neck may be involved in a disease process, 95% of the abnormalities usually seen are related to disorders of the thyroid gland, the veins, the carotid arteries and the lymph nodes. This should be borne in mind while inspecting the neck for diagnostic clues. Congenital legacies take the major share of the remaining 5% of the cervical abnormalities.

The shortness of the neck can be recognized by looking at the distance between the ear lobules and the shoulder (6.1), then by comparing it with that of a normal subject of the same sex and height (6.2). A *short neck* is an important feature in many patients with gross obesity; the associated small and narrow pharyngeal cavity collapses during sleep, resulting in ineffectual thoracoabdominal movements which causes snoring, particularly when the patient sleeps on his or her back (the **sleep apnoea sysndrome**). Recurrent episodes of apnoea lead to chronic hypercapnia and hypoxaemia known as the **Pickwickian syndrome** (6.1). On the other hand, an excessively long, elongated neck such as the one in **Marfan's syndrome** can be detected by the same method of comparison (6.3).

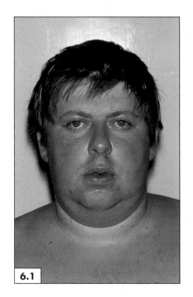

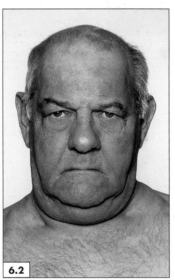

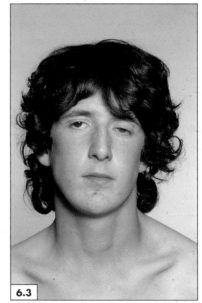

6.1
Pickwickian syndrome: a short neck and facial plethora

6.2
Somewhat overweight subject with hypothyroidism

6.3
Marfan's syndrome. Note the long neck and a partial ptosis of the left eye due to long-standing dislocation of the lens and myopia

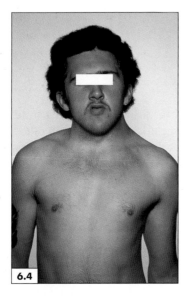

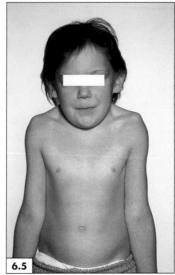

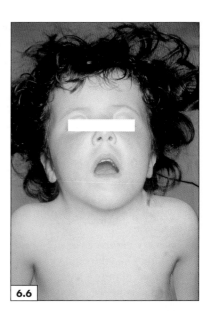

6.4, 6.5 and 6.6
Klippel–Feil
syndrome with a
short, webbed neck

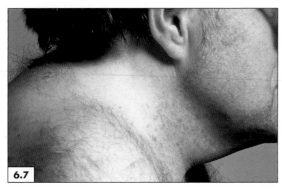

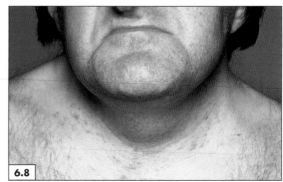

6.7 and 6.8
Klippel–Feil
syndrome: short
neck with low-set
ears

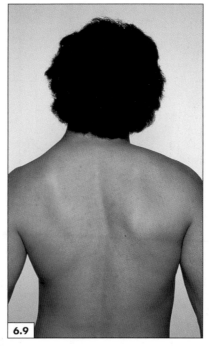

6.9
Thoracic scoliosis

In **craniovertebral anomalies** there is often a dispropor-tion between the clinical manifestations and the structural derangement. Congenital fusion of the cervical vertebrae is the reason for the short neck (6.4) in the **Klippel–Feil syndrome**. The appearance is very striking and the condi-tion can be diagnosed in early childhood (6.5, 6.6). Some-times the vertebrae are not only fused but also deficient in number, thereby producing a very short neck with the ears nearly touching the shoulders (6.7, 6.8). Other vertebrae may also be involved and there may be an associated tho-racic scoliosis (6.9).

The presence of a **cervical rib** (a fibrous band or an enlarged seventh cervical transverse process) produces a complex clinical picture (i.e. sensory, motor, vascular or mixed). Numbness and paraesthesiae usually occur along the ulnar border of the forearm and hand and, in some cases, there may be weakness and wasting of the small muscles of the hand. There is often nothing to see in the neck but sometimes there is a little prominence, as can be seen in the right supraclavicular fossa in this patient (6.10, 6.11). Pressure on the palpable cervical rib may produce pain and tingling in the ulnar border of the hand and forearm.

Webbing of the neck, although not always present, is a characteristic feature of **Turner's syndrome** (6.12). It is more likely to be associated with congenital cardiac abnor-malities such as *coarctation of the aorta*, atrial or ventricu-lar septal defect and aortic stenosis. These patients with XO sex chromosomes have gonadal agenesis with primary amenorrhoea, poorly developed secondary sexual charac-teristics, short stature, a shield-like chest, shortening of one or more of the metacarpals (see 9.144) and an increased carrying angle at the elbow (6.13). Some patients with the Klippel–Feil syndrome also have webbed necks (6.5, 6.6).

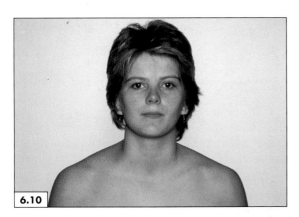

6.10

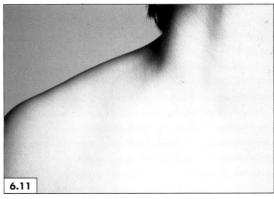

6.11

6.10 and 6.11
Right cervical rib suggested by a prominent area in the right supraclavicular fossa

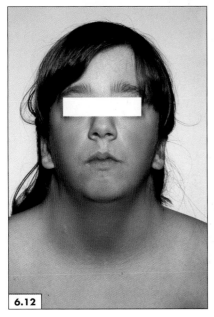

6.12

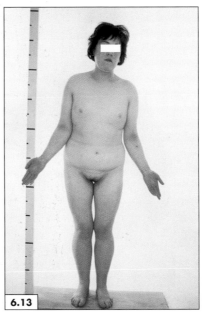

6.13

6.12
Turner's syndrome with a short, webbed neck

6.13
Turner's syndrome: short stature, broad, shield-like chest, absent pubic hair and increased carrying angles

There is another form of Turner's syndrome (**pseudo-Turner's, Ullrich's, Noonan's syndrome**) (6.14) in which there is webbing of the neck with associated short stature, ptosis, congenital heart disease (pulmonary stenosis, atrial septal defect, etc.), hypogonadism, triangular facies, promi-nent brow and hypertelorism. The patient is usually a phenotypic male with testicular aplasia.

A short neck and small stature are also characteristic features of the **growth hormone deficiency syndrome** (6.15).

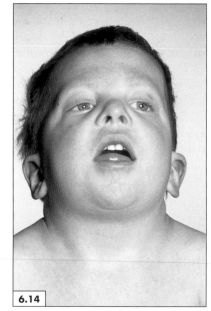

6.14
Noonan's syndrome with a short, webbed neck and hypertelorism

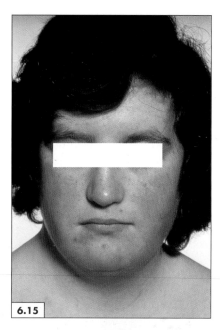

6.15
Growth hormone deficiency syndrome

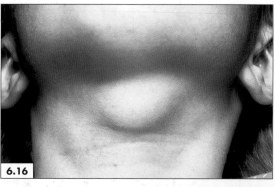

6.16
Thyroglossal cyst

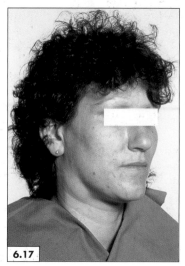

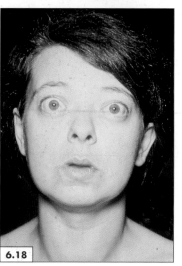

6.17
Branchial cyst

6.18
Graves' disease with diffuse enlargement of the thyroid gland

A **thyroglossal cyst** is the commonest congenital neck swelling. It is a painless, smooth, midline swelling between the thyroid isthmus and the hyoid bone (6.16), that usually makes its appearance at adolescence. The swelling moves upwards when the patient swallows or protrudes the tongue.

A **branchial cyst** arises from the vestigial remnant of the second branchial cleft. Although it is present at birth, it usually only becomes visible at adolescence. It appears at the anterior border of the sternomastoid muscle at the level of the hyoid bone (6.17). It is deep-seated, painless, fluctuant and transluminant unless infected when it becomes tense and painful.

Enlargement of the **thyroid gland (goitre)** is by far the commonest neck swelling with important clinical implications as it may be associated with a normal, hyperactive or underactive thyroid status. Patients with **Graves' disease** have diffuse enlargement of the thyroid gland often with associated eye signs (6.18). A **toxic multinodular goitre** may produce unequal enlargement of the two lobes and the swelling may reach as high as the submandibular gland (6.19). The boundaries of the enlarged thyroid gland can be better appreciated if viewed when the patient swallows a sip of water. There are usually no eye signs (6.20) unless the patient also has Graves' disease.

Both the toxic multinodular goitre and the **toxic adenoma** (6.21–6.23) are more common in areas of iodine deficiency. Hyperthyroidism may be readily precipitated by iodine ingestion in iodine-deficient patients and in those with goitres (*Jod–Basedow phenomenon*). An isolated small swelling may mimic a thyroglossal cyst as in this patient (6.24) with autoimmune thyroiditis.

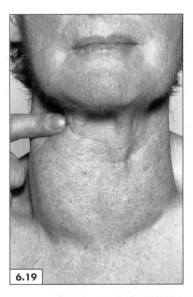

6.19

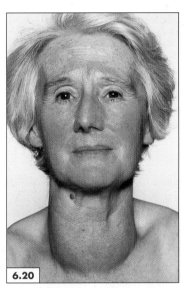

6.20

6.19 and 6.20
Multinodular goitre unassociated with eye signs

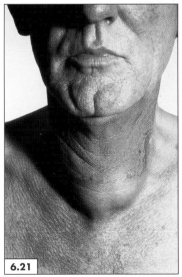

6.21

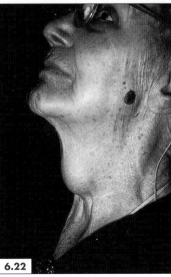

6.22

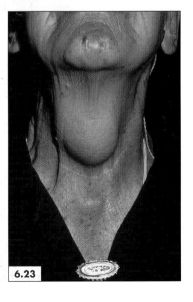

6.23

6.21
Multinodular goitre

6.22 and 6.23
Toxic adenoma with the swelling in the isthmus of the thyroid gland

Endemic iodine deficiency and the ingestion of goitrogens are common causes of a goitre in certain areas. Cassava is a well-known goitrogen in some areas of iodine deficiency. Such patients often have large goitres (6.25) without any clinical or biochemical evidence of hypothyroidism.

A multinodular goitre may be **malignant**, in which case one or more nodules may be hard and *fixed* to the deep tissues and to the skin. There may also be associated features such as lymphadenopathy or *spread* to the deep tissues and the skin. Figure 6.26 shows a malignant multinodular goitre that has spread retrosternally, causing obstruction of the superior vena cava.

Lymph node enlargement, which is either easily palpable or visible, is almost always clinically significant, since infection, lymphoma and metastasis are all possible causes. Asymptomatic, gross, nontender lymphadenopathy of the neck (6.27) may be the only manifestation of a lymphoma at presentation. In some cases, there may be coexisting mediastinal involvement (6.28). Figure 6.28 shows the telangiectasis and the maculopapular lesions secondary to radiotherapy.

Tuberculous adenitis usually affects one group of glands, most frequently along the upper jugular chain (6.29, 6.30). The majority of patients are either children or young adults in whom the organism gains access through the tonsils. The likely source of infection is either exposure to a patient with open tuberculosis or ingestion of contaminated milk. In most patients, the infection is limited to the cervical glands but the urine should be examined for acid-

6.24
Localized swelling confined to the isthmus of the thyroid gland

6.25
A large goitre associated with endemic iodine deficiency

6.26
Thyroid malignancy with tethered, erythematous overlying skin. Note the bluish, engorged veins due to superior vena caval obstruction

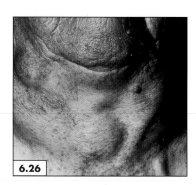

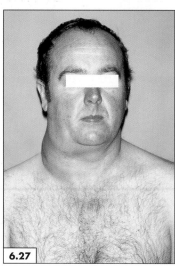

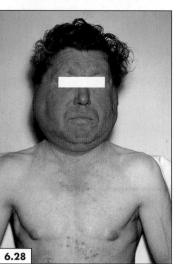

6.27
Lymphoma

6.28
Lymphoma with plethora, telangiectasis and maculopapular lesions on the chest

6.29
Tuberculous adenitis

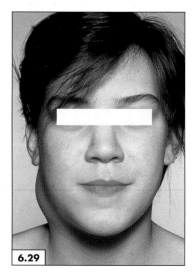

fast bacilli and the chest should be X-rayed, since there may be a primary focus in the lungs and the kidneys may also be involved.

In untreated cases, the infection progresses to a *cold abscess* (6.31, 6.32) and the caseating material may liquify and break through the capsule producing a nonhealing sinus (6.33).

The neck is an area where more than one structure may be affected simultaneously. The clinician, after finding one abnormal sign (e.g. a goitre), must be careful not to abandon the search for other abnormalities such as lymphadenopathy (6.34).

Cervical lymphadenopathy is also a frequent manifesta-tion of **infectious mononucleosis** and **toxoplasmosis** (6.35), sometimes in association with AIDS.

Most of the vascular signs in the neck are dynamic phe-nomena, for example the large upstroke and a sharp fall of the carotid pulse wave (*Corrigan's sign*) in **aortic incom-petence**, the associated nodding movements of the head (*de Musset's sign*), and the giant *v* wave oscillating the ear lobe in patients with **tricuspid incompetence** and **conges-tive cardiac failure**. The *engorged* and *static* neck veins, without an oscillating column of blood even on standing, and the suffused face suggest **superior vena caval obstruc-tion** (6.36, 6.37).

A careful inspection of the neck can reveal clues that

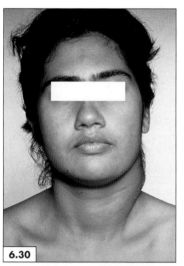

6.30

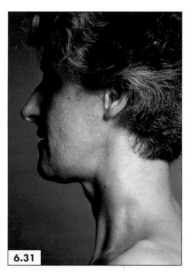

6.31

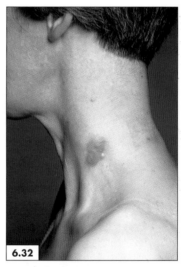

6.32

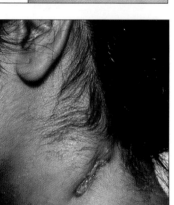

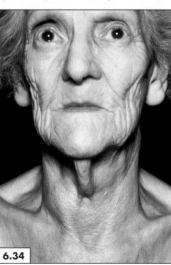

6.33

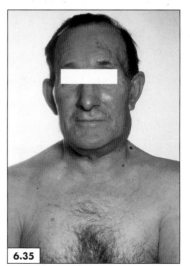

6.34

6.35

6.30
Tuberculous adenitis of the left jugular chain

6.31 and 6.32
A cold, tuberculous abscess

6.33
A nonhealing tuberculous sinus

6.34
A nodular goitre on the right side and enlarged lymph nodes in the left anterior cervical triangle. Note associated wasting

6.35
Cervical lymphadenopathy: toxoplasmosis

may be of profound clinical significance. Figure 6.38 shows an emaciated man with grossly reduced cricomanubrium distance suggestive of a wasting condition and chronic obstructive airways disease. In such thin patients the surface contour of the trachea is better seen than felt, and a closer look suggests that it is deviated to the right (6.39). This patient had a **bronchogenic carcinoma** in the right lung causing collapse of a part of the upper lobe.

The skin of the neck may be involved in skin diseases affecting other parts of the body but there are a few disorders of particular importance to the neck. For example, **herpes zoster** may be localized to the cervical spinal nerves and the vesicles may be seen only on the neck along the cutaneous distribution of C2–C4 (6.40). **Contact dermatitis** caused by a metal is seen on the neck along the areas of contact with a necklace (**nickel dermatitis**) in sensitive

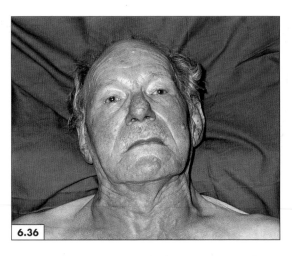

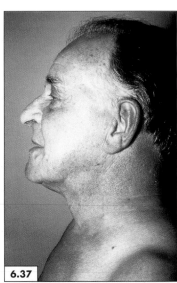

6.36 and 6.37
Superior vena caval obstruction: engorged jugular veins and suffused face

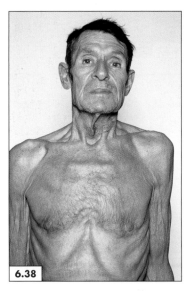

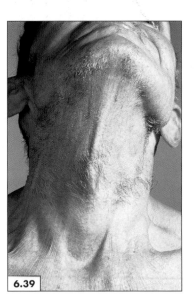

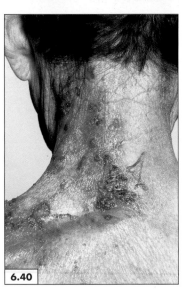

6.38 and 6.39
Chronic obstructive airways disease and bronchogenic carcinoma. Note reduced cricomanubrium distance and right-deviated trachea

6.40
Herpes zoster with ruptured, crusted vesicles

patients (6.41, 6.42). A similar reaction occurs when nickel-containing jewellery is worn on the ear lobes, wrists and fingers of nickel-sensitized individuals.

There are some skin conditions that have a predilection for other areas but, when present on the neck, they produce a striking appearance. Among these are the brownish, crusted papules of **Darier's disease** (6.43, see also p. **44**), and the polygonal, flat-topped, white papules of **lichen sclerosis atrophicus** (6.44). In the former, the severity differs from person to person; in severe cases the skin may be widely affected, causing much discomfort and embarrassment, since the abnormality remains for life. In the latter, the lesions may involve genitalia causing dysuria, dyspareunia, phimosis and recurrent balanitis.

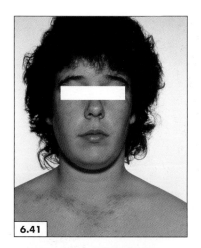

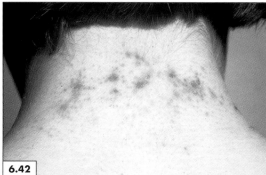

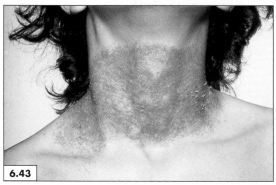

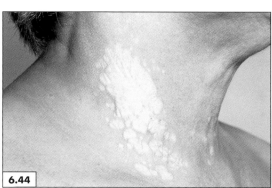

6.41
Nickel dermatitis

6.42
Small, darkish-red, confluent papules with indistinct margins along the line of contact with a necklace containing nickel

6.43
Darier's disease: small, brownish confluent papules with scales, coalescing into a large patch

6.44
Lichen sclerosus atrophicus: porcelain-white, confluent papules

The neck is a characteristic site for the yellowish papules of **pseudoxanthoma elasticum**, which give the 'plucked chicken skin' appearance (6.45, 6.46). Once suspected, the axillae can be examined for further supportive evidence where similar cutaneous lesions (6.47) and the redundant, loose, inelastic skin folds, caused by the changes in the connective tissue in this condition, can be seen (6.48). The cutaneous lesions are usually seen in childhood but the most devastating complications are the vascular manifestations, which appear later and include hypertension, gastrointestinal and cerebral haemorrhages, peripheral vascular insufficiency and coronary artery occlusion.

6.45
Scattered yellowish papules and the underlying defective elastin and collagen giving a 'plucked chicken' appearance

6.46
Multiple, confluent, yellowish and brownish papules forming a pebbled plaque. Note a tendency to formation of folds laterally

6.47
Yellowish (pseudoxanthomatous) papules

6.48
Loose, excessive folding in the skin

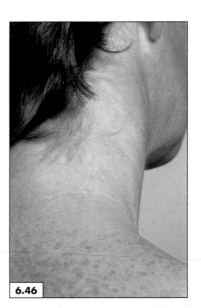

6.45

6.46

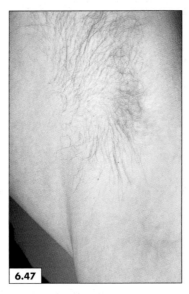

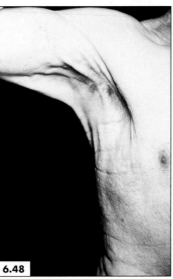

6.47

6.48

Lichen simplex chronicus, as circumscribed areas of lichenification, occurs on the neck (6.49) as it does on other areas of friction (e.g. arms, legs, ankles and anogenital areas). The lesions are caused by repeated rubbing or scratching, either as a habit or due to stress (localized neurodermatitis).

The neck and the upper part of the trunk may be involved in the localized **scleroderma of Buschke**; here the neck looks hidebound with nonpitting, tight, indurated skin (6.50). The condition is often associated with diabetes mellitus and correlates with the duration of the disease and the presence of microangiopathy. In **systemic sclerosis**, the neck may not only show the telangiectasia, which

is usually seen on the face, but it is also a suitable place to see the tethered skin (6.51) so characteristic of this condition.

Neuromuscular and joint disorders can cause abnormal postures that provide clues to an underlying condition. A lesion of the eleventh cranial nerve, which supplies the sternomastoid and trapezius muscles, can be suspected from the absence of the muscle fold between the neck and the shoulder, giving the affected side a flatter appearance (6.52). A reduction in the bulk of the supraspinatus muscle (6.53) is often the result of an injury to the suprascapular nerve (C5), which also supplies the infraspinatus muscle (6.54). This can be suspected from the frontal appearance

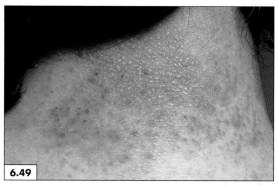

6.49

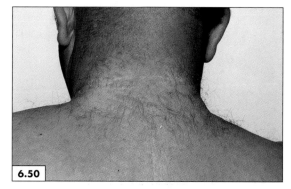

6.50

6.49
Lichen simplex chronicus: confluent, papular, follicular eczema forming a plaque with lichenification

6.50
Scleroderma of Buschke with a poorly defined induration of the skin

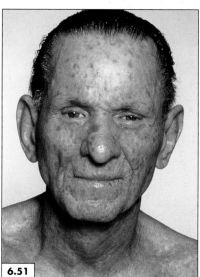

6.51

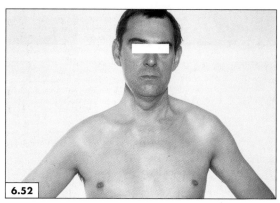

6.52

6.51
Systemic sclerosis. Note the stretched, wrinkled skin over the neck and perioral furrowing

6.52
Right eleventh cranial nerve palsy

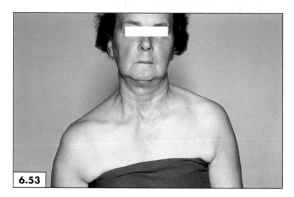

6.53

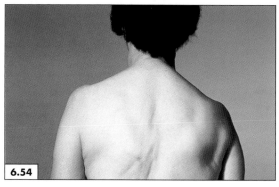

6.54

6.53 and 6.54
Injury to the suprascapular nerve causing wasting of the supraspinatus and infraspinatus muscles. Note the dimples at the back caused by the wasting of the infraspinatus muscle

because of the steep line between the neck and the shoulder, which drops straight onto the point of the shoulder joint due to the flattening caused by the atrophy of the supraspinatus muscle (6.53).

Ankylosing spondylitis distorts the spinal curvatures producing a *fixed thoracic kyphosis*, with compensatory extension of the cervical spine to maintain a horizontal visual axis; also, the patient is unable to look up at the ceiling (6.55). There is also loss of the lumbar lordosis and the anterior abdominal wall is squeezed out by the extreme thoracic kyphosis (6.56).

In cases of **attempted hanging** the neck should be examined for the critical ligature marks, with deeper chemotic impression in the front and suffused skin above the mark (6.57, 6.58). The question can be of great medicolegal importance, particularly when the subject with the ligature mark (6.59) is accusing someone else for the attempted hanging.

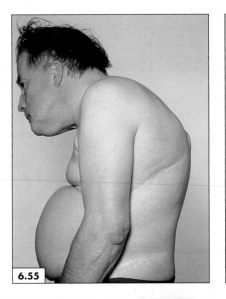
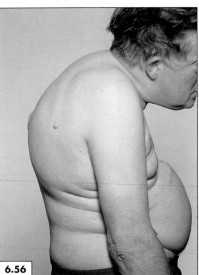

6.55 and 6.56 Ankylosing spondylitis: fixed, severe thoracic kyphosis producing a question-mark appearance

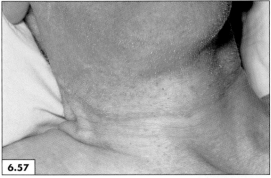
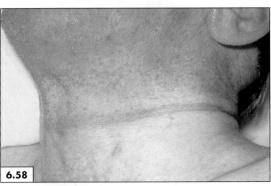

6.57 and 6.58 Attempted hanging with a well-defined ligature mark

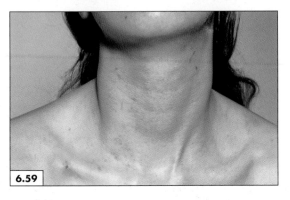

6.59 A self-inflicted, ill-defined ligature mark

7 THE CHEST

A clinician's inspection of a patient's bare chest has to yield three major objectives. First, the chest offers a large surface area where abnormalities (e.g. cutaneous, vascular, glandular, muscular and bony) relevant to the chest, the organs within and to other systems of the body may be found. Second, the movements of the rib cage during inspiration, whether expanding outwards (normal), or mainly upwards (chronic airways obstruction), their symmetry, fullness or indrawing of the rib spaces (*rib recession*), and any precordial pulsations should all be carefully noted. Third, a competent clinician always *listens* to the patient's breathing while observing the chest. As the information likely to be gained from the breath sounds is so valuable, it is worth placing the bell of the stethoscope in front of the patient's mouth and listening through it. Particular note should be taken of the relative length of the inspiration and expiration, and of any noises accompanying each. This is a dynamic exercise and cannot be treated with any detail in an atlas.

The inspection of the chest is best carried out by standing a few feet in front of the subject so that the overall shape of the rib cage, its various dimensions, and the apices and their symmetry can be assessed. *Deformities of the rib cage* are very informative, not only about the conditions that caused them but also because they may alter the findings obtained during the subsequent parts of the examination. Both *pectus carinatus* (pigeon chest) (7.1) characterized by a prominent anterior sternal ridge with the ribs falling steeply away on either side, and the *pectus excavatus* (funnel chest) (7.2) may displace the apex beat and give an erroneous impression of cardiomegaly. In most cases the main symptom is the embarrassment because of the deformity but some patients may complain of dyspnoea, palpitations and recurrent bronchopulmonary infections.

Harrison's sulcus (7.3, 7.4) is a horizontal groove on either side of the chest lying a few centimetres above the costal margin. It is usually caused by recurrent respiratory infections complicating childhood **rickets.**

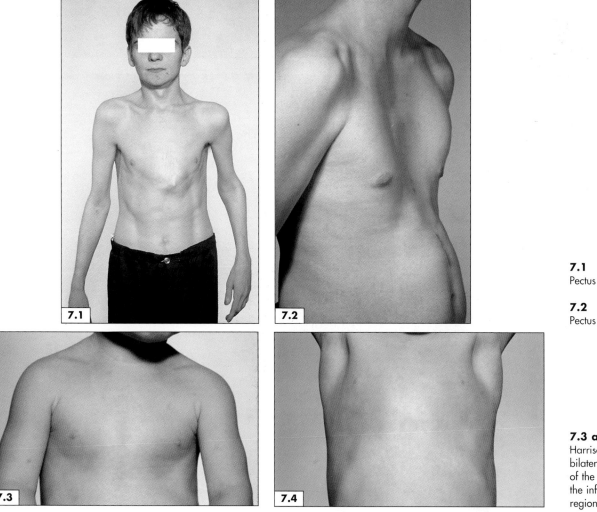

7.1
Pectus carinatus

7.2
Pectus excavatus

7.3 and 7.4
Harrison's sulcus: bilateral depression of the rib cage in the inframammary regions

Ankylosing spondylitis (7.5) distorts the shape of the chest, reduces the movements of the rib cage, and is sometimes associated with *apical fibrosis* of the lungs.

It is unsafe to conclude that any altered shape of the chest is caused by some intrinsic lung disease without prior inspection of the spine, looking for scoliosis or kyphosis and for the possible effects of previous surgery.

Scoliosis (7.6), **kyphosis** (7.7) and **kyphoscoliosis** (7.8) may result from a congenital abnormality (with or without vertebral defects), disorders affecting the vertebral bodies (e.g. tuberculosis, rickets, osteomalacia, trauma), neuromuscular disease (e.g. poliomyelitis, Friedreich's ataxia) or a thoracoplasty. In scoliosis, the spine is curved convex to the side of the scoliosis, and the rib cage on the

7.5
Ankylosing
spondylitis:
kyphoscoliosis

7.6
Scoliosis with
convexity on the
right side

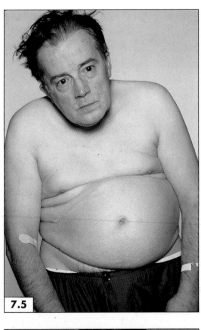

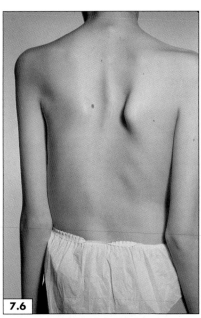

7.7
Kyphosis

7.8
Congenital
kyphoscoliosis

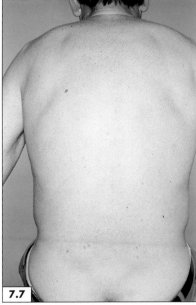

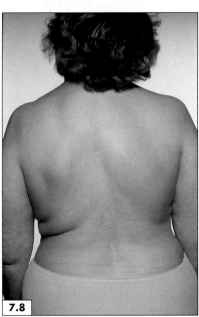

opposite side appears unsupported and compressed, raising up one or more folds of the skin (7.9, 7.10). The principal clinical features of severe kyphoscoliosis, apart from the deformity, are dyspnoea on effort, often leading to **cor pulmonale**. This results from the *rigidity* of the rib cage, which increases the work of breathing, decreases the vital capacity and tidal volume (with rapid shallow breathing), and eventually leads to *hypoxaemia* and *hypercapnia*.

Apical flattening on one side may be the result of an old **thoracoplasty** (the recommended treatment for tuberculosis before the era of effective chemotherapy). There will be a scar of the operation (7.11) and a closer look may show that the trachea is deviated to that side (7.12). A somewhat flatter chest wall on one side without an obvious scar should induce one to look at the back of the chest, where the large scar of a previous thoracoplasty may be easily visible (7.13).

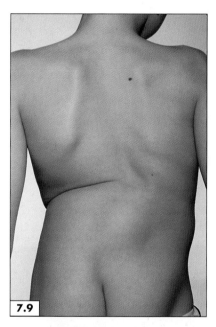

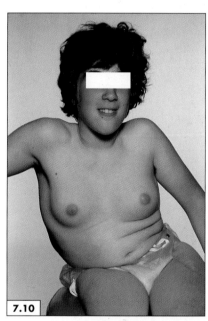

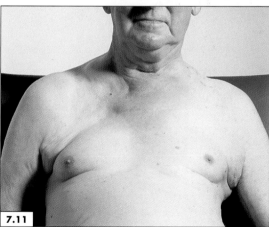

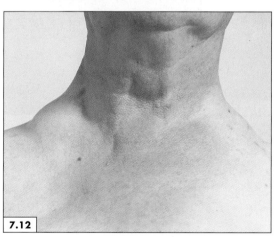

7.9 and 7.10
Marked scoliosis affecting thoracoabdominal posture

7.11
Scar of previous thoracoplasty and consequent flattening of the upper chest

7.12
Thoracoplasty scar and deviation of the trachea to the right

Cystic fibrosis should be suspected in any patient who is an underachiever in weight and height for their age (7.14), who has a deformity of the rib cage (7.15), clubbing of the fingers (7.16) and who presents with cough and purulent expectoration suggestive of **bronchiectasis.** Nasal polyps (7.17) occur in approximately one-half of these patients. In most cases, there is also evidence of pancreatic insufficiency.

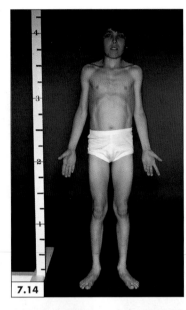

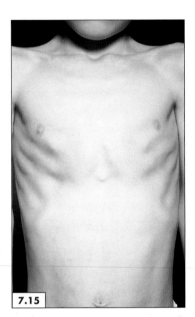

7.13
Thoracotomy scar

7.14
Cystic fibrosis

7.15
Marked rib recession with carinatus deformity

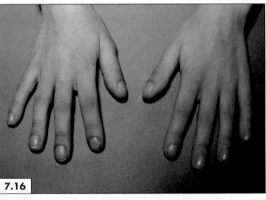

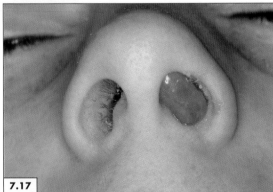

7.16
Clubbing and cyanosis of the fingers

7.17
A nasal polyp

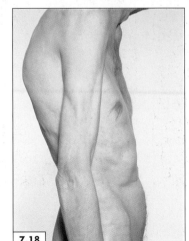

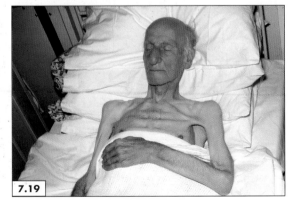

7.18
Crohn's disease: a bare rib cage and thin abdomen

7.19
Bronchogenic carcinoma: cachexia

The overall nutritional status of a patient can be assessed by looking at the chest. In wasting disorders, the loss of muscle bulk and subcutaneous fat makes the normally rounded rib cage look square, as in this patient with **Crohn's disease** (7.18). The ribs become prominent and the rib spaces show marked guttering, as seen in this man with a **carcinoma of the lung** (7.19).

A scar of a previous **mitral valvotomy** (7.20) will often explain a patient's symptoms and give some insight into the possible auscultatory findings. It is not ususual for a patient to forget to mention this operation; the benefit and timing of it having been obscured by a galaxy of worsening symptoms. A midline scar (7.21) suggests that the patient has either had a valve replacement or coronary artery bypass surgery.

Multiple dilated veins on the chest together with *static engorgement* of the neck veins (7.22) point to **superior vena caval obstruction**. The offending lesion may either be a carcinoma of the bronchus, as in this patient (7.23) with visible radiation markings; a lymphoma involving the mediastinal glands; mediastinal fibrosis; aortic aneurysm; a retrosternal goitre or carcinoma of the thyroid gland with mediastinal extension.

The normal anatomical structures on the anterior surface of the chest are the nipples in a male and the breasts in a female. These should be inspected carefully for any enlargement in the male, and for underdevelopment or asymmetry in the female. A broad, shield-like chest with widely spaced nipples and underdeveloped breasts (7.24) are seen in females with **Turner's syndrome**. These patients are short (usually less than 1.5 m) in stature, with gonadal agenesis (chromosomes 45, XO) and often have cardiovascular abnormalities (see p. **131**).

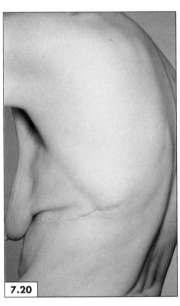

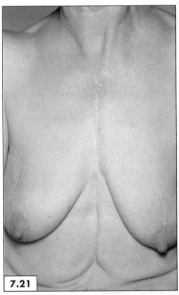

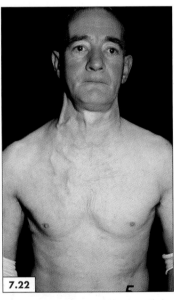

7.20
Scar of a previous mitral valvotomy

7.21
A midline scar of major cardiac surgery

7.22
Superior vena caval obstruction: dilated veins on the neck and over the chest and facial suffusion

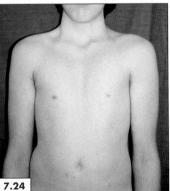

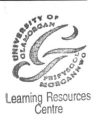

7.23
Radiation marks on the chest of a patient with carcinoma of the bronchus

7.24
Turner's syndrome: a broad, shield-like chest with underdeveloped breasts

Gynaecomastia (7.25, 7.26) has many causes and associations:

- Age-related (e.g. puberty, senile – rise in oestrogens and fall in androgens);
- Endocrine (e.g. thyrotoxicosis, hypothyroidism, pituitary disease, Addison's disease, testicular tumours, adrenal carcinoma, isolated gonadotrophin deficiency);
- Chromosomal (e.g. Klinefelter's syndrome – 47, XXY);
- Metabolic (e.g. hepatic failure);
- Neoplastic (e.g. carcinoma of the lung);
- Drug-induced (e.g. oestrogen therapy, aldactone, digoxin, alkylating agents, griseofulvin, methyldopa, phenothiazines, tricyclics, anabolic and adrenocortical steroids, isoniazid, etc.).

Approximately 5% of patients with carcinoma of the lung develop gynaecomastia, sometimes associated with hypertrophic pulmonary osteoarthropathy. The presence of gynaecomastia must not be accepted on inspection alone, particularly in an obese subject. The swelling must be palpated for the presence of *glandular tissue*, thereby distinguishing it from adipose tissue.

Puckering and indrawing of a part of the breast (7.27), with or without apparent induration, is a serious sign and suggests the presence of a neoplasm.

Almost all of the skin disorders can involve the chest, although in some cases the lesions are missed because of inadequate undressing before clinical examination of the patient. *Telangiectasia* are by far the most important of the **cutaneous lesions** to look for, since these are seldom found below the transnipple line. Sometimes they occur in crops on the upper chest, as in this patient with the **Budd–Chiari syndrome** (7.28).

Psoriasis (7.29) and **drug eruptions** (7.30) are two good

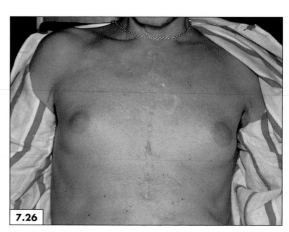

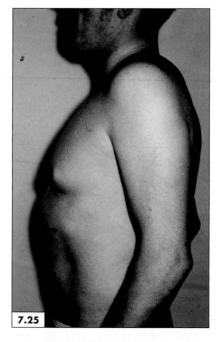

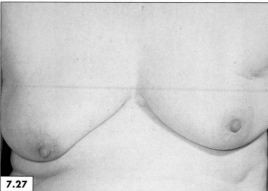

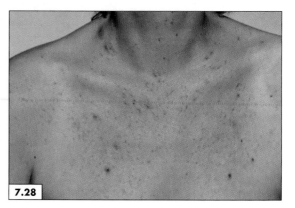

7.25
Gynaecomastia

7.26
Gynaecomastia with prominent breasts and unassociated with confounding obesity

7.27
Malignancy: puckering and indrawing of the left breast

7.28
Diffuse telangiectasis

examples where an unwary clinician either ignores or forgets to look at the trunk. In **guttate psoriasis**, numerous papular lesions appear on the trunk (7.31), sometimes well before any appear on the extremities. This condition usually follows, within 1–3 weeks, an upper respiratory tract infection.

In **chicken pox**, *pruritic* vesicles and pustules are present mainly on the face and trunk (7.32, 7.33). The initial lesion is a papule but by the time of presentation the papules have changed into vesicles, which develop into pustules. In a typical eruption, all these successive stages (vesicles, pustules and crusts) may be seen together.

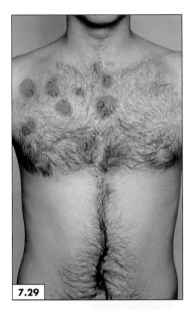

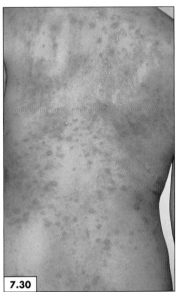

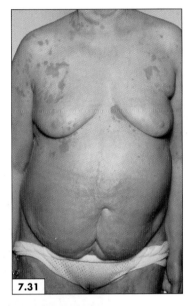

7.29
Psoriasis: well-circumscribed, erythematous, scaling plaques

7.30
Drug eruption: diffuse maculopapular rash

7.31
Guttate psoriasis: confluent, erythematous, scaling papules and plaques

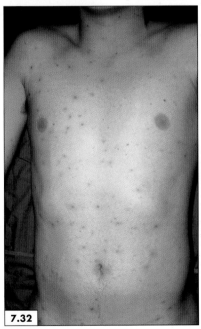

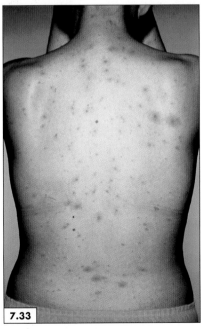

7.32 and 7.33
Varicella: a papulovesicular eruption with crusting over ruptured vesicles

Tinea versicolor, a chronic fungal (*Pityrosporum orbiculare*) infection, has a predilection for the trunk. The lesions are sharply defined, red, white or brown macules with fine scaling, usually in clusters, and are scattered both on the back (7.34) and the front (7.35) of the chest. This infection occurs mostly in warmer climates and also in susceptible patients who may have had prolonged treatment with corticosteroids.

Inspection of the chest can provide further supportive evidence in many cases where diagnosis is suspected after looking at the exposed parts of the body. In the **Ehlers–Danlos syndrome** (see also p. **64**), paper-thin scars may be seen on the chest (7.36) which are caused by the constant trauma of the clothes rubbing on the skin. *Café-au-lait* spots can be the earliest sign of **von Recklinghausen's disease** (**neurofibromatosis**). These spots, usually found on the trunk (7.37), appear in early childhood and become bigger and more numerous with advancing age. Unilateral pigmentation, usually in a nerve root pattern on the trunk, occurs in **Albright's syndrome** (7.38). This condition usually affects females who have *sexual precocity* and *polyostotic fibrous dysplasia* (deformity of the upper part of the femur, asymmetry of the long bones and of the skull, etc.).

7.34 and 7.35
Pityriasis versicolor: sharply marginated, scaling, light-brown macules

7.36
Thin, 'cigarette paper' scars

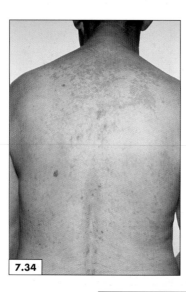

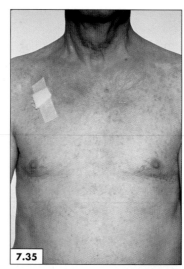

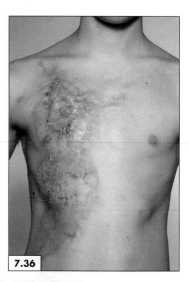

7.37
Café-au-lait spots: sharply demarcated, hypermelanosis macules

7.38
Albright's syndrome: pigmented patches over the C4 and C5 dermatomes

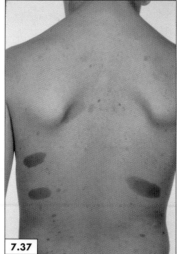

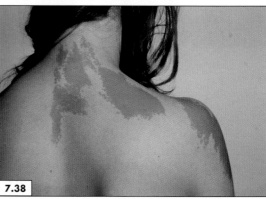

Both *axillae* should be looked at for a glandular swelling or a cutaneous lesion as part of the *visual survey* of the chest. **Acanthosis nigricans** has a predilection for the axillae, groins and other body folds. In this condition, there is *hyperpigmentation* with diffuse velvety *thickening* of the skin (7.39, 7.40). In its *juvenile* form (below 40 years), it may be familial or be associated with a variety of endocrine disorders (e.g. noninsulin-dependent diabetes mellitus, acromegaly, Addison's disease, hypothyroidism, hyperthyroidism, Cushing's syndrome and hyperandrogenic states often associated with obesity and polycystic ovaries).

Seborrhoeic warts may be seen in the axillae (7.41) and may develop rapidly on the legs (*Leser–Trélat sign*), associated with internal malignancy. In elderly patients, acan-

thosis nigricans is often a sign of an underlying malignancy, usually adenocarcinoma of the stomach, large and small bowel and uterus, less commonly ovary, breast, prostate and lung. Sometimes, it precedes the neoplasm by some years. Verrucous lesions appearing in a nonobese adult merit a vigorous search for an underlying neoplasm, mostly in the stomach.

Erythrasma (Greek for 'red spot'), a chronic bacterial infection caused by *Corynebacterium minutissimum*, affects the intertriginous areas such as the axillae, groins and between the toes. The lesions are red or brownish-red, sharply marginated macules, which are seen either scattered or in confluent patches (7.42). The lesion fluoresces coral-red under Wood's lamp.

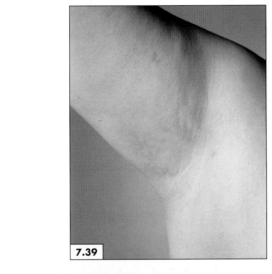 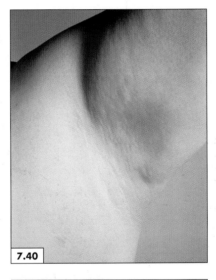

7.39 and 7.40 Acanthosis nigricans: poorly defined, hyperkeratotic verrucous changes

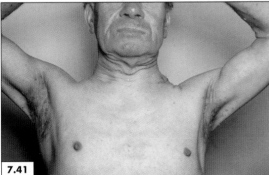 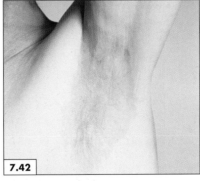

7.41 Seborrhoeic warts: multiple, 'stuck on', keratotic warts

7.42 Erythrasma: sharply marginated, reddish-brown macular patch

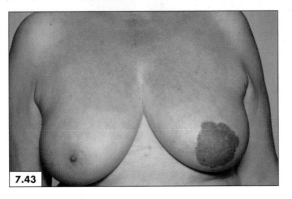

7.43 Bowen's disease: sharply demarcated, scaly, erythematous plaque

Bowen's disease, or an **intraepidermal epithelioma** (7.43), appears as a small, rounded or oval plaque with erythema and scaling. Although its course tends to be benign, metastases are known to occur.

Vitiligo, a circumscribed hypomelanosis resulting from enlarging and coalescing white macules, appears in a mirror-image distribution (see 9.99) around body orifices, over the bony prominences (e.g. knees, elbows, hands), in the axillae (7.44) and groins. It is familial in over one-third of cases and is often associated with a variety of auto-immune disorders (see Table 9.2, p. **176**).

Pemphigoid (7.45) and the *papular exanthem* of **secondary syphilis** (7.46) are some of the other skin conditions that involve the trunk. **Tuberculoid leprosy** may present as one or more asymmetrical, well-defined, slightly scaly hypopigmented areas on the chest (7.47). There is always loss of sensation in these lesions, which helps to distinguish them from pityriasis versicolor. The loss of sensation usually affects light touch and temperature, but sometimes appreciation of pain is lost as well.

7.44
Depigmented, sharply demarcated macular patch

7.45
Erythematous papules and ruptured bullae with crusted tops

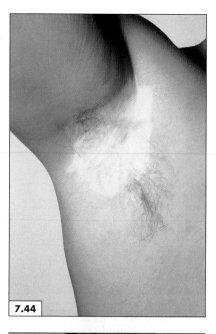

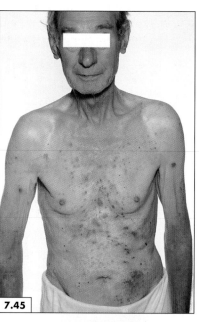

7.46
Secondary syphilis: maculopapular eruption

7.47
Tuberculoid leprosy: well-defined, hypopigmented, anaesthetic macule

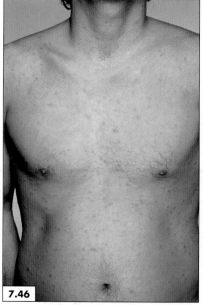

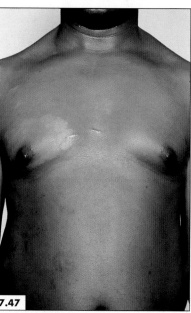

8 THE ABDOMEN

Although in many cases inspection of the abdomen may have less to offer than palpation and percussion, a good visual scan is still essential to obtain the most from the subsequent examination. For example, the question of whether an abdomen is protuberant because of obesity and/or ascites may be difficult to resolve, without first scanning the patient both in the standing and lying positions. In **simple obesity**, fat is laid down over many years and it tends to gravitate in the suprainguinal and suprapubic folds (8.1). This *chronic fixed dependence* can be better

appreciated by looking at the side view of the patient (8.2) which also reveals fat-laden skin folds at the back.

In contrast, the patient with **ascites** shows *mobile dependence* of the ascitic fluid, which, on standing, protrudes in the middle and overhangs the pubis (8.3). The suprainguinal areas on either side show a furrow instead of a fold and the umbilicus looks stretched, sometimes everted, under the pressure of the fluid (8.4). These points are reinforced by looking at the side view of this patient with **ascites** (8.5) compared with Figure 8.2. The ascitic

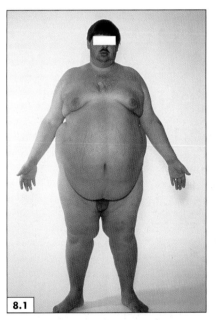

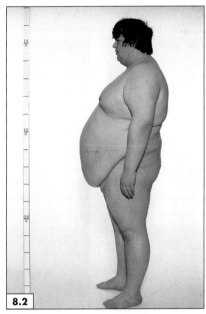

8.1 and 8.2
Simple obesity: deposition of fat in suprainguinal, suprapubic and lateral abdominal skin folds

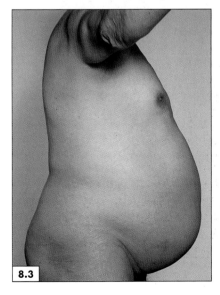

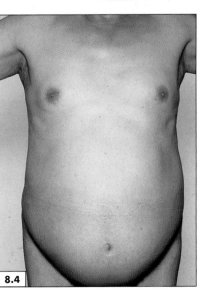

8.3 and 8.4
Ascites: central protuberance with a stretched umbilicus

fluid has gravitated to the suprapubic region, leaving a furrow in the left suprainguinal region where a redundant fold of fat is seen in the obese patient (8.2). In addition, *gynaecomastia* and *dilated veins* can be seen in Figure 8.5, which are helpful clues about this patient's underlying **portal cirrhosis.** The lateral furrow is also seen when the abdominal swelling is caused by a retroperitoneal cyst or hydronephrosis (8.6, 8.7).

Only after attention to these details can a clinician proceed to further examination with ample confidence. Sadly, many postgraduate students let themselves down in higher examinations by proceeding with palpation and percussion of the abdomen without first *looking* at it. This is the chief reason why they miss polycystic kidneys in an obese subject.

The abdomen and the chest provide a large area for looking for the various stigmata of **liver disease** such as *jaundice, gynaecomastia, telangiectasia* and *scratch marks* (8.8). In bright natural light, jaundice can be detected easily by looking at the skin, as in this patient with a **cholangiocarcinoma** (8.8).

Looking at a standing patient with suspected intra-abdominal pathology should not be omitted in those with no ascites, since a fullness caused by an enlarged liver (8.9) or spleen, or both (8.10), may be made obvious by this procedure. A lateral view will also reveal the scar of a previous operation and a surface impression of a transplanted kidney (8.11).

Dilatation of the abdominal wall veins (8.12) occurs in **portal hypertension** and in **inferior vena caval obstruction**. The flow of blood within the veins can be determined by blanching the dilated vein (8.13) and then by releasing the pressure at each end to see the refilling in the direction of the flow (8.14). In *intrahepatic* portal hypertension,

8.5
Ascites: gravitation of fluid centrally, leaving a furrow in the suprainguinal region. Note gynaecomastia and dilated veins due to underlying hepatic cirrhosis

8.6 and 8.7
Bilateral hydronephrosis associated with a large, retroperitoneal cyst

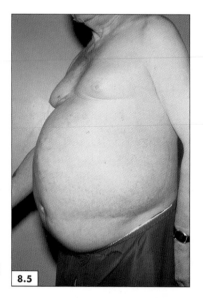
8.5

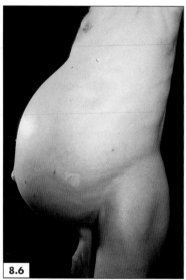
8.6

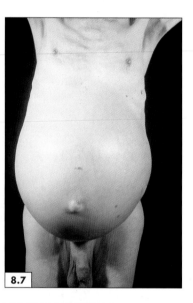
8.7

8.8
Cholangiocarcinoma: jaundice, telangiectasis and gynaecomastia

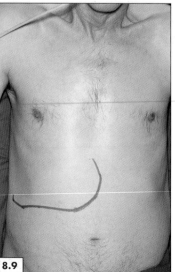
8.8

8.9
Hepatomegaly

8.9

paraumbilical veins are enlarged and the flow is away from the umbilicus towards the caval system (8.5, 8.15, 8.16). In inferior vena caval (IVC) obstruction, the collateral venous channels carry blood upwards to reach the superior vena caval system (8.17). The interpretation regarding the flow should be made with caution in *tense ascites*, which may cause functional obstruction of the inferior vena cava (8.18). Rarely, a number of prominent collateral veins may

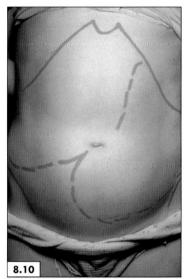

8.10

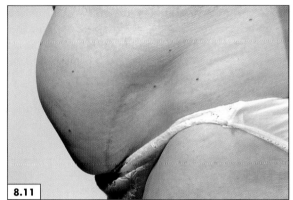

8.11

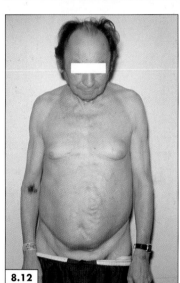

8.12

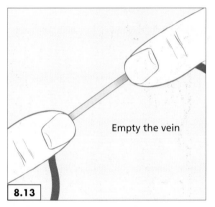

8.13 Empty the vein

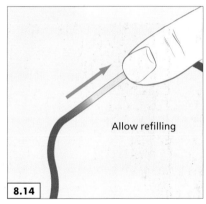

8.14 Allow refilling

8.10
Hepatosplenomegaly

8.11
Transplanted kidney

8.12
Portal hypertension: gynaecomastia and dilated surface veins

8.13 and 8.14
Testing for the direction of venous flow

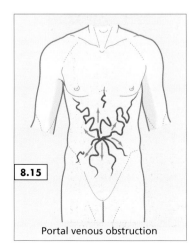

8.15 Portal venous obstruction

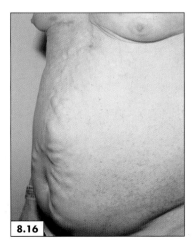

8.16

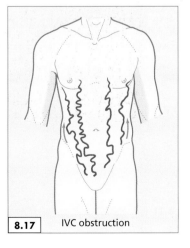

8.17 IVC obstruction

8.15 and 8.16
Portal hypertension: dilated veins drain away from the umbilicus to the caval circulation

8.17
Dilated veins drain to superior vena cava

be seen radiating from the umbilicus *(caput medusae)* (8.19). Attention should be directed to the other clinical features associated with chronic liver disease (8.20).

The umbilicus should be inspected for the presence of **umbilical** and **periumbilical herniae** (8.21, 8.22), which usually occur in obese subjects particularly after abdominal surgery. **Nickel dermatitis** (8.22) may be seen around the umbilicus in sensitive subjects wearing nickel buckles next to the skin.

The umbilicus is also a site of predilection for the dark red papules of angiokeratoma corporis diffusum (**Fabry's disease**; 8.23), which is an X-linked recessive disease. This

is an inborn error of metabolism in which there is a deficiency of alpha-galactosidase A, leading to an accumulation of glycosphingolipid ceramide in endothelial cells, and fibrocytes in the dermis, heart, kidneys and autonomic nervous system. Progressive renal failure occurs in adult life. Most patients have attacks of excruciating, unexplained pain in their hands.

A valuable but rare sign of **acute haemorrhagic pancreatitis** is a bruise or pigmentation near the umbilicus termed *Cullen's sign* (8.24). This occurs when retroperitoneal blood dissects its way anteriorly towards the umbilicus, where the colour of the overlying skin depends on the age

8.18
Portal hypertension with tense ascites: the dilated veins are draining towards the superior vena cava

8.19
Caput medusae

8.20
Clinical features of chronic liver disease

8.21
Umbilical hernia

8.22
Periumbilical hernia. Note maculopapular eruption caused by nickel buckles

8.23
Fabry's disease: periumbilical rosette of dark red papules

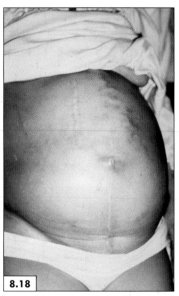

8.18

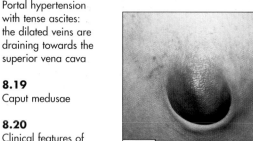

8.19

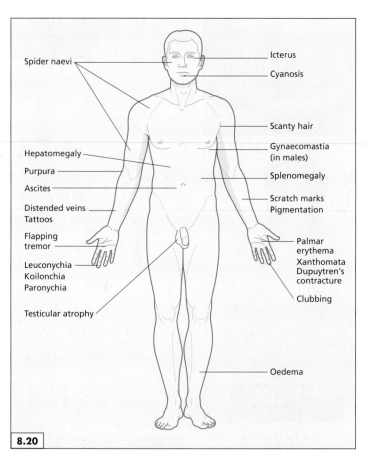

8.20

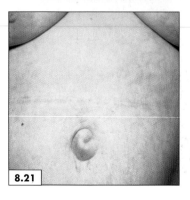

8.21

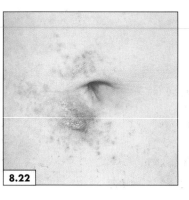

8.22

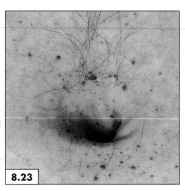

8.23

of the resulting bruise. The blood may also dissect into the flanks where a similar discolouration may be seen called the *Grey Turner's sign* (8.25).

As for the axillae, the groins should be inspected for increased or decreased pigmentation, glandular swellings, intertriginous infections, and for herniae. Small glands may be palpable in normal subjects but visible large glandular masses (8.26) are mostly pathological (e.g. suggestive of infection, lymphoma or secondaries). Tuberculous adenitis may involve the inguinal glands and form a **cold abscess** (8.27). **Lymphogranuloma venereum** (8.28) is a sexually

transmitted disease caused by *Chlamydia trachomatis.* Among heterosexuals, primary infection produces a rarely observed genital ulcer 2–3 weeks after exposure, followed later (2–4 weeks) by painful inguinal lymphadenopathy, often associated with signs of systemic infection. It heals spontaneously. It must be distinguished from a tumour, chancroid, syphilis and other granulomatous diseases.

An **inguinal hernia** (8.29) is not difficult to recognize in a standing patient but it may regress in a recumbent position.

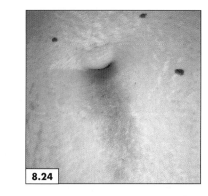
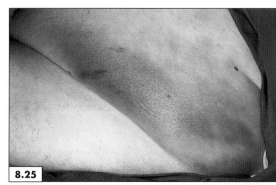
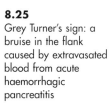
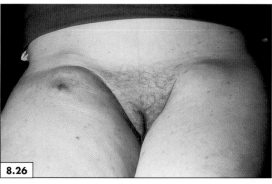
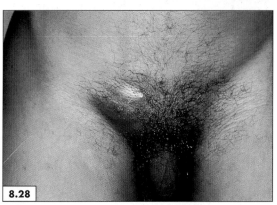
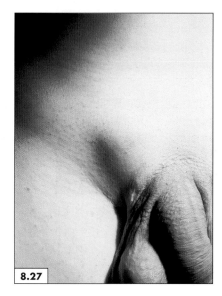
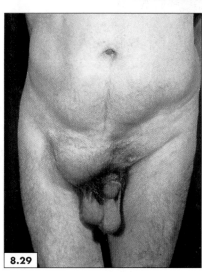

8.24
Cullen's sign. Note the coincidental presence of Campbell de Morgan (cherry angiomas) spots

8.25
Grey Turner's sign: a bruise in the flank caused by extravasated blood from acute haemorrhagic pancreatitis

8.26
Bilateral inguinal lymphadenopathy. Note a reddened, inflamed area overlying an infected lymph node

8.28
Lymphogranuloma venereum; enlarged inguinal and femoral lymph nodes separated by a groove made by the inguinal ligament (*groove sign*)

8.27
Tuberculous adenitis forming an inguinal mass

8.29
Right inguinal hernia

It would seem logical to extend the examination of the groins to that of the genitalia as part of the overall clinical assessment. However, most clinicians limit this practice to those occasions when they expect to find an abnormality. Thus, testicular bulk would be assessed in **chronic liver disease** and **myotonia dystrophica**, whereas under-developed and *infantile genitalia* would be looked for in **Klinefelter's syndrome** (8.30) and in the **growth hormone deficiency syndrome** (8.31).

A dermatologist may look routinely for genital lesions when he or she has already diagnosed **scabies** (8.32) or **lichen planus** (8.33).

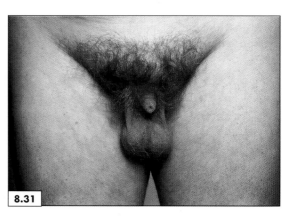

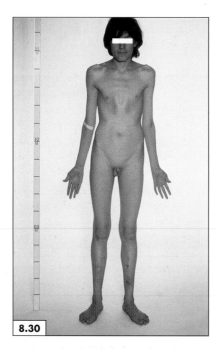

8.30
Klinefelter's syndrome

8.31
Growth hormone deficiency disease: infantile genitalia

8.32
Scabies: crusted papules on the penile shaft and erythematous scrotum

8.33
Lichen planus: flat-topped papules with white, shiny surface (Wickham's striae) in an annular formation on the proximal edge of the glans and under the prepuce

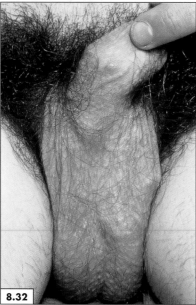

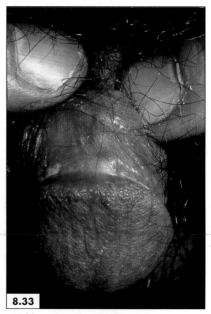

9 THE HANDS

Inspection of the hands is next only to that of the face in yielding a plethora of useful clinical signs. The task of clinically scrutinizing the hands is vast and needs a logical approach. The *visual survey* should address *five* questions.

1. Is there an **arthropathy**? (e.g. rheumatoid, osteoarthrosis, gout, psoriasis, septic);
2. Is there a **skin lesion**? (e.g. dermatoses, systemic disorders);
3. Is there a **neuromuscular disorder**? (e.g. wasting, deformity, fasciculation);
4. Is there a **sign supporting those found elsewhere**? (e.g. ulcers, erythema, cyanosis, pigmentation, acropachy, etc.);
5. Is there a **fundamental sign suggesting a systemic disorder**? (e.g. clubbing, xanthomata, erythema nodosum, etc.).

These questions can be summarized as looking for *swelling, deformity, wasting, skin lesions*, and normal and abnormal movements. A diagnostic hypothesis can be synthesized from any one or a combination of these signs as illustrated in the following five sections.

Arthropathies

The hands should be looked at for any signs of **arthritis** such as swelling, deformity, wasting, subluxation or ankylosis of the joints. **Rheumatoid arthritis** is by far the commonest of the arthritides (1–5%) afecting females at least three times more often than males, and with a peak incidence between the fourth and sixth decade, although it may develop for the first time in patients even in their seventies. *Morning stiffness* is one of the earliest symptoms and *spindle swelling* of the proximal interphalangeal joints, tightening of the skin and a slight flexion deformity (9.1) may be seen in such patients. In many early cases the metacarpophalangeal joints (particularly the second and third) are swollen with a characteristic prominence of the knuckles (9.2), and there may be rheumatoid nodules over

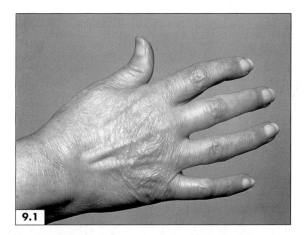

9.1
Rheumatoid arthritis

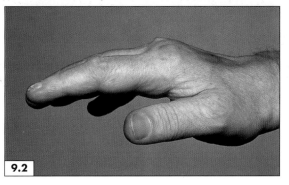

9.2
Rheumatoid arthritis with swelling of the metacarpophalangeal joints

the tendons and wasting of the interossei (9.3), which are suggestive of a severe and progressive disease.

Long-standing disease leads to a variety of deformities caused by wasting of the small muscles, subluxation or ankylosis of the joints. *Ulnar deviation* of the fingers (9.4, 9.5) results from subluxation and dislocation of the metacarpophalangeal joints. *'Swan-neck' deformity* (hyperextension of the proximal interphalangeal joint with fixed flexion of the metacarpophalangeal and terminal interphalangeal joints) (9.6); *Boutonnière deformity* (flexion deformity of the proximal interphalangeal joint with extension contracture of the terminal interphalangeal and metacarpophalangeal joints) (9.7); *flexion contracture* of the fingers (9.8); and *Z-deformity* (flexion deformity of the metacarpophalangeal joint and hyperextension of the proximal interphalangeal joint) of the thumb (9.9) are all well-recognized features of chronic rheumatoid arthritis.

9.3
Rheumatoid arthritis: erythematous nodules and guttering caused by wasting of the interossei

9.4
Swelling of the metacarpophalangeal and proximal interphalangeal joints with ulnar deviation

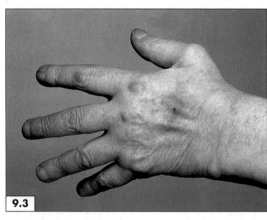

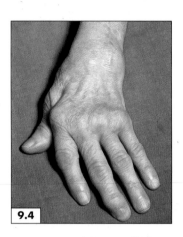

9.5
Marked subluxation of the metacarpophalangeal joints and ulnar deviation

9.6
Rheumatoid nodules, swelling, subluxation and ulnar deviation. Note *'swan-neck' deformity* in the right second and left fifth fingers

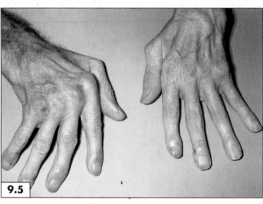

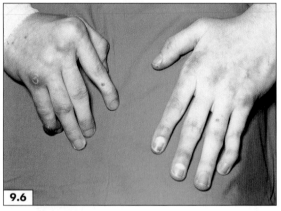

9.7
Boutonnière deformity in the right fourth finger and *swan-neck deformity* in the left fifth finger

9.8
Flexion contracture and *palmar erythema*

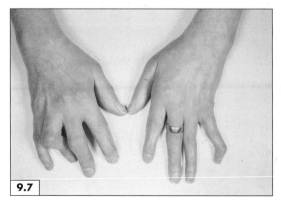

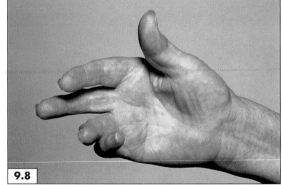

Cutaneous changes in rheumatoid arthritis may be the result of the disease or caused by the treatment. Atrophic, *thin* skin and *purpura* in association with severe arthritis (9.10) often results from corticosteroid treatment. *Skin nodules* (9.11) occur in approximately one-quarter of patients. They are usually associated with severe disease and a high titre of *rheumatoid factor*. *Palmar erythema* may occur with both the mild (9.12) as well as the severe forms of the disease (9.13).

Nailfold infarcts (9.14) are an external expression of digital arteritis, and are the result of inflammation which eventually leads to thrombosis of tiny end-arteries. Extensive digital arteritis may result in a complete loss of perfusion and gangrene of the finger (9.15).

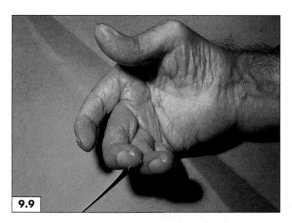

9.9

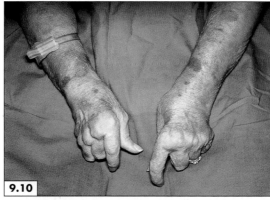

9.10

9.9
Z-deformity of the thumb

9.10
Advanced rheumatoid arthritis: bilateral deforming arthropathy and purpura from corticosteroid therapy

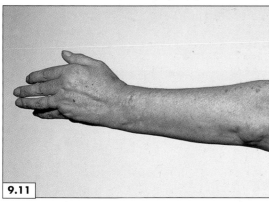

9.11

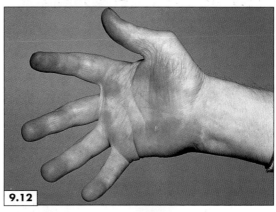

9.12

9.11
Rheumatoid arthritis. Note a nodule with erythematous surface on the elbow

9.12
Palmar erythema

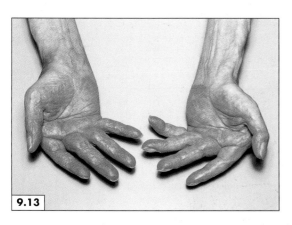

9.13

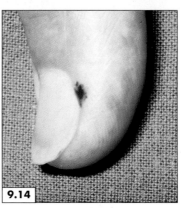

9.14

9.13
Rheumatoid arthritis with marked ulnar deviation and palmar erythema

9.14
Nailfold infarct

9.15
Digital arteritis resulting in a gangrene

9.16
'Burnt-out' rheumatoid arthritis

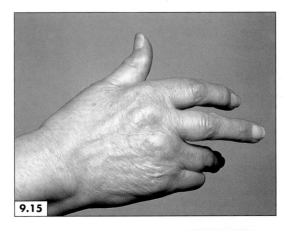

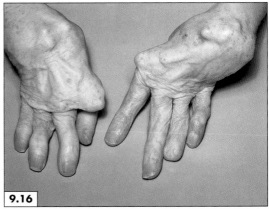

9.17 and 9.18
'Burnt-out' grossly deforming rheumatoid arthritis

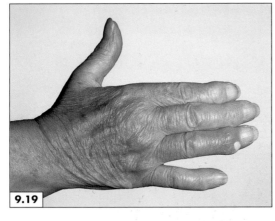

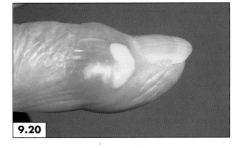

9.19
Chronic gouty arthritis with an ulcerated tophus

9.20
An ulcerated tophus revealing a yellowish-white urate deposit

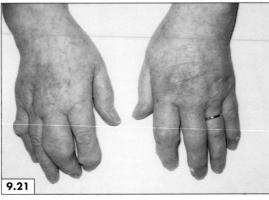

9.21 and 9.22
Chronic gouty arthritis with asymmetrical, nodular swellings

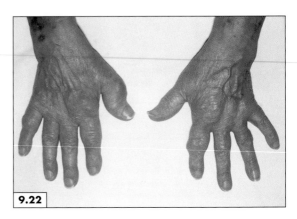

Unlike in a neuromuscular disorder, many patients with rheumatoid arthritis, even with gross muscular wasting, retain a reasonable degree of power and function in the hands. Nevertheless, end-stage or 'burnt-out' arthritis severely distorts the hands (9.16, 9.17), and sometimes only short and disfigured stumps of fingers (9.18) remain, with very little useful function.

Chronic gouty arthritis (9.19) sometimes resembles rheumatoid arthritis at first sight but it may be betrayed by the presence of *tophaceous urate deposits*, which may produce a yellowish-white, hard swelling on one or more of the fingers (9.20). As a result of these tophaceous deposits, the joint deformities in gout, unlike those in rheumatoid arthritis, are neither predictable nor symmetrical (9.21, 9.22). In gout, one joint may be much more swollen with an irregular tumescence compared with its neighbour (9.23, 9.24), and the urate deposits may ulcerate through the stretched shiny skin (9.25). The tophi are usually painless and nontender but their presence causes stiffness, ache and *decreased mobility* of the affected joint.

Subcutaneous deposits of urate on the finger tips can show through the skin as yellowish-white granular swellings (9.26).

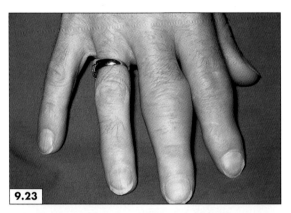

9.23

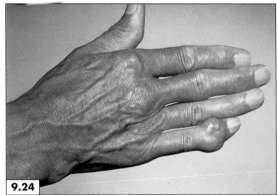

9.24

9.23 and 9.24 Chronic gouty arthritis with tophaceous, nodular swelling of some fingers while sparing the others

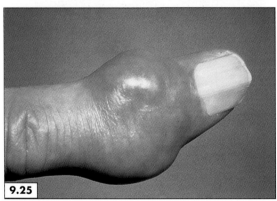

9.25

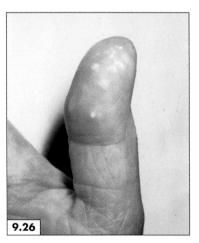

9.26

9.25 A urate tophus ulcerating through the skin

9.26 Yellowish-white granules of urate deposits

Acute gout should always be considered in the differential diagnosis of a sudden monoarthritis (three-quarters of initial attacks affect a single joint). Although over half the attacks affect the lower extremity, a sudden appearance of an inflamed, painful elbow (9.27) should alert the clinician to the possibility of acute gout.

In **osteoarthrosis**, the hands present a characteristic picture of a 'square hand' with adduction of the first metacarpal, bony enlargements, subluxation of the meta-carpophalangeal joints, wasting of the small muscles and deformity of the terminal interphalangeal joints (9.28). Women are more commonly affected than men (in a ratio of 3:2) and are particularly liable to develop the **nodular form of osteoarthrosis** (9.29).

Heberden's nodes (nodular swellings of the terminal inter-phalangeal joints) (9.30), often associated with flexion (9.31) or lateral deformity (9.32) of the terminal phalanges, are the characteristic features of osteoarthrosis of the hands.

9.27
Acute gout of the elbow

9.28
Osteoarthrosis with flexion deformity of the terminal interphalangeal joints

9.29
Nodular osteoarthrosis with a typical 'square hand' deformity

9.30
Heberden's node

9.31
Heberden's nodes on the terminal interphalangeal joints with flexion deformity

9.32
Heberden's nodes with lateral deformity of the terminal phalanges

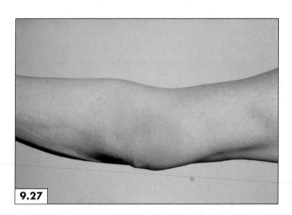
9.27

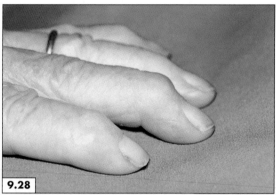
9.28

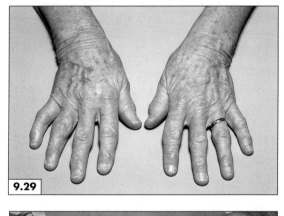
9.29

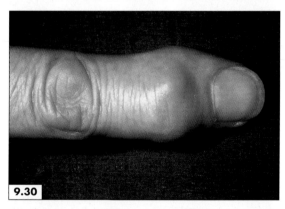
9.30

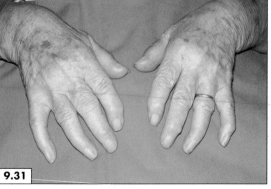
9.31

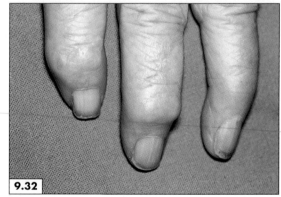
9.32

Bony swellings may also occur at the proximal interphalangeal joints (*Bouchard's nodes*) (9.33). Deformity of the distal interphalangeal joints may also occur in gout (see 9.24) and in psoriasis (9.34); however, neither condition is difficult to distinguish from osteoarthrosis.

The shoulder joint is less likely to be involved in osteoarthrosis than the weightbearing hip and knee joints. However, a rapidly destructive osteoarthrosis with a blood-stained effusion may occur in the shoulder joint (9.35) and in other sites.

Psoriatic arthropathy characteristically affects the distal interphalangeal joints and there may be associated pitting of the nails (9.36). In advanced cases, there may be an extremely destructive arthropathy resulting in absorption of the phalanges, giving rise to telescoping of the fingers and the '*main-en-lorgnette*' phenomenon in which the fingers can be lengthened or shortened by the examiner (9.37, 9.38). Fortunately, most cases of psoriatic arthritis are benign and do not progress to such mutilation (*arthritis mutilans.*)

Septic arthritis usually affects bigger joints in patients who have other evidence of septicaemia. The arthritis may appear in more than one joint as in this patient, who

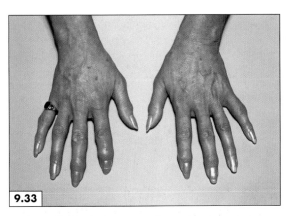

9.33 Bouchard's and Heberden's nodes

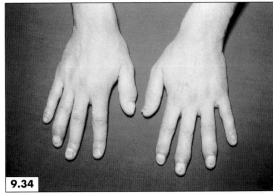

9.34 Psoriatic arthropathy affecting distal interphalangeal joints. Note the associated nail dystrophy

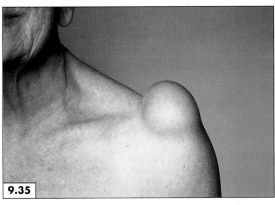

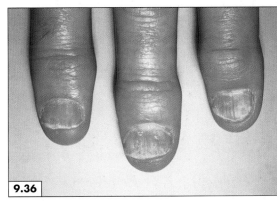

9.35 Osteoarthrosis with effusion of the shoulder joint

9.36 Psoriasis: pitting of the nails

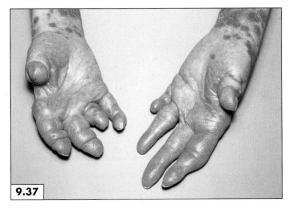

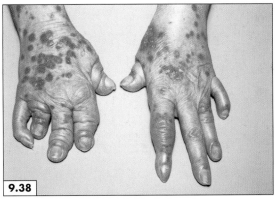

9.37 Arthritis mutilans with telescoping of the right fourth finger

9.38 Arthritis mutilans with telescoping and 'pencil and cup' sign. Note the multiple psoriatic plaques

developed septic arthritis of the left wrist (9.39) 3 days after cellulitis, septicaemia and septic arthritis of the right knee. Nevertheless, this diagnosis should always be considered when there is arthritis of a single joint (9.40), as urgent treatment is mandatory.

Clinical diagnosis

The correct diagnosis depends upon obtaining a good history, having some knowledge of the specific appearances and matching these with the observed findings, and on carrying out several relevant tests. All the arthritides have a typical appearance and the diagnosis is not usually difficult. Some knowledge of what and where to look for obtaining supplementary evidence is necessary for making an accurate diagnosis. For example, rheumatoid *disease* involves almost any part of the body (9.41) and a comprehensive clinical examination will yield some helpful clues to support the impression gained by looking at the hands.

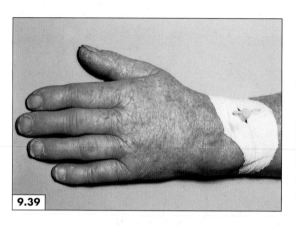

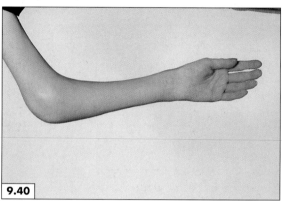

9.39
Septic arthritis of left wrist

9.40
Septic arthritis with swollen, inflamed left elbow joint

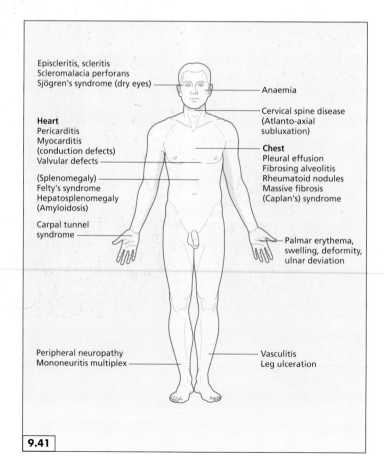

9.41
Clinical features of rheumatoid disease

The elbows and the tendon sheaths along the ulnar border of the forearm must be inspected for the presence of *rheumatoid nodules* (9.42), some of which may bear *vasculitic lesions* (9.43) characteristic of the disease. The fingers and nailfolds should also be examined for the presence of vasculitic lesions (9.44).

The asymmetrical, nodular swellings of tophaceous gout (9.45) are not difficult to recognize and the diagnosis can be reinforced by locating tophi on the fingertips and the ear (9.46).

An **acute monoarthritis** often poses a major diagnostic problem because a delay in providing the appropriate treatment may have consequences not only for the joint but also for the patient, particularly if an acute septic

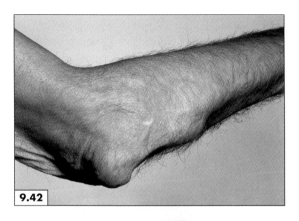

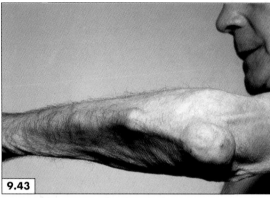

9.42 and 9.43 Rheumatoid nodules. Note the vasculitic lesions on the surface of the nodules

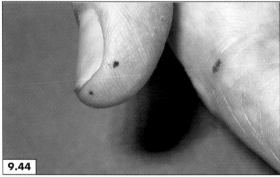

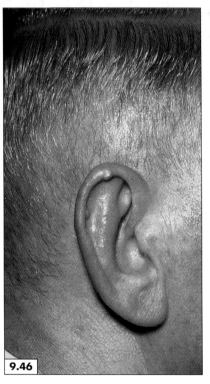

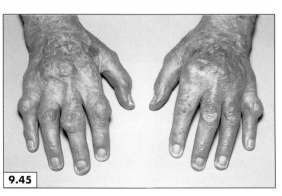

9.44 Rheumatoid arthritis with vasculitic lesions

9.45 Chronic tophaceous gouty arthritis

9.46 A gouty tophus on the helix of the ear

arthritis is missed. Acute gout, pseudogout, haemarthrosis (usually in a haemophiliac patient), osteoarthrosis and septic arthritis must all be considered in the differential diagnosis of acute monoarthritis. The joint is inflamed, swollen, painful and immobile in septic arthritis (9.47) but these characteristics can also apply to the other arthritides mentioned above.

Although certain features including a past history of monoarthritis, the patient's age and gender (gout and haemophilia) and the associated conditions (pseudogout with hyperparathyroidism, haemochromatosis, acromegaly, diabetes mellitus, Wilson's disease, hypothyroidism, etc.) are important pointers, the definitive diagnosis can only be made by microscopic examination and culture of the fluid aspirated from the joint. The immune status of the patient should be investigated; those with **hypogammaglobulinaemia** are prone to developing septic arthritis (9.48), and approximately one-third of the patients with this condition develop a rheumatoid-type arthritis.

Skin lesions

The correct diagnosis of a dermatological condition on the hands requires a two-step approach. First, attention should be concentrated on a single lesion to make a descriptive diagnosis (e.g. macule, papule, nodule, vesicle, plaque, tumour, ulcer, etc.). Second, the rest of the body should be examined for the distribution of the lesions and for the presence of any associated signs. Skin lesions of the hands, like those of the face, can be subdivided broadly into two subgroups: (i) dermatoses; and (ii) lesions related to systemic disorders. The commonly encountered dermatoses are listed in Table 9.1.

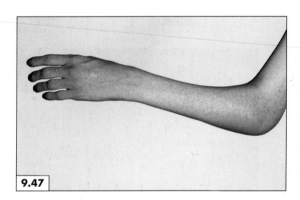

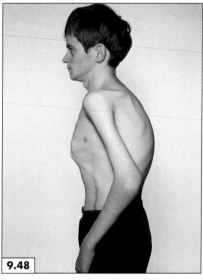

9.47
Septic arthritis with inflamed, swollen and immobile joint

9.48
Septic arthritis and wasting in an immunocompromised patient

Table 9.1 Skin lesions in the hands

Lesions	Dermatoses	Systemic disorders
Macules, papules, plaques	Erythema multiforme, solar keratosis, scabies, psoriasis, lichen planus, erysipeloid	Vitiligo, lupus erythematosus, secondary syphilis, granuloma annulare, mycosis fungoides
Nodules, tumours	Squamous cell carcinoma, melanoma, verruca, pyogenic granuloma	Granuloma annulare
Vesicles, bullae, pustules, ulcers, erosions, scars	Scabies, herpes simplex, erythema multiforme, infections	Porphyria, lupus erythematosus, secondary syphilis

Dermatoses

Common conditions

Scabies is caused by a mite, *Sarcoptes scabiei*. It predominantly affects the hands and the perineum, usually spreads by skin-to-skin contact, and causes generalized and intractable *pruritus*, with frequent secondary bacterial infection. The characteristic lesions are skin-coloured or grey ridges overlying *burrows*. They are approximately 1 cm long, with a vesicle or a papule at the end (9.49, 9.50). More often vesicles, crusted papules, or small urticarial papules occur on the hands (9.51). Even in the absence of burrows, crusted lesions and denuded vesicles on the dorsum and the inner sides of the fingers (9.52) provide a characteristic appearance suggestive of scabies. These lesions are scattered throughout the body (9.53), over the arms (9.54), over and under

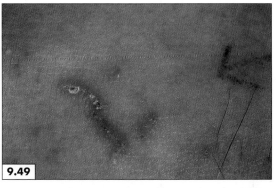

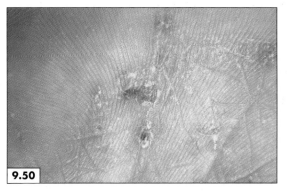

9.49
Scabies: greyish and erythematous linear ridges with ruptured vesicles

9.50
Skin-coloured ridges with ruptured vesicles

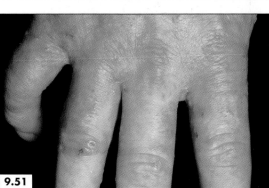

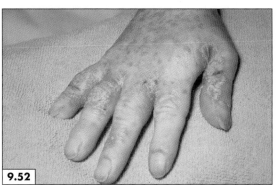

9.51
Scabies: interdigital burrow, papules and vesicles

9.52
Scabies with scratch marks and crusting

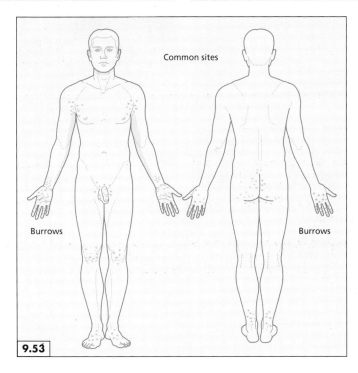

Common sites

Burrows

Burrows

9.53
Distribution of scabies

the breasts (9.55), on the buttocks and in the pubic area (9.56).

Eczematous plaques, indurated nodules, excoriations and crusts of superimposed bacterial infection are seen on the arms (9.57) and hands. The clinical diagnosis is often suspected on circumstantial evidence. Poverty, overcrowding and sexual promiscuity encourage skin-to-skin spread in epidemic proportions. *Intense itching*, particu-

larly at night, is suggestive of the condition. The diagnosis can be confirmed by detecting typical burrows through a magnifying lens and by finding the mite.

Psoriasis may involve the elbows (9.58), hands and nails (9.59) as well as the trunk and the legs which makes the diagnosis easy. However, the palms and soles may be the only areas affected and the diagnostic clues are the sharp demarcation of the lesions and the presence of silvery-

9.54
Scabies: papulovesicular lesions

9.55
Papulovesicular plaques of scabies under the breast

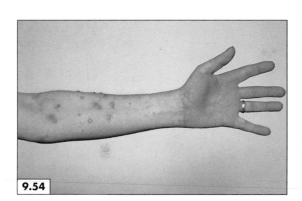

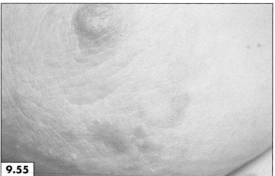

9.56
Scabies: papules on the glans and the penile shaft

9.57
Papulonodular lesions with superimposed infection

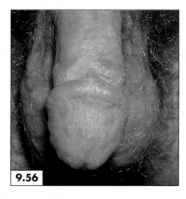

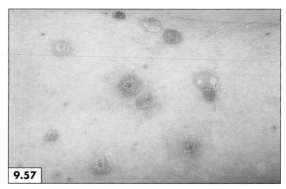

9.58
A psoriatic plaque with silvery scales

9.59
Pitting of the nails and psoriatic plaques on the dorsum of the hand

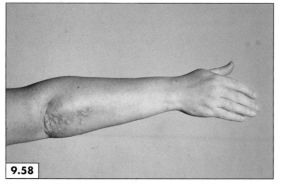

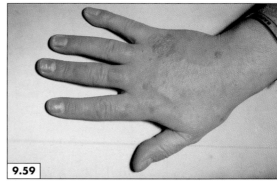

white scales (9.60). This form of the disease is often intractable and may require PUVA photochemotherapy and retinoids. The areas affected by psoriasis are shown in Figure 9.61.

Lichen planus often affects the flexor aspect of the wrists (9.62) with flat-topped, umbilicated and violaceous papules, some of which are discrete and some coalescent. A closer look shows the characteristic central umbilication of the flat, violaceous papules with thin, lacy, white lines known as *Wickham's striae* (9.63, 9.64). These striae are

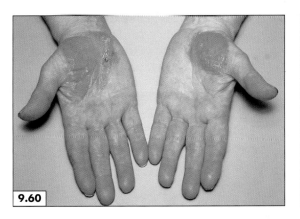

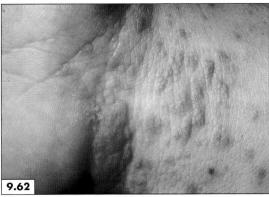

9.60
Sharply demarcated, erythematous plaques with silvery scales

9.62
Lichen planus: flat-topped, oval and polygonal, grouped, violaceous papules

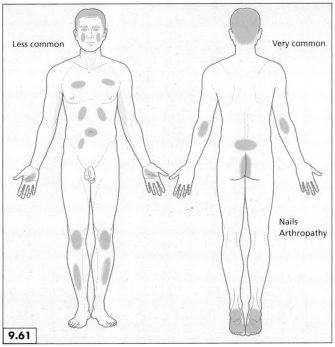

9.61
Areas of the body affected by psoriasis

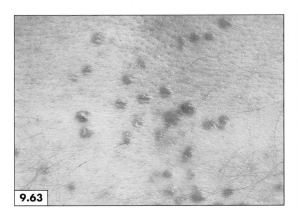

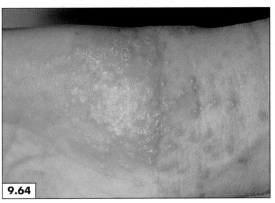

9.63
Flat-topped, violaceous, grouped papules with a shiny surface and lacy pattern (*Wickham's striae*)

9.64
Erythema multiforme: erythematous skin, papules and ruptured vesicles with crusting

better seen with a hand lens. *The papules are shiny and can be shown to reflect light.*

Erythema multiforme is characterized by a symmetrical eruption of erythematous, iris-shaped papules ('*target*' lesions) (9.65), erythematous macules and papules (9.66), and vesicobullous lesions. Although in approximately one-half of the cases there may be no cause, the rash often follows an infection (e.g. herpes simplex, mycoplasma) or the ingestion of a drug (e.g. penicillin, sulphonamides).

Pompholyx (dyshidrotic eczematous dermatitis) is a deep-seated vesicular type of recurrent eczema on the feet and hands. The tapioca-like eruption occurs mostly on the fingers (9.67), palms and soles. The vesicles are deep and pruritic. The cause is unknown although sometimes it may be caused by either a fungal infection, chromium or nickel.

The hands, like other exposed areas (face, ears, neck), have a tendency to develop **solar keratosis**. The lesions are discrete, dry, scaly and adherent multiple or single nodules (9.68). There is excessive folding of the skin in exposed areas. Outdoor workers, such as farmers and sailors, in sunny climates are particularly vulnerable.

9.65
Iris-shaped target lesions with a tendency to bullous formation in the peripheral rim

9.66
Erythema multiforme: a maculopapular eruption

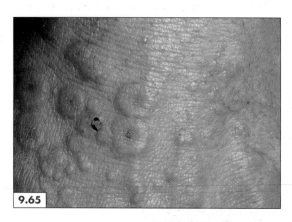

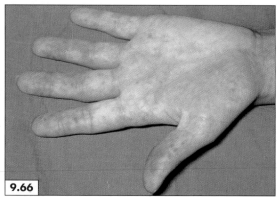

9.67
Pompholyx: sharply demarcated vesicular patches with irregular margins

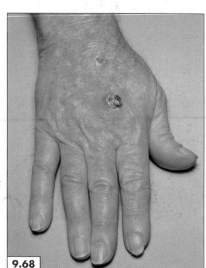

9.68
Solar keratosis: papules with hyperkeratotic crusts and increased folding of the skin

9.69
Pyogenic granuloma

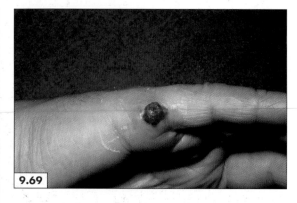

The fingers and face are common sites for **pyogenic granuloma**, which is a rapidly developing, red or brownish-red nodule (9.69). The lesion is benign but may bleed and is sometimes mistaken for a melanoma.

Infections

Erysipeloid is an acute infection of the hands caused by *Erysipelothrix insidiosa*. It is an occupational hazard to fishermen, meat processing workers, poultry workers, poachers, abattoir workers, veterinarians and butchers. The lesions are usually red, sharply defined plaques on the back of the hands and fingers (9.70, 9.71). Like an acute cellulitis, the lesions look red, angry and indurated but, unlike cellulitis, erysipeloid is neither very hot nor very tender. Blood cultures should be performed in every patient as the infection can become disseminated.

Another infection related to fish is a granuloma caused by an **atypical mycobacterium** in those who handle and look after fish in tanks. This so-called **fish-tank granuloma** is a raised, skin-coloured or erythematous plaque on the back of the hands and fingers (9.72, 9.73).

Dermatophyte, or **fungal**, **infections** are caused by fungi that thrive on the nonviable tissues of the skin or hair, and mostly occur in children or young adults, particularly in immunocompromised patients. These are usually superficial infections and may be well-demarcated as in this patient with **tinea** (**ringworm**) infection of the hand (9.74).

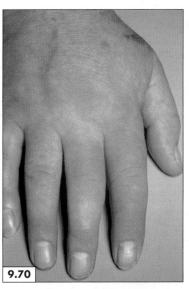

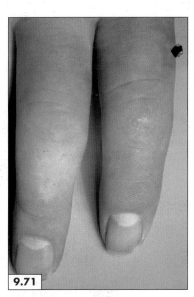

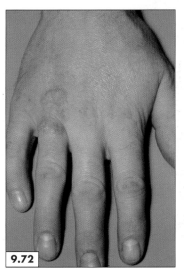

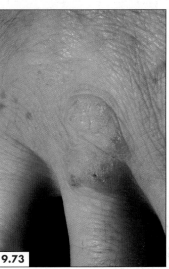

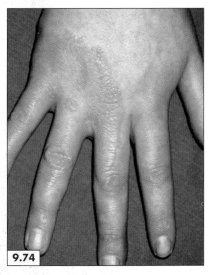

9.70 and 9.71
Erysipeloid: purplish-red, cellulitic plaques

9.72 and 9.73
Fish-tank granuloma: skin-coloured and darkish-red, verrucous plaques

9.74
Tinea: well-demarcated, red, scaling plaque with a raised border and central clearing

The palms become erythematous (9.75) and often show exaggerated creases, fine *scaling* and some degree of *hyperkeratosis* (9.76).

Orf starts as a small, firm papule and then changes into a flat-topped pustular nodule with a violaceous or erythematous periphery (9.77). The original infection is **contagious pustular dermatitis** in lambs, caused by a pox virus, and is transmitted to those handling infected animals. Orf may be complicated by lymphadenitis and erythema multiforme. It clears up spontaneously in about a month.

Cutaneous **anthrax** usually occurs in the upper extremities or on the face and neck, which are likely to be exposed to the contaminated animal product or soil. The initial lesion starts, at the site of an abrasion, as a pruritic papule, which changes into a vesicle and finally ulcerates. The black eschar (9.78) characteristically evolves over several weeks and it gradually separates leaving a scar. The black eschar accounts for the name 'anthrax' (from the Greek word for coal). The lesion may progress with nonpitting, gelatinous oedema with a larger, erythematous, brawny area with the black eschar within (9.79).

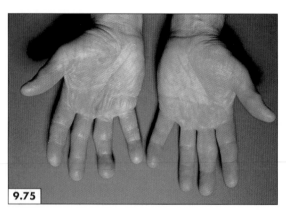

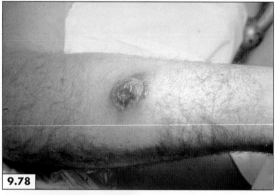

9.75 and 9.76
Tinea manuum: erythema and scaling (best seen in the skin folds) with hyperkeratosis

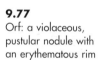

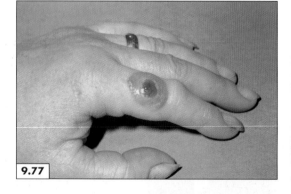

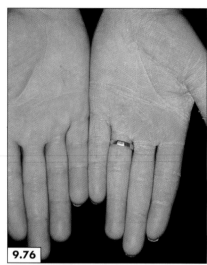

9.77
Orf: a violaceous, pustular nodule with an erythematous rim

9.78
Anthrax: a slowly healing ulcer with an erythematous rim and black eschar

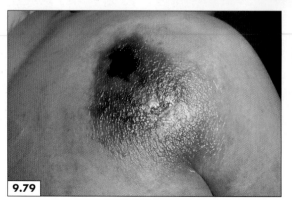

9.79
Anthrax: a large, ill-defined, erythematous, oedematous area. Note the black eschar within the lesion

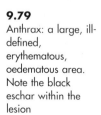

Systemic disorders

Although many skin lesions have some relationship with a systemic disorder, there are some lesions that are either a usual, specific, chief or sole manifestation of a systemic disease; these will be discussed in this section.

Systemic lupus erythematosus (SLE) is suspected by its characteristic 'butterfly' rash (see p. **46**) but the hands also show some helpful clues such as *nailfold infarcts* (9.80) and vasculitic lesions on the tips of the fingers (9.81).

The characteristic changes of the skin on the face and hands are the most distinctive diagnostic features of **systemic sclerosis**; here the skin is smooth, shiny and taut and may be peppered with telangiectases (9.82). The soft tissues atrophy and the overlying skin becomes thin and shiny, particularly over the pulps and the bony prominences of the fingers (9.83, 9.84). These hidebound and tapering fingers (*sclerodactyly*) lose their free mobility at the interphalangeal joints and the fingertips become fixed in flexion (9.85). In a few patients, these changes are associated with typical rheumatoid-like arthritis affecting

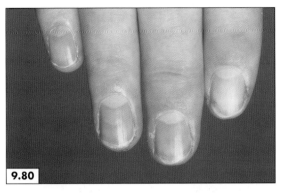

9.80

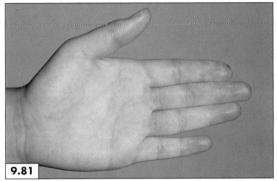

9.81

9.80 and 9.81 Systemic lupus erythematosus: nailfold infarcts and vasculitic lesions on the fingertips. Note the characteristic *striate leuconychia* in the nails of the middle and ring fingers (see also 10.77)

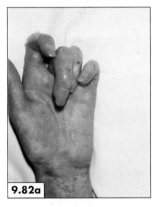

9.82a

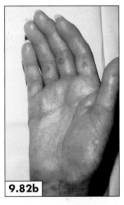

9.82b

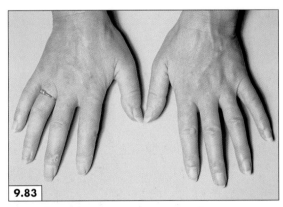

9.83

9.82 and 9.83 Systemic sclerosis: telangiectases and taut skin

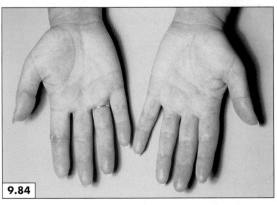

9.84

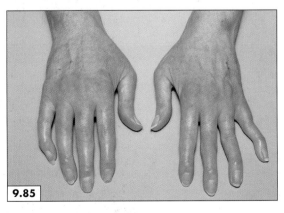

9.85

9.84 and 9.85 Systemic sclerosis: sclerodactyly – tapering, shiny fingers with flexion deformity of distal phalanges

the metacarpophalangeal joints (9.86). Frequent attacks of Raynaud's phenomenon and vasculitis lead to digital ulcerations and fingertip calluses (9.87, 9.88).

Raynaud's phenomenon (spasm of the arteries supplying the fingers and toes, usually provoked by exposure to the cold) occurs without any underlying disorder in approximately 5% of young women (**Raynaud's disease**). An attack can be precipitated by immersing the hand in tepid water. The submerged finger becomes pale and blanched due to vasoconstriction (9.89), followed by cyanosis caused by a sluggish circulation.

Evidence of chronic *Raynaud's phenomenon* (cyanosed, tapering, sometimes gangrenous fingertips, with shiny and flattened pulps) (9.90, 9.91) may be seen as a feature of systemic sclerosis. However, in the absence of any of the other features of this condition, other causes of Raynaud's phenomenon must be considered as follows:

- Idiopathic Raynaud's disease;
- Occupational causes (e.g. vibrating tools, drills, etc.);
- Systemic sclerosis;
- Connective tissue diseases (e.g. SLE, polymyositis, Sjögren's syndrome, rheumatoid arthritis);
- Cervical rib;
- Cryoglobulinaemia;
- Hypothyroidism.

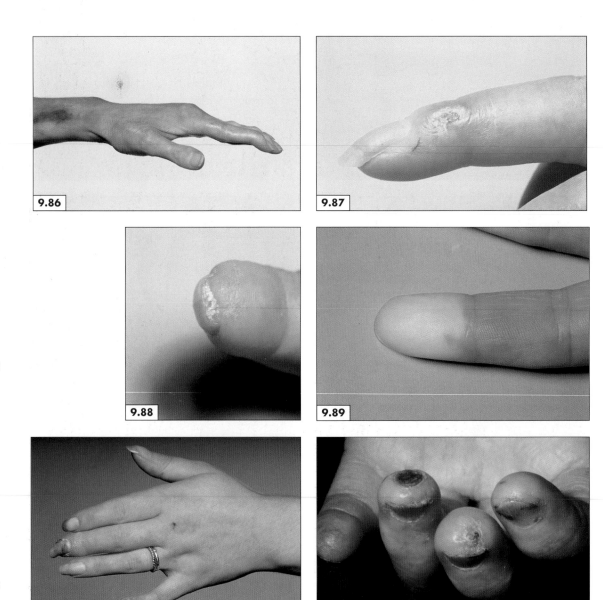

9.86
Sclerodactyly

9.87
Digital ulceration

9.88
Subungual callus

9.89
Raynaud's phenomenon: vasospasm causing pallor of the fingertip after immersion in tepid water

9.90 and 9.91
Raynaud's disease: tapering fingertips with gangrenous areas in the pulps

Mixed connective tissue disease, a variant of systemic sclerosis, may be suspected if there are additional musculoskeletal signs such as a myositis and an inflammatory arthritis. Such patients may complain of morning stiffness, muscle pains, weakness and also of general malaise. In addition to sclerodactyly, nailfold infarcts (9.92) and atrophied, shiny finger pulps (9.93), there may be evidence of synovial thickening and erythema over the knuckles and interphalangeal joints (9.94).

In **dermatomyositis**, the characteristic heliotrope rash seen on the eyelids and face (see 1.246; p. **48**) is often also found on the knuckles and on the back of the interphalangeal joints (9.95).

Vitiligo on the hands is a striking clinical finding (9.96) and occurs in approximately 1% of the population. It causes considerable psychological stress because of its cosmetic effects, particularly in racially pigmented subjects among whom it is commoner than in Caucasian subjects. The lesions start as white macules (9.97), which coalesce into circumscribed, milky-white patches and invade the

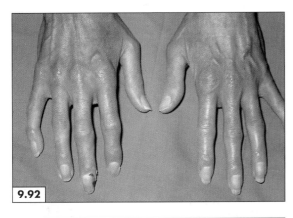

9.92

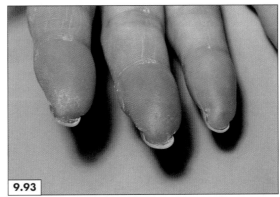

9.93

9.92 and 9.93
Mixed connective tissue disease: sclerodactyly, nailfold infarcts and shiny finger pulps

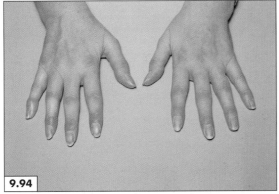

9.94

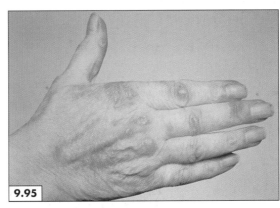

9.95

9.94
Erythema over the finger joints

9.95
Dermatomyositis: lilac, atrophic papules (Gottron's papules) over the knuckles and finger joints

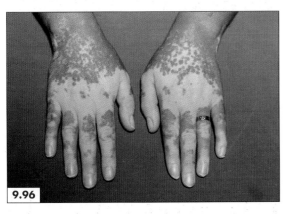

9.96

9.97

9.96
Vitiligo: macular patches of hypomelanosis

9.97
Hypomelanosis macules

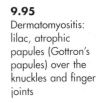

normally pigmented skin (9.98). Sites that are subject to friction and trauma are often affected in a symmetrical distribution (9.99).

The lesions are sometimes difficult to see in an untanned, fair-skinned person (9.100). Exposure to sunshine not only makes them easily recognizable (9.101, 9.102) but also provokes pruritus and may cause sunburn. Vitiligo can be associated with several clinical disorders (Table 9.2), although often it is the only abnormality in an otherwise healthy subject.

In **neurofibromatosis (von Recklinghausen's disease)**, the pedunculated or sessile tumours of varying size may occur on the hands (9.103, 9.104) as elsewhere (see 1.267; p. **52**). It is one of the commonest autosomal dominant conditions. The disorder is associated with neurological tumours (glioma of the optic nerve and chiasm) and various skeletal and endocrine disorders (e.g. kyphoscoliosis, dysplasia of the skull, phaeochromocytoma). Hypertension may result from renal artery dysplasia and female patients commonly develop it during pregnancy.

The hands may show numerous telangiectasia in **Osler–Weber–Rendu syndrome** (9.105, 9.106). This finding is of particular importance when there are no stigmata on the face.

Table 9.2 Conditions associated with vitiligo	
Endocrine disorders	Hyperthyroidism, hypothyroidism, diabetes mellitus, Addison's disease, hypoparathyroidism
Skin diseases	Morphoea, lichen sclerosus, alopecia areata, malignant melanoma
Other conditions	Pernicious anaemia, myasthenia gravis, etc.

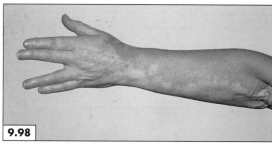

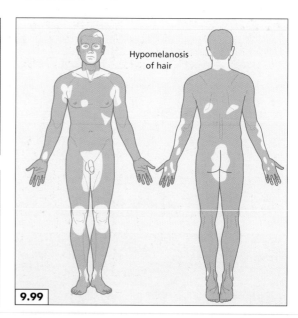

9.98
Hypomelanosis spreading into the normal, pigmented skin

9.99
Vitiligo: sites of predilection

9.100
Vitiligo in a fair-skinned forearm

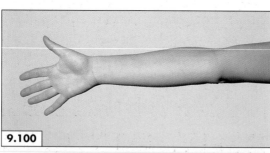

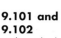

9.101 and 9.102
Vitiligo: the lesions become more obvious in sun-exposed, tanned skin

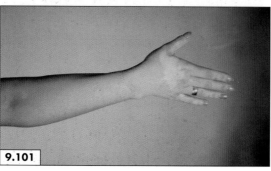

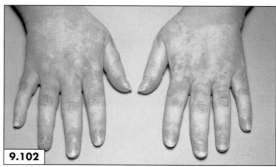

Tylosis, or hyperkeratosis of the palms (9.107) and soles, is a genetic disorder (autosomal dominant trait). The hyperkeratotic change does not cross the wrist line or involve the extensor surface. In some cases it precedes **oesophageal carcinoma** but sporadic cases have been described in which there was no link between tylosis and cancer.

Neuromuscular disorders

Wasting, *deformity* and *fasciculation* are the three markers of neuromuscular involvement of the hands and should be looked for carefully. Wasting of the small muscles of the hand may be caused by a lesion affecting the anterior horn cells at the C8/T1 level (e.g. motor neurone disease, syringomyelia, Charcot–Marie–Tooth disease, cord compression, poliomyelitis), by a lesion affecting the C8/T1 roots (e.g. cervical spondylosis, tumour), by injury to the brachial plexus (e.g. cervical rib, Pancoast's tumour, violent traction of the arm), or by injury to the median and ulnar nerves that supply the muscles of the hand.

In all conditions that involve the ventral horn cells supplying C8/T1 nerve roots, there is *wasting* of the small muscles of the hand with *dorsal guttering*. *Global wasting* only occurs in **muscular dystrophy** and in **motor neurone disease** (9.108). The diagnosis cannot be made by looking at the hands alone either in these two conditions or in

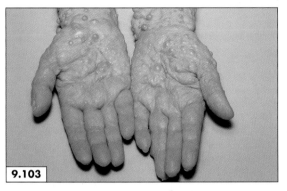

9.103

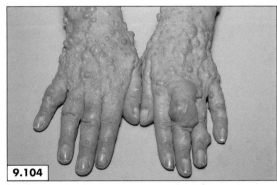

9.104

9.103 and 9.104
Von Recklinghausen's disease (neurofibromatosis I): myriads of skin-coloured and pink-tan, soft papules and nodules

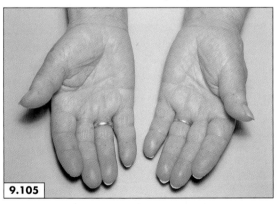

9.105

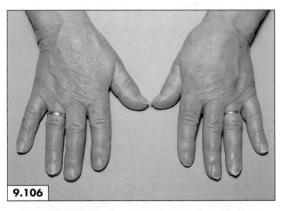

9.106

9.105 and 9.106
Osler–Weber–Rendu syndrome: multiple telangiectasia

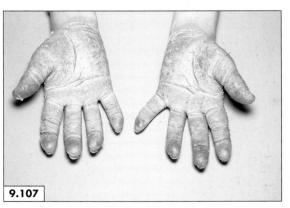

9.107

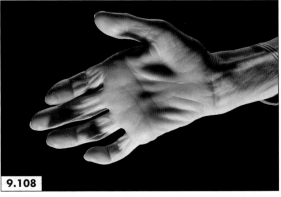

9.108

9.107
Tylosis (keratoderma): thickly keratotic skin with painful fissuring

9.108
Motor neurone disease with global wasting of the muscles of the hand

Charcot–Marie–Tooth disease (9.109), in which there is usually a positive family history (autosomal dominant trait), and a characteristic distal wasting of the arms and legs (*'inverted champagne bottle'*) with pes cavus (see 11.86, 11.87; p. **232**). The muscles do not waste in a global manner (9.110) and the degree of disability is often slight. The condition is now referred to as **hereditary motor and sensory neuropathy**. In some cases the common peroneal and ulnar nerves are palpable. The patients walk with a high-stepping gait because of bilateral foot drop.

Patients with the **cervical rib syndrome** (see also p. **131**) are likely to be young or middle-aged females who complain of pain, weakness and numbness in the hand or forearm (in the area of C8/T1), particularly after using the affected limb. The resulting muscular atrophy is seldom uniformly global; it predominantly involves the radial side of the thenar eminence caused by wasting of the abductor pollicis brevis and the opponens pollicis (9.111). In some cases there is only slight wasting of these muscles, which can best be appreciated by comparing the two hands, as in this patient with a left **cervical rib syndrome** (9.112).

There is no good explanation for the selective sensitivity of these two muscles to the effects of nerve compression at the level of the first rib. There is hyperextension at the metacarpophalangeal joints and flexion at the interphalangeal joints (caused by the action of the long extensors of the fingers unopposed by the lumbricals) producing a claw hand or *main-en-griffe* (9.113, 9.114).

9.109 and 9.110
Charcot–Marie–Tooth disease: wasting affecting principally the lateral aspect

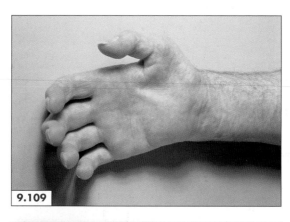
9.109

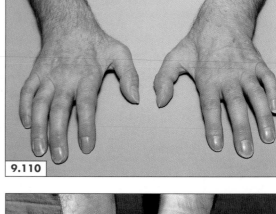
9.110

9.111 and 9.112
Left cervical rib syndrome: wasting of the thenar eminence

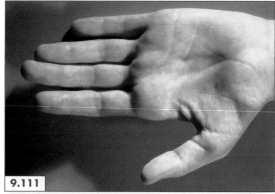
9.111

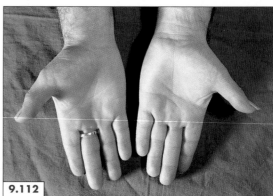
9.112

9.113 and 9.114
Claw hand: unopposed action of the long extensors causing resting hyperextension at the metacarpophalangeal joints

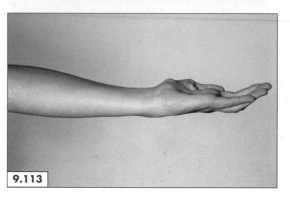
9.113

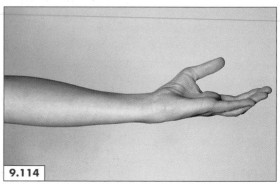
9.114

Cervical myelopathy caused by spondylosis is a capricious condition with a lack of correlation between the range of symptoms (headache, giddiness, drop attacks, numb or 'useless hands', muscle wasting, etc.), their severity, and the radiological severity of the spondylosis. In many patients there are a number of symptoms but few neurological signs. In a few patients, there may be a paraparesis or segmental muscle wasting, as in this patient with spinal subluxation at the level of C6/7 (9.115). Some patients (usually the elderly) with normal power in the hands complain of a loss of feeling, of awkwardness, and of difficulty in performing daily activities, such as dressing, shaving and using toilet paper. Their hands are strong and show no muscle wasting but, when the patient's eyes are closed, the fingers tend to wander ('*pseudoathetosis*' or *sensory wandering*) and the patient is unable to maintain a stationary position of the affected arm (9.116, 9.117). The sensory loss is usually confined to posture and vibration; the objects placed in the patient's hand (with the eyes closed) cannot be identified by touch (*astereognosis*).

The *claw hand* caused by an injury to the ulnar nerve differs from that described already (see 9.113, 9.114) in that the clawing predominantly affects the fourth and fifth fingers of the hand (9.118, 9.119), which also show a slight degree of abduction. This deformity is a result of paralysis

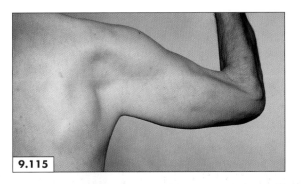

9.115
Wasting of some of the muscles supplied by C6/7 roots

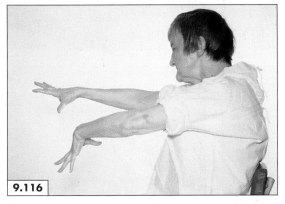
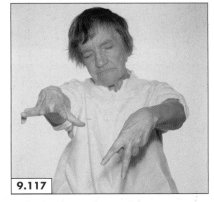

9.116 and 9.117
Pseudoathetosis: the patient is unable to keep the affected hand in the same posture after closing her eyes, when the visual input is lost

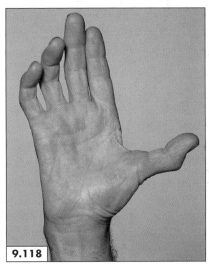
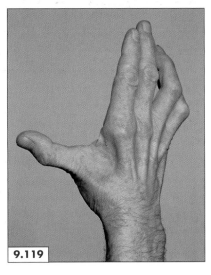

9.118 and 9.119
The ulnar claw hand affecting principally the fourth and fifth fingers. Note wasting of the muscles supplied by the ulnar nerve

9.120
The ulnar claw hand

9.121
Ulnar nerve palsy with flattening of the hypothenar eminence

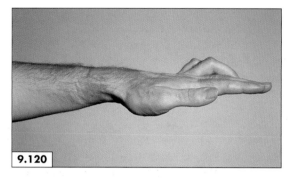
9.120

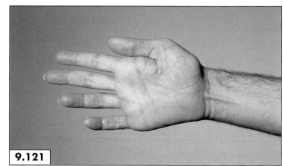
9.121

9.122
Right ulnar nerve injury at the elbow: flattening and hollowing of the right hand

9.123
Dorsal guttering

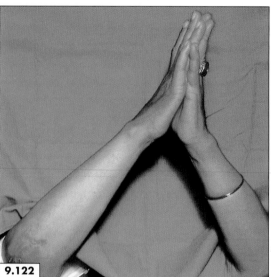
9.122

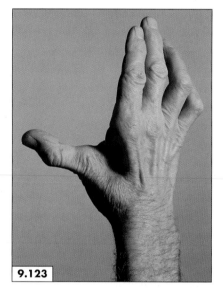
9.123

9.124
Flattening of the right palm

9.125
The journal test of Froment: the patient has to pinch to hold on to the paper

9.126
A long, linear scar of surgery in the elbow joint. Note dorsal guttering and clawing of the hand

9.127
Osteoarthrosis of the elbow: the patient can only touch his head by lifting the arm higher at the shoulder joint. Note the claw hand

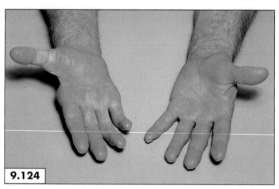
9.124

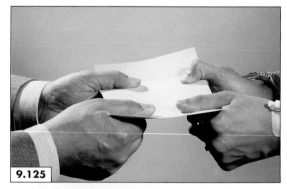
9.125

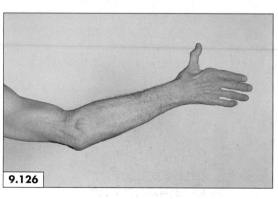
9.126

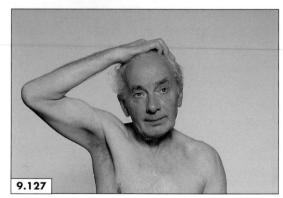
9.127

of the interossei and the medial two lumbricals, which, in combination, flex the fingers at the metacarpophalangeal joints with the distal joints extended. When these muscles are paralysed (caused by an injury to the ulnar nerve) the unopposed action of the long flexors (from the median nerve) and extensors of the fingers (from the radial nerve) produces hyperextension at the metacarpophalangeal joints and flexion of the distal phalangeal joints (9.120). Since the two lateral lumbrical muscles are supplied by the median nerve, the clawing occurs only in the two medial (ulnar lumbricals) fingers.

The hypothenar eminence is flattened (9.121) with loss of the ulnar contour, which can be readily revealed by asking the patient to fold their hands in the manner of the Indian greeting (9.122). Note the evidence of injury at the right elbow showing the cause of the ulnar nerve palsy. There is *guttering* of the spaces between the metacarpals on the dorsum of the hand (9.123) caused by paralysis of the interossei, which are supplied by the ulnar nerve. The palm is hollowed out (9.124) and there is a zone of cutaneous anaesthesia along the ulnar border of the hand, the fifth finger and the inner half of the fourth finger.

The patient with an ulnar nerve palsy is unable to flex the little finger at the interphalangeal joints (using the short flexor), adduct (using the palmar interossei) or abduct (using the dorsal interossei) the fingers in the affected hand. The thumb is also affected because of paralysis of the adductor and short flexor muscles. The weakness of these two muscles can be revealed by the *journal test* of Froment (9.125). The patient and the examiner hold the opposite ends of a piece of paper between the thumb and index finger and, as the examiner pulls gently the patient tries to hold on to the paper by *pinch-flexing the thumb at the interphalangeal joint* ('pinch-grip'), using flexor pollicis longus (the median nerve, C8J.

The corresponding elbow must be examined in every patient with an ulnar nerve palsy for any evidence of injury, fracture, dislocation, scar (9.122, 9.126) or arthritis. A patient with **osteoarthrosis** of the elbow joint will be unable to touch his head with the hand, while keeping his arm straight at the shoulder joint (9.127). The ulnar nerve may be involved in **Hansen's disease** (**leprosy**) producing a typical claw hand (9.128). In this condition the thickened ulnar nerve may be palpable in the ulnar groove at the elbow joint. The nerve may also be injured by penetrating wounds, and as a late sequel to callus or scar formation at any point along its course. Certain occupations such as roofing, carpentry and bricklaying are associated with osteoarthrosis of the elbow and injuries to the nerve in its shallow olecranon groove (9.127).

The **carpal tunnel syndrome** is the commonest cause of a median nerve palsy and is caused by compression of the nerve, as it traverses the tunnel under the thick and inelastic transverse carpal ligament. *Flattening of the thenar eminence* (9.129) is the hallmark of a median nerve palsy. Scalding of the index and middle fingers (9.130) resulting from loss of sensory perception is seen rarely today. The diagnosis is made early on the strength of a good history (pain and numbness over the median nerve distribution, which is worse at night, often relieved by rubbing and hanging the arm out of bed) and by functional evaluation of the thumb and the outer two fingers (weak abductor pollicis and opponens pollicis). This condition is usually seen in middle-aged, obese females. It may be associated with pregnancy, myxoedema, acromegaly, rheumatoid arthritis, tophaceous gout and primary amyloidosis.

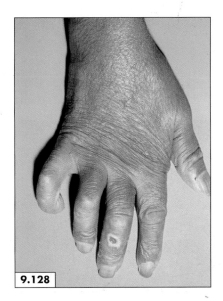

9.128

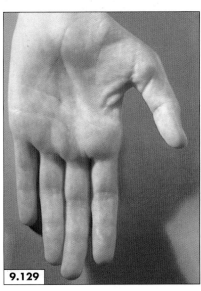

9.129

9.128
Hansen's disease: ulnar nerve damage resulting in a claw hand

9.129
The carpal tunnel syndrome: atrophy of the thenar eminence

The extended thumb and index finger, hollowing of the thenar eminence with the thumb on a level with the fingers, and the flat, even appearance of the palm, produce the *monkey* (or *simian*) *hand* (9.131).

In complete palsy of the median nerve in the forearm, the appearance of the hand and the forearm is characteristically flat on the flexor aspect, with slight ulnar deviation and loss of pulp in the affected fingers. The patient can bend the middle finger but not the terminal phalanx of the thumb and index finger (9.132), which requires the use of flexor digitorum profundus and flexor pollicis longus. Abduction of the thumb is weak and can be easily overcome (9.133) from paralysis of the abductor pollicis brevis.

Inability to make a complete fist by flexing the terminal phalanges of the thumb and index finger (9.134) is caused by an injury to the **anterior interosseous nerve**, which arises from the median nerve in the forearm. This nerve supplies the radial half of the flexor digitorum profundus and flexor pollicis longus.

A lesion of the **posterior interosseous nerve** (a major motor branch of the radial nerve), which supplies the supinator and the long extensors of the wrist and fingers, will result in a wrist drop predominantly affecting the fingers and the thumb, which remain flexed and partially curled. When the forearm is supported in the supine position on a table, the patient will be unable to extend the thumb and fingers at the carpometacarpal and metacarpophalangeal joints (9.135). There is no sensory loss if the wrist drop is

9.130
The carpal tunnel syndrome: scalding of the anaesthetic fingers. Note the flattening of the thenar eminence

9.131
Bilateral carpal tunnel syndrome: the simian hand with atrophic thenar eminence and extended thumb and index finger

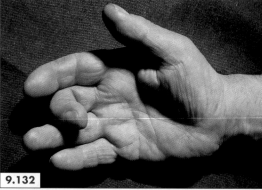

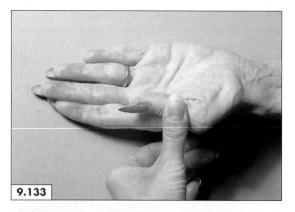

9.132
Median nerve injury in the forearm: can only bend the middle finger when asked to bend the first three fingers

9.133
Median nerve palsy: unable to abduct the thumb against resistance. Note flattening of the thenar eminence

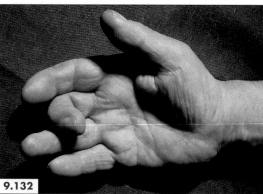

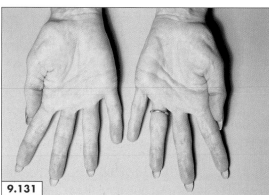

9.134
Anterior interosseous nerve palsy: loss of flexion at the terminal interphalangeal joints

9.135
Right posterior interosseous nerve palsy: unable to extend the thumb and fingers

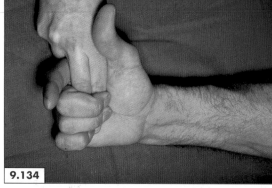

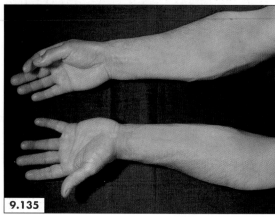

caused by a lesion (injury, compression) of the posterior interosseous nerve. Both the interossei nerves are liable to entrapment and trauma at the elbow and upper forearm.

Wrist drop (9.136), or a complete inability to extend the hand and fingers, is a cardinal feature of **paralysis of the radial nerve**. Even when the wrist is passively held straight, the fingers remain flexed at the metacarpophalangeal joints owing to paralysis of the long extensors (9.137). The patient is, however, able to straighten the interphalangeal joints (9.138) since these movements are affected by the lumbricals and interossei (the ulnar nerve). The grip is weak (9.139) because of the loss of synergistic extension of the wrist; however, it improves if the hand is passively dorsiflexed. Despite extensive cutaneous distribution of the radial nerve over the dorsum of the hand, the sensory loss resulting from the lesion of this nerve may be limited to the space between the first two metacarpals. This is due to the overlapping supply from the adjacent median and ulnar nerves.

Additional signs of systemic disorders

In some systemic diseases, helpful signs are found in the hands, which confirm the diagnostic significance of other features present elsewhere on the body. For example, in **hepatic failure**, there can be palmar erythema (9.140), periungual erythema (9.141) and clubbing (9.142), which add

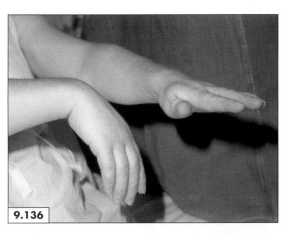

9.136
Radial nerve palsy: wrist drop; unable to extend the wrist or the fingers

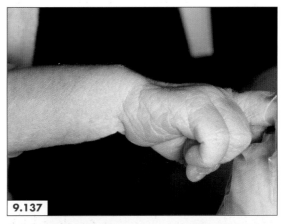

9.137
Radial nerve palsy: unable to extend the fingers

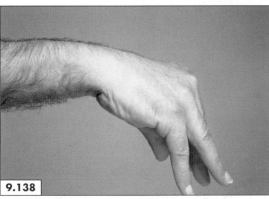

9.138
Radial nerve palsy: the patient can straighten the fingers (ulnar nerve) but not extend at the metacarpophalangeal joints

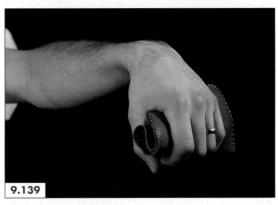

9.139
Radial nerve palsy: unable to extend the wrist to grip tightly

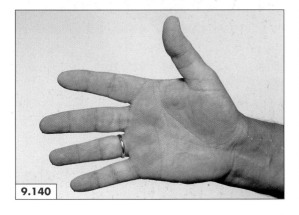

9.140
Hepatic failure: palmar erythema

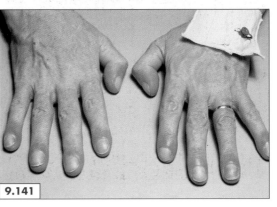

9.141
Periungual erythema

to the diagnostic weight of the jaundice and spider naevi already seen on the face. In such cases, the hands are examined with a predetermined objective and care should be taken in *scrutinizing* the expected signs. Sometimes it is easy to believe that a sign, which is needed to support a suspected diagnosis, is present. In cases of doubt and, wherever possible, the abnormal part should be compared with the normal to look for any difference, as in this example of periungual erythema (9.143).

When the diagnosis of **Turner's syndrome** is made in a short-statured female with a *short, webbed neck*, the hands should be examined looking for hypoplastic nails and short fourth and fifth metacarpals. In normal subjects the fourth finger is almost always either equal to or longer than the index finger. In this patient with Turner's syndrome (9.144), the right fourth finger is shorter than the index finger because of the shorter metacarpal in the former, and the proximal phalanx can be seen to arise at a lower level than the other corresponding phalanges.

The syndrome of **pseudohypoparathyroidism** (tissue unresponsiveness to parathyroid hormone) may be suspected from the facial features (e.g. mental retardation, short stature, short neck, round face and abnormal teeth) but the hands can offer reassuring clues (9.145). The third, fourth and fifth metacarpals, or any one or two of them, are short, which can be readily demonstrated by comparing the abnormal hands with the (left) hand of a normal subject placed on the right in Figure 9.146. The shortness

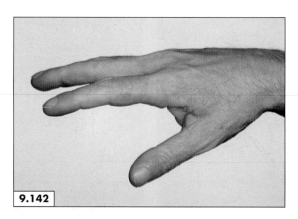

9.142
Hepatic failure: clubbing of the fingers

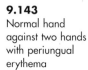

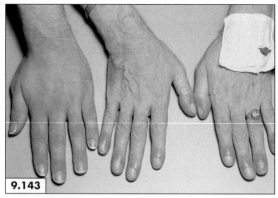

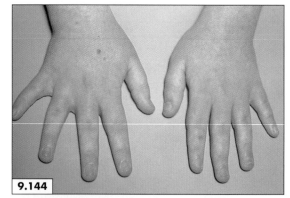

9.143
Normal hand against two hands with periungual erythema

9.144
Turner's syndrome: a shorter right fourth finger

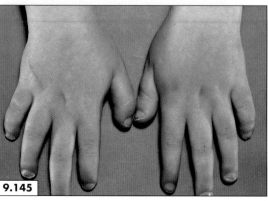

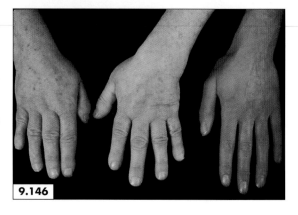

9.145 and 9.146
Pseudohypoparathyroidism: shorter fourth and fifth fingers compared with the normal hand on the extreme right

of the metacarpal can be revealed by asking the patient to make a fist (9.147).

In the **Lawrence–Moon–Biedl syndrome**, the presence of *polydactyly* (9.148) is associated with obesity, mental retardation and hypogonadism. It is important to look for these additional features because polydactyly can be present in a normal subject as an incidental finding (9.149).

Patients with **Marfan's syndrome** may be recognized by their tall stature, *dislocated lenses* and a high-arched palate; nevertheless, hands with *arachnodactyly* (long

webbed fingers) (9.150) provide convincing supportive evidence.

The dominant biochemical feature of **hypoparathyroidism** is *hypocalcaemia*, which is responsible for its symptoms of neuromuscular hyperactivity and, in the long term, for many of its clinical features (9.151).

Hypocalcaemia causes a decreased threshold of excitation in nervous tissues (latent tetany), which can be detected by several simple procedures. *Chvostek's sign* is elicited by *percussing* the facial nerve just anterior to the ear lobe, or just below the zygomatic arch, where it

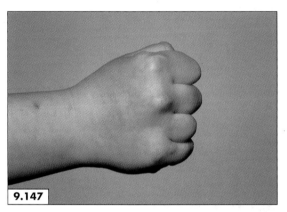

9.147

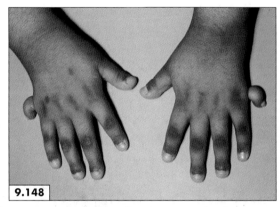

9.148

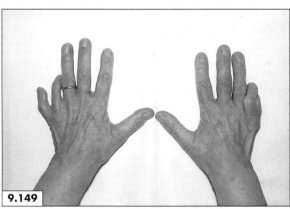

9.149

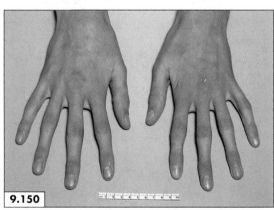

9.150

9.147
The dimple caused by the shorter fourth metacarpal bone

9.148
Lawrence–Moon–Biedl syndrome: polydactyly

9.149
Polydactyly in a normal subject

9.150
Arachnodactyly

emerges from the parotid gland. This may result in twitching at the corner of the mouth (which sometimes occurs in normal subjects), or in a more extensive contraction of the facial muscles.

Trousseau's sign is elicited with a sphygmomanometer cuff inflated around the arm to just above the systolic blood pressure for approximately 5 min (9.152). A typical carpal spasm (painful flexion of the metacarpal joints and adduction of the thumb across the palm) (9.153), which relaxes approximately 5 s after the cuff is deflated (and not instantly), constitutes a positive response.

The clinical features found in the hands of patients with endocrine disorders have been referred to earlier (**Chapter 1**). When an endocrine disease is suspected, the entire

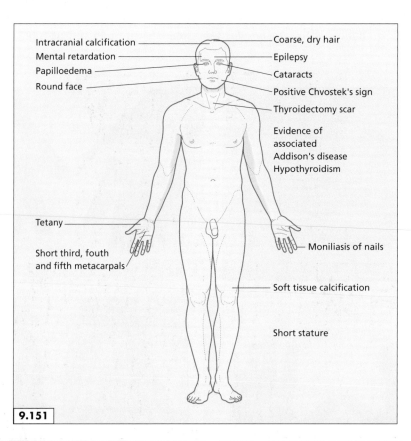

9.151
Clinical features of hypoparathyroidism

9.152 and 9.153
Tetany in hypoparathyroidism: eliciting Trousseau's sign

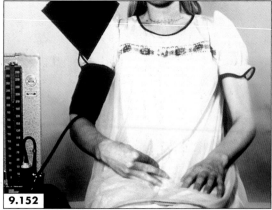

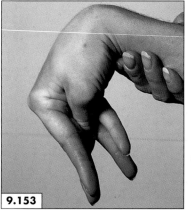

upper limbs should be inspected for helpful clues. For example, areas of friction and scars (9.154) should be examined for the presence of pigmentation in **Addison's disease**.

Thyroid acropachy (9.155) may resemble clubbing of the fingers but there is no thickening and swelling of the nail bed.

Purpura seen on the thin and transparent skin of the dorsum of the hands (9.156) is an important feature of **Cushing's syndrome**. The diagnosis of **acromegaly** is

strengthened by the demonstration of the thickened skin on the dorsum of the large and square, spade-like podgy hands (9.157).

Diabetic patients can develop specific skin lesions as discussed in Chapter 11 (see p. **217**). While *necrobiosis lipoidica diabeticorum* occurs chiefly on the legs, *granuloma annulare*, which is not specific to diabetes mellitus, occurs both on the upper (9.158) and lower extremities. A generalized form of granuloma annulare has been associated with diabetes mellitus, and the cutaneous lesions

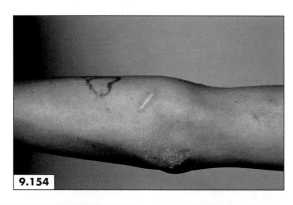

9.154
Addison's disease: pigmentation around an old scar

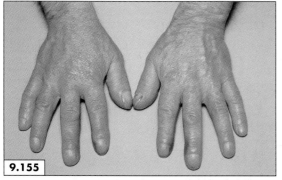

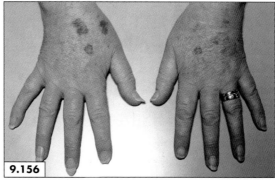

9.155
Thyroid acropachy with periungual tufting

9.156
Cushing's syndrome: purpura and thin, transparent skin

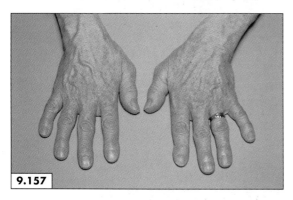

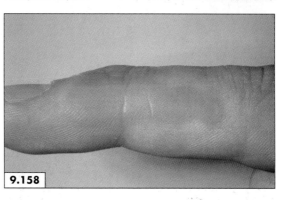

9.157
Acromegaly: large, square, spade-like hands

9.158
Granuloma annulare: a well-defined darkish-red dermal plaque

(9.159) may precede the diagnosis of the disease. *Diabetic dermopathy* (maculopapular lesions) may occur anywhere on the body (see 11.20; p. **219**) but these spots often remain undiagnosed in busy diabetic clinics. Rarely, diabetic patients can develop blisters on exposed areas (*epidermolysis bullosa*), and these may be confused with porphyria. For this reason, it is sometimes referred to as **pseudoporphyria** (9.160). The blister is usually preceded by erythema, leaks serous fluid and collapses leaving a parched, whitish membrane covering the denuded area (9.161, 9.162).

Raynaud's disease has been referred to earlier in this section. Raynaud's phenomenon must be distinguished from **acrocyanosis** in which sustained cyanosis of the whole hand, rather than pallor or cyanosis of the digits, is a characteristic feature (9.163). Acrocyanosis is a rare primary disorder of unknown aetiology, characterized by persistent cyanosis of the hands (less frequently of the feet) with reduced temperature. The cyanosis is intensified with exposure to the cold. Trophic changes and ulcerations are uncommon but may occur (9.163, 9.164).

9.159
Generalized granuloma annulare: multiple, annular, arciform or single reddish papules

9.160
Pseudoporphyria: erythema and a blister containing serous fluid

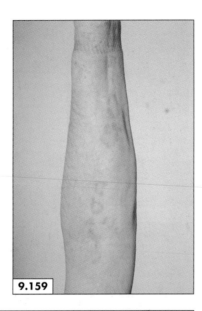

9.159

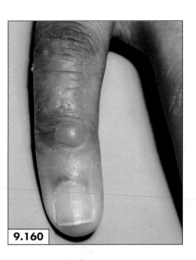

9.160

9.161 and 9.162
Pseudoporphyria in diabetes mellitus: erythematous skin and ruptured blisters

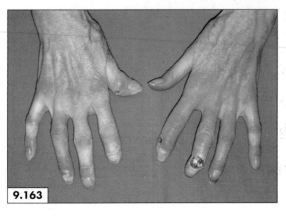

9.161

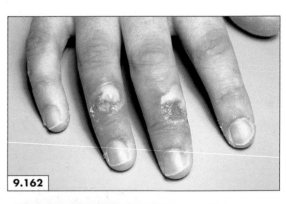

9.162

9.163 and 9.164
Acrocyanosis: dusky skin with ulceration in terminal digits

9.163

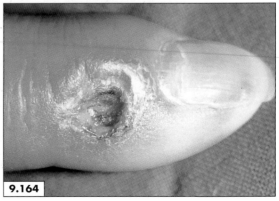

9.164

The presence of unequivocal *clubbing of the fingers* can be used as strong support for diagnosing an associated condition; however, care must be taken not to accept the diagnosis with insufficient evidence. The primary condition should be diagnosed on sound clinical grounds, and the presence of clubbing should be taken as an additional feature, as in this case of cystic fibrosis (9.165).

Miliary sarcoidosis consists of groups of dusky red papules, 1–5 mm in diameter, on the face and arms (9.166) and is usually associated with pulmonary involvement.

Dupuytren's contracture, particularly in association with palmar erythema (9.167), is usually linked with alcoholic cirrhosis but can also occur in diabetes mellitus, gout and epilepsy. It is usually bilateral, favours Caucasian males, and occurs more frequently in some occupations such as gardening and shoemaking.

A dusky-red colour of the skin may be particularly noticeable on the face (see 1.293; p. **58**) and the hands (9.168), due to high haematocrit in cutaneous circulation in **polycythaemia rubra vera**. Patients with the **Ehlers–Danlos syndrome**, because of their excessive joint laxity, can perform circus tricks with their hands (9.169).

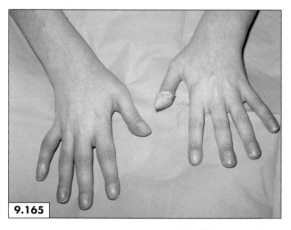

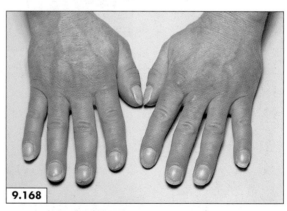

9.165
Cystic fibrosis with clubbing of the fingers

9.166
Miliary sarcoidosis: multiple, brownish-red papules

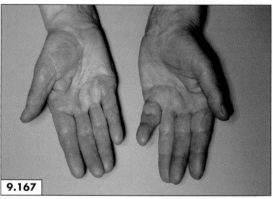

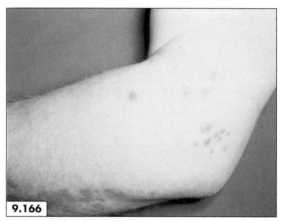

9.167
Dupuytren's contracture with palmar erythema

9.168
Polycythaemia rubra vera: diffuse, dusky-red skin

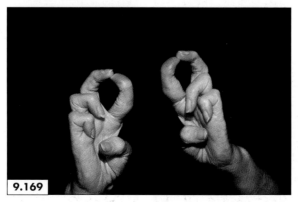

9.169
Ehlers–Danlos syndrome: demonstration of joint laxity

Fundamental signs

Fundamental signs are those clinical features that are invariably associated with one or more diseases; for example central cyanosis *suggests* a cardiopulmonary disorder or an arteriovenous fistula, an extensor plantar *suggests* an upper motor neurone lesion, and pale conjunctiva *suggests* anaemia or a low cardiac output state. This section discusses those critical signs in the hands that point to abnormalities present elsewhere in the body. Such signs should be accepted only after applying very stringent criteria: self-criticism and not self-congratulation should be the guiding principle in the critical evaluation of a fundamental sign. Equivocal and doubtful findings should not be regarded as a basis for a diagnosis, nor should a fundamental sign be assumed to be present just because a related primary disorder has been diagnosed by other means.

Clubbing of the fingers is one of the many fundamental signs found in the hands and the one most abused by 'expert' clinicians. One constantly hears of 'early', 'slight' and 'mild' clubbing but never that 'early' has become 'late' clubbing, or that the slight beaking of the nails noted initially has become drumstick clubbing. The hands should be viewed from the front (9.170) as well as from the side (9.171), and clubbing should never be accepted unless there is a definite swelling of the nail bed (9.172). It is the thickening and oedema of the nail bed that lifts the nail, thereby obliterating the angle between the proximal nailfold and the nail (9.173) over which *fluctuation* can be elicited.

Clubbing of the fingers can become a stronger suggestive sign, for example, in **fibrosing alveolitis**, when it is asso-

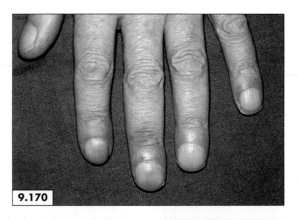

9.170
Clubbing. Note the raised nail plates at proximal nailfolds

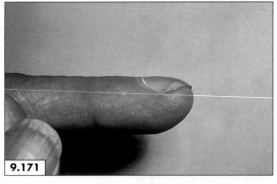

9.171
Clubbing: thickened nail bed raising the root of the nail which is in a straight line with the finger

9.172
Clubbing: thickened nail bed giving the thumb a bulbous appearance

9.173
Clubbing: curved nails obtusely set at the proximal nailfold. Note the rounded appearance of the thumb caused by a thickened nail bed

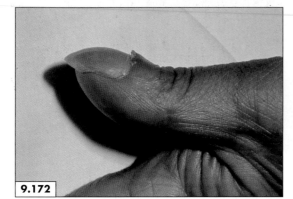

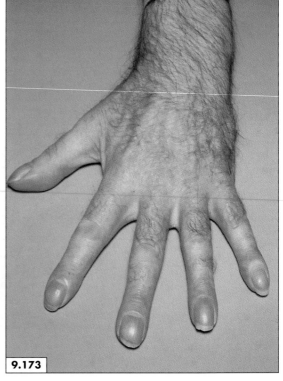

ciated with cyanosis of *warm* fingers (9.174, 9.175). The presence of cyanosis can be confirmed by looking at the tongue and by comparing it with a normal tongue (see 2.72, 2.73; p. **81**). Similarly, *nicotine staining* of the fingers in association with clubbing (9.176) may be a strong pointer when a diagnosis of a **bronchogenic carcinoma** is being considered.

Tuberous xanthomata over the tendons of the knuckles (9.177, 9.178) suggest that the patient has **familial hyper-**cholesterolaemia. Further search over the extensor tendons may prove rewarding and similar swellings may be found over the elbows (9.179). A positive family history of hypercholesterolaemia and/or of coronary heart disease in a first-degree relative before the age of 50 years is usually found.

A change in the normal pink colour of the palmar creases in a Caucasian subject is significant. Pallor of the creases, demonstrable by blanching, suggests anaemia, and

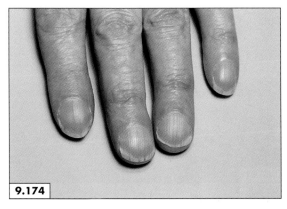

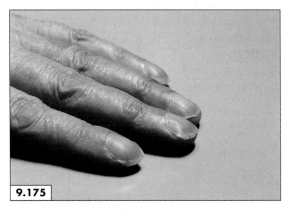

9.174 and 9.175
Fibrosing alveolitis: clubbing of the cyanosed fingers

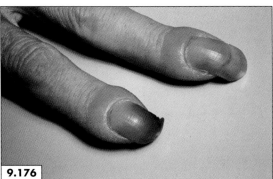

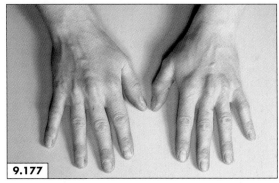

9.176
Nicotine-stained fingers and clubbing

9.177
Familial hypercholesterolaemia: tuberous xanthomata

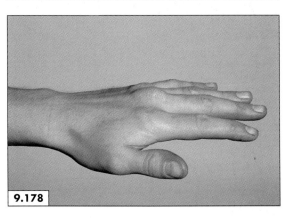

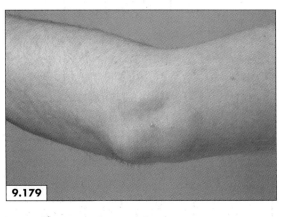

9.178 and 9.179
Tuberous xanthomata: reddish-yellow, subcutaneous nodules attached to the tendons

the discovery of pigmentation (9.180, 9.181) may suggest **Addison's disease**. Some Caucasian patients with this disease or Nelson's syndrome (an adrenocorticotrophic hormone (ACTH)-producing pituitary tumour that develops after bilateral adrenalectomy for Cushing's syndrome) develop a brownish discolouration of the nails.

If the creases show a yellowish hue (9.182), they should be inspected more closely for the presence of planar xan-

thomas (9.183, 9.184), which are a valuable sign of **type III hyperlipidaemia**, and also sometimes of **chronic obstructive liver disease**. In the former condition there is a defective conversion from very low-density lipoprotein (VLDL) remnants to low-density lipoproteins (LDL), where both cholesterol and triglycerides accumulate in the blood. In the absence of planar xanthomata, a yellowish tinge of the palms may be caused by **carotenaemia** (9.185). This is

9.180 and 9.181
Addison's disease with pigmentation of the fingers and palmar creases

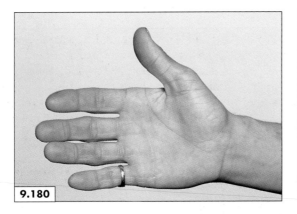

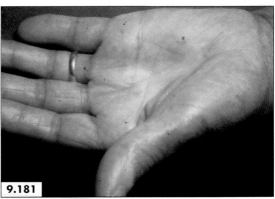

9.182
Palmar creases with faint, yellowish tint

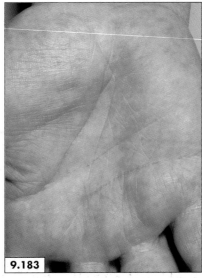

9.183 and 9.184
Type III hyperlipidaemia: planar xanthomatosis

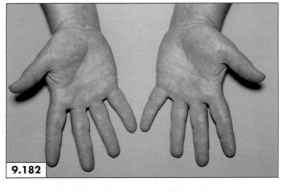

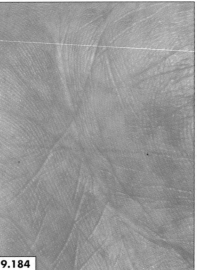

caused by the presence of carotene in the circulating blood from excessive carrot consumption. Unlike in jaundice, this yellow discolouration does not affect the sclerae.

Erythema nodosum (9.186) and **nodular panniculitis (Weber–Christian disease)** (9.187) are both *fundamental signs* since they have associations with systemic disorders. They are difficult to distinguish from each other since they both arise in deep subcutaneous fat as tender red nodules; usually both occur on the legs, although erythema nodosum has a predilection for the pretibial areas. Erythema nodosum is discussed further in Chapter 11 (see 11.120–11.124; pp. **239–41**).

Weber–Christian disease affects subcutaneous and visceral fat in the lungs, kidneys, liver, intestines, bone marrow and adrenal glands. Patients may present with arthralgia, malaise, fatigue, cutaneous nodules and abdominal pain. Anaemia, leucopenia, hepatomegaly, steatorrhoea and intestinal perforation have all been reported. The mouth should always be examined as there may be ulcerated nodules on the tongue (9.188).

The hands and arms should be carefully viewed for the well-known cutaneous stigmata of various systemic disorders (e.g. infective endocarditis, vasculitis, coeliac disease, porphyria, mycosis fungoides, syphilis, etc.) in which the skin lesions may be the only manifestation or may precede the systemic disease. The signs that follow are included in this section because of their relative specificity for the diseases with which they are associated.

Osler's nodes are red, *tender*, cutaneous nodules that occur on the pads of the fingers (9.189, 9.190) and toes, palms (9.191) and soles (see 11.129, 11.130) in **bacterial endocarditis**. Although first described in association with infective endocarditis, and always looked for in this disease, Osler's nodes are not pathognomonic of this condition since they also occur in typhoid fever, gonococcal infection and systemic lupus erythematosus.

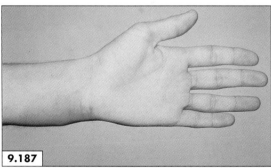
9.185

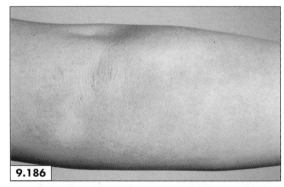
9.186

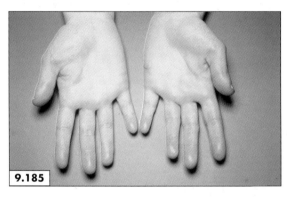
9.187

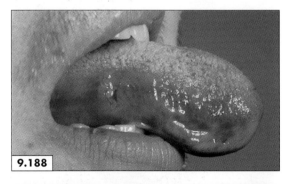
9.188

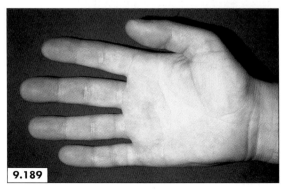
9.189

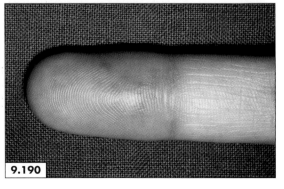
9.190

9.185
Carotenaemia: global yellowish tint

9.186
Erythema nodosum: subcutaneous nodules with ill-defined erythema of the overlying skin

9.187 and 9.188
Weber–Christian disease: subcutaneous nodules with erythema of the overlying skin and lingual ulers

9.189
Infective endocarditis: reddish nodules on the finger pulps

9.190
A collection of small cutaneous nodules representing microemboli

Vasculitic lesions (9.192) occur in a variety of **vasculitides** (see p. **56**). Macules, papules, purpura and even urticarial lesions are seen in association with these disorders. Small, nodular lesions may be seen on the pads of the fingers in a patient with **systemic lupus erythematosus** (9.193).

Erythematous lesions, blisters, scabs over collapsed vesicles (9.194) and a history of itching that precedes the appearance of the eruption are all strongly suggestive of **dermatitis herpetiformis**. In approximately two-thirds of cases a duodenal biopsy may show the mucosal changes resembling gluten enteropathy. Although the **malabsorption syndrome** with all its manifestations develops in only a few patients, a low body weight, low serum folate and/or iron level with concomitant episodic diarrhoea occur in most patients.

The hands, because of their constant exposure to sunshine and trauma, are one of the principal sites that exhibit the cutaneous manifestations of the **porphyrias** (see 1.249–1.255; pp. **49–50**). Cutaneous photosensitivity, unusual fragility of the sun-exposed skin, bullae, shallow ulcers, disordered pigmentation and hypertrichosis occur in almost all varieties. Disfiguring scars with loss of parts of the fingers (9.195) from repeated trauma are seen in **congenital erythropoietic porphyria**.

Blisters, when present, are easy to see on chronically fragile skin (9.196) but more often they may have ruptured

9.191
Tender, brownish-red cutaneous nodules

9.192
Vasculitis: multiple maculopapular lesions ('palpable purpura')

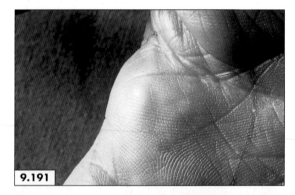
9.191

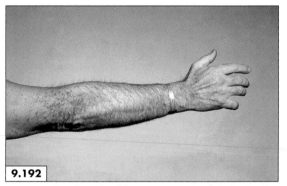
9.192

9.193
Small, bluish, faded, erythematous nodules

9.194
Dermatitis herpetiformis: grouped erythematous lesions and ruptured blisters with scabs

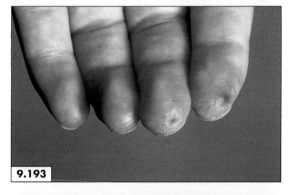
9.193

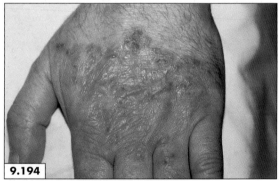
9.194

9.195
Congenital erythropoietic porphyria: scarring, hypopigmentation and loss of fingertips

9.196
Porphyria cutanea tarda: intact and ruptured blisters on sun-exposed hands

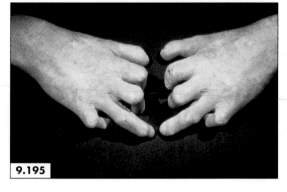
9.195

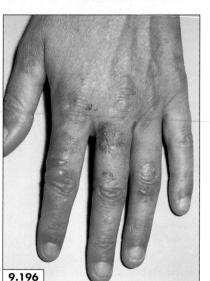
9.196

leaving behind ulcers at various stages of healing (9.197, 9.198) and scars with indurated, white papules (*milia*) (9.199, 9.200). These changes occur in both **variegate porphyria** and **porphyria cutanea tarda** but are more common, and often more severe, in the latter where the skin usually shows evidence of chronic trauma, hypo- and hyperpigmentation (9.201). As in other forms of **hepatic porphyrias** (e.g. acute intermittent porphyria, hereditary coproporphyria), the occurrence of acute neurological attacks is the most important clinical feature in variegate porphyria.

The cutaneous changes of porphyria cutanea tarda also occur in association with hepatoma, renal failure with haemodialysis, systemic lupus erythematosus, haemochromatosis and diabetes mellitus. In many of these cases, no increase in tissue porphyrins has been reported, thus the syndrome is termed **pseudoporphyria** (see 9.160–9.162).

Mycosis fungoides is a type of **T-cell lymphoma** that

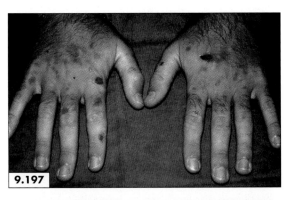

9.197

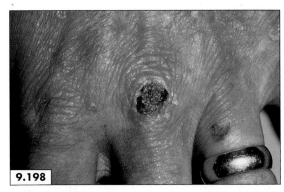

9.198

9.197
Ruptured blisters with denuded red areas

9.198
Thin, wrinkled skin and a ruptured blister

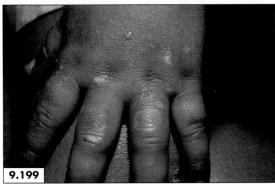

9.199

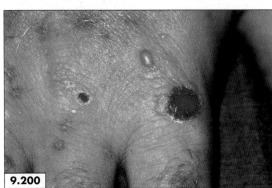

9.200

9.199
Milia: scars with indurated white papules

9.200
Porphyria cutanea tarda: intact and ruptured blisters and milia

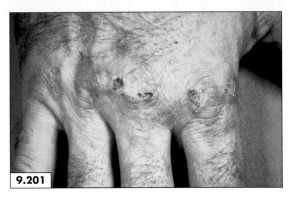

9.201

9.201
Ruptured blisters, hypopigmentation and hyperpigmentation

begins in, and remains limited to, the skin for many years. The lesions are usually *pruritic* and appear as well-circumscribed, reddish or brownish, circular, annular, or arciform in shape (9.202, 9.203). At a later stage, which may be as long as 40 years, ulcers and tumours appear. Extra-cutaneous disseminated disease initially involves the lymph nodes and then, in advanced stages, the liver, spleen and other internal organs.

In **secondary syphilis**, a characteristically polymorphic maculopapular rash appears all over the body, but more particularly on the palms and soles, approximately 4–8 weeks after the appearance of the primary chancre. The papules are pink, dusky, brownish-red or coppery, indurated, oval or round and often scaling. They are usually scattered on the palms (9.204) but may also be present on the face (9.205).

9.202 and 9.203
Mycosis fungoides: patch stage – generalized, flat, reddish-brown plaques with some scaling

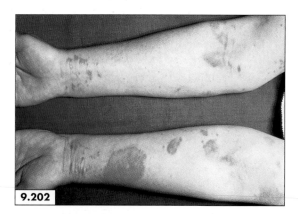

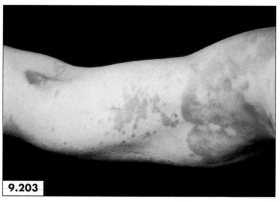

9.204 and 9.205
Secondary syphilis: papulosquamous lesions on palms, fingers and face – discrete, copper-coloured, keratotic papules

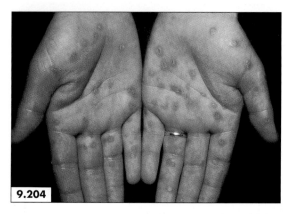

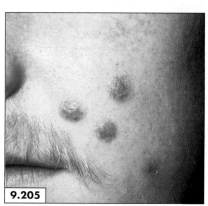

10 THE NAILS

The nails are involved in many dermatological and systemic disorders, and therefore they should be scrutinized carefully at the same time as examination of the hands. Some anatomical considerations of the nail and its associated parts are necessary for the understanding of its disorders. The nail plate is composed of many layers of flattened, keratinized and fused cells; it is attached to, and protects, the pink nail bed (10.1, 10.2).

The half-moon shaped lunula is white because the surface cells of the underlying nail bed in this proximal area are only partially keratinized; the distal pink area is not keratinized at all. The lunula is of variable size in different fingers (10.3) and sometimes absent altogether (10.4) without any clinical significance. The nail plate is enveloped at its origin by the *proximal nailfold*, which is continuous with the *lateral nailfold* on either side of the nail (10.2). The nail plate is attached firmly to the nail bed except distally where it separates from the underlying *hyponychium* (10.5). Healthy nails protect the fingertips, enhance their fine tactile appreciation, and are used as instruments to relieve itching and to open tightly fitting lids of containers.

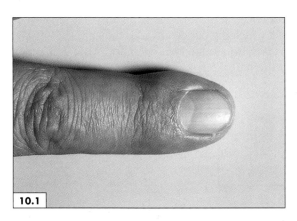

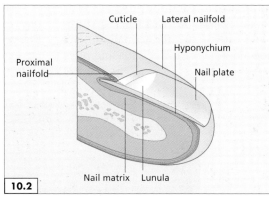

10.1
A normal nail

10.2
Components of a normal nail

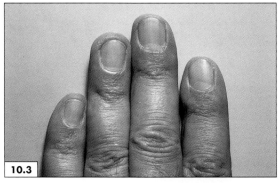

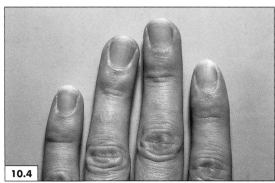

10.3
Nails: variable sizes of crescentic lunulae

10.4
Absent lunulae

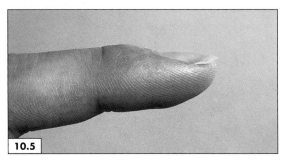

10.5
Lateral view of a nail plate and hyponychium

Disorders of the nails

The nails are expected to share some of the skin diseases because of their close embryological and anatomical relationship to the skin. They can also be affected in some generalized systemic disorders.

Dermatological diseases

The commonest skin diseases to cause abnormalities of the nails are **psoriasis** followed by **lichen planus**; in either case the nails may be affected in the *absence* of any skin lesions. The commonest infections affecting the nails are *Candida* spp. and tinea.

Psoriasis, during its entire course, affects the nails in over 80% of cases. *Pitting* (*onychia punctata*), *discolouration* and *onycholysis* (10.6, 10.7) are by far the commonest nail abnormalities. The changes in the nail plate depend on the location and extent of the parakeratotic process, which can cause gross abnormalities in colour, shape and texture. The pits vary in size and often spare the toenails. Other causes of pitting include alopecia areata, eczema and pity-

riasis rosacea but diffuse and deep pitting is almost exclusive to psoriasis.

Parakeratotic lesions may involve the nail bed and hyponychium, producing reddish spots of varying sizes. There may also be splinter haemorrhages (10.8), which are seen in over one-third of the cases. Thickening and onycholysis (separation of the nail plate from its bed) (10.6, 10.9) are common findings; the whitish colour is indicative of the presence of air under the separated part of the nail.

The nails are affected in approximately 10% of patients with **lichen planus**. The most characteristic feature is vertical ridging of the nail caused by small foci of lichen planus in the matrix, producing depressions or bulges (10.10, 10.11). This bulging may be seen more proximally in the skin, while the nails may also show pigmentation, longitudinal ridging and dystrophy (10.12). Thinning of the nail plate, with atrophy of the matrix (*onychatrophy*) and subungual hyperkeratosis with onycholysis (10.13) also occur. These changes may lead to complete atrophy of the nail, spontaneous shedding and permanent *anonychia*. A characteristic change of lichen planus of the nails is *pterygium* in which the cuticle invades the nail bed (10.14). Pterygium is also found occasionally with ischaemic atrophy of the nail.

10.6
Psoriasis: discrete, multiple pits with distal onycholysis

10.7
Diffuse pitting with streaks of onycholysis

10.8 and 10.9
Psoriasis: splinter haemorrhages, pitting and dystrophic changes

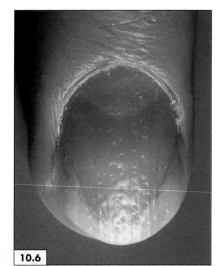

10.6

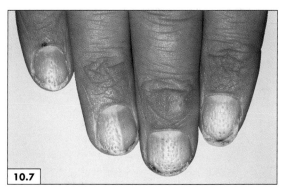

10.7

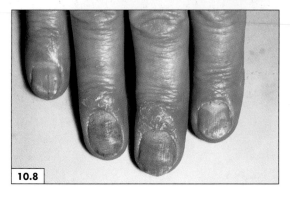

10.8

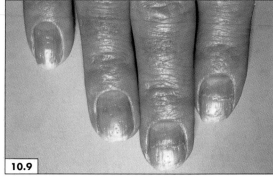

10.9

Fungal infection of the nails (onychomycosis) is largely an opportunistic invasion associated with the conditions that are favourable to these normal inhabitants of the body, such as diabetes mellitus, immunosuppressive states and the use of antibiotics, steroids and cytotoxic drugs. A pre-existing onycholysis and excessive moisture also encourage the fungal invasion. *Candida albicans* (*monilia*) is a normal inhabitant of the gastrointestinal tract (not usually found on the skin), and affects the mucous membranes (see 2.95–2.97; pp. **85–6**) the nails and the moist flexural surfaces. *C. albicans* usually invades the skin around the base of the nails (**chronic paronychia**) (10.15) and may involve a part of the nail plate (sometimes without the preceding paronychia), causing a dark brown pigmentation, ridging and dystrophy (10.16, 10.17).

The infection caused by tinea (**ringworm**) is limited to hair, nails and the horny layer of the epidermis (see 9.74–9.76; p. **171–2**), since these organisms are unable to penetrate the deeper living cells. Ringworm of the nails is common, especially in the great toes (10.18, 10.19); it is usually caused by a species of *Trichophyton* (e.g. *Trichophyton rubrum, T. interdigitale, T. unguium* or *T. mentagrophytes*). In **distal and lateral subungual onychomycosis** (10.20), the fungus reaches the underside of the plate via

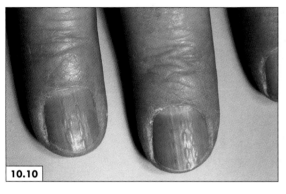

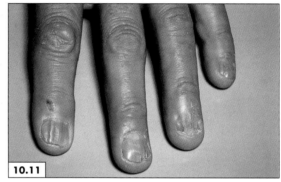

10.10 and 10.11
Lichen planus: vertical ridging and distal dystrophy

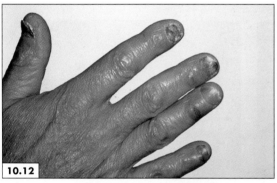

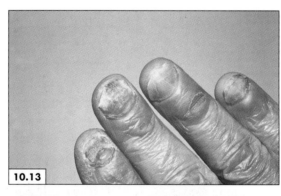

10.12 and 10.13
Lichen planus: ridging, pigmentation, onycholysis and onychoatrophy

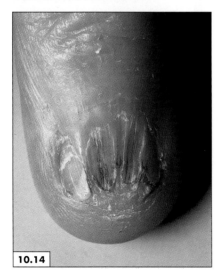

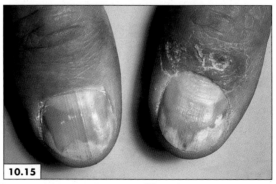

10.14
Pterygium: cuticle invasion and distal onychoatrophy

10.15
Onychomycosis: distal onycholysis with subungual hyperkeratosis. Note the associated fungal infection of the proximal nailfold with erythema and crusting

the hyponychium or the lateral nailfold, raising the free edge of the nail plate, with thickening and opacification. The disease spreads proximally and the whole nail plate becomes opaque (10.21, 10.22). During this process there is progressive dystrophy and onycholysis with the distal parts of the nails separating and falling off (10.23, 10.24).

The clinical appearances of nail dystrophies are seldom diagnostically distinctive for the different fungi; however, hyperkeratosis accompanying onycholysis is a common feature of dermatophyte (*Trichophyton*) infections. Con-versely, in *Candida* **onychomycosis**, gross hyperkeratosis of the entire nail plate is usually seen in patients with chronic mucocutaneous candidiasis.

All the nails may become involved in a chronic, gener-alized dermatophytosis, with simultaneous invasion of the distal ends of the nail plates (10.25, 10.26). As the infection progresses, the distal end of the plate becomes hyperkera-totic and opaque, lifting off the nail bed (10.27). This process separates the entire nail plate from the dead keratinized tissue on the nail bed (10.28). In advanced

10.16
Distal and lateral subungual onychomycosis

10.17
Onycholysis and hyperkeratosis (distal and lateral subungual types)

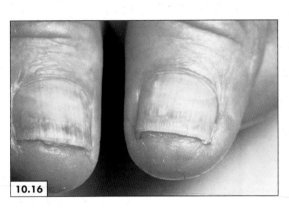

10.16

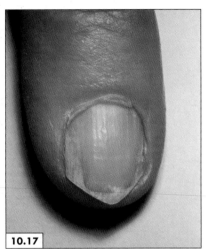

10.17

10.18 and 10.19
Tinea unguium: distal onycholysis with subungual hyperkeratosis

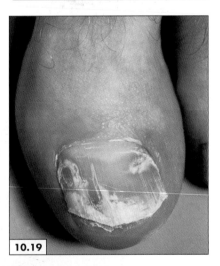

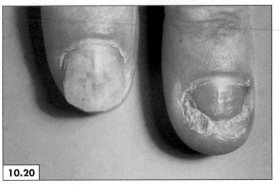

10.18

10.19

10.20
Onycholysis and distal onychatrophy

10.20

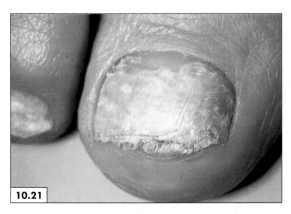

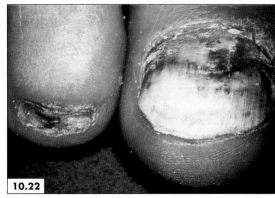

10.21 and 10.22
Total dystrophy: onycholysis with diffuse hyperkeratosis (yellowish and chalk-white discolouration)

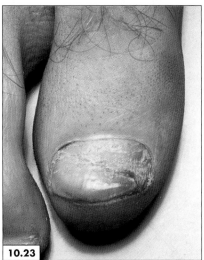

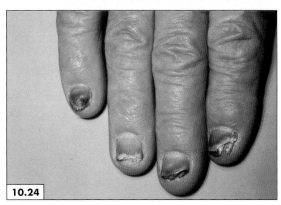

10.23
Hyperkeratosis with fracture of the nail plate

10.24
Distal subungual hyperkeratosis

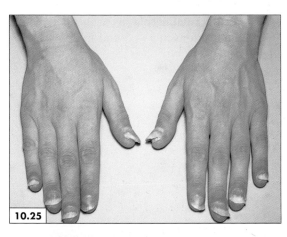

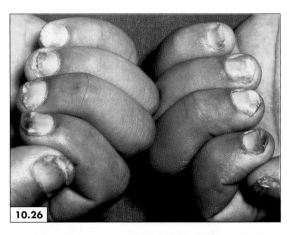

10.25 and 10.26
Distal onycholysis and hyperkeratosis

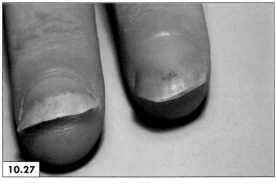

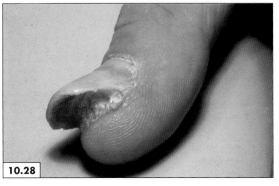

10.27
Distal onycholysis

10.28
Subungual hyperkeratosis with separation of the nail plate

untreated cases, there results a **total dystrophic ony-chomycosis** whereby the nail disappears leaving behind a thickened nail bed.

Congenital and systemic disorders

Before linking any abnormality of the nail to a particular disease, the clinician should take into consideration *three* important preliminaries. First, the abnormality may be congenital and may have attracted attention only because the patient sought advice about an *apparently* related complaint. Hereditary and congenital nail disorders may be associated with almost any deformity of the nail. Congenital nail deformities may be summarized as follows:

- Pachyonychia congenita;
- The nail–patella syndrome;
- Anonychia;
- Congenital ectodermal dysplasia;
- Racket nails;
- Leuconychia totalis;
- Congenital pitting/ridging/dystrophy;
- Hereditary koilyonychia;
- Congenital clubbing;
- Macronychia/micronychia.

A thorough personal and family history and a search for the associated findings are essential for relating a nail change to a systemic disorder.

Second, the nails are cosmetically important and their condition (e.g. dirty, overgrown, bitten, discoloured, stained, unusually painted, etc.) gives important informa-tion about the patient's personal hygiene and about his or her psychological and economic status.

Third, the nails should be examined as critically as any other system. Clinicians often look at the nails as an after-thought when they have already suspected a systemic dis-order and then hope to find some well-known associated signs (e.g. clubbing, splinter haemorrhages, white nails, etc.) to confirm their diagnosis. An uncritical application of this practice in time assumes a procrustean fervour, when nonexistent signs are accepted with compromising qualifi-cations such as 'slight', 'mild' and 'early'. A more orthodox, and invariably safer, approach is to examine the nails as part of the *general examination* looking for any abnormal-ities of shape, colour and size of the nails, nailfolds and nail beds. Any clues detected at this stage will form the basis on which a diagnosis can be constructed after completion of the *systemic examination*.

As already mentioned, the nails can be affected by many congenital abnormalities some of which (e.g. hereditary ectodermal dysplasias) are clinically important in their own right. In **anonychia congenita** (10.29), all or part of the nails may be absent, and some of these underdeveloped plates may be thin and ridged, resembling the *onychatro-phy* of lichen planus (10.30). It may be impossible to make the distinction between the two, particularly as the nail changes may precede the other cutaneous manifestations in lichen planus. Figure 10.30 also shows the pterygium so characteristic of lichen planus.

Koilonychia, or *spoon nails*, may be familial (10.31) or acquired (10.32). The former may be a lone finding or asso-ciated with other **ectodermal dysplasias** or the **nail–patella syndrome**. Acquired koilonychia is found in many condi-tions as follows:

10.29
Congenital deficiency of the nail plates

10.30
Congenital onychatrophy. Note the cuticle invasion of the nail plate (pterygium)

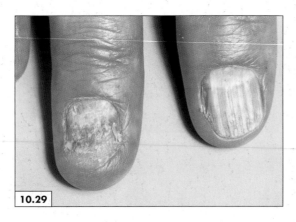
10.29

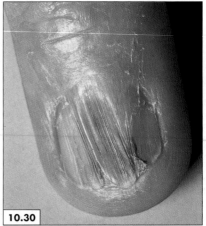
10.30

■ **Hereditary and congenital forms**
— Ectodermal dysplasias;
— Adenoma sebaceum;
— Osteo-onychodysplasias (the nail–patella syndrome).
■ **Acquired forms**
— Iron deficiency states (e.g. Plummer–Vinson syndrome, polycythaemia rubra vera);
— Haematological (e.g. haemoglobinopathy, haemochromatosis);
— Infections (e.g. fungal diseases);
— Endocrine disorders (e.g. acromegaly, hypothyroidism);
— Traumatic;
— Malnutrition;
— Dermatoses (e.g. lichen planus, acanthosis nigricans, psoriasis);
— Connective tissue diseases;
— Carpal tunnel syndrome.

Koilonychia is easy to recognize because the nails are concave (normally convex) with everted edges (10.33). It usually affects several fingers, especially the thumbs. Some clinicians use the *water-drop test* (10.34) as a criterion for accepting koilonychia. This is not necessary as the nails clearly look concave and abnormal. The concavity can be best appreciated when the affected thumbs are held tip-to-tip and viewed laterally, compared with the similarly held thumbs of the examiner (10.35, 10.36).

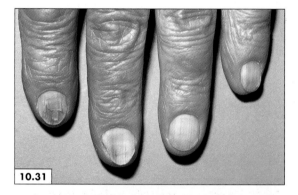
10.31

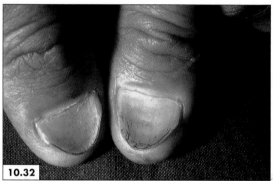
10.32

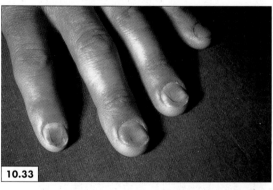
10.33

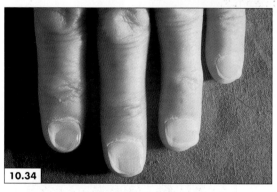
10.34

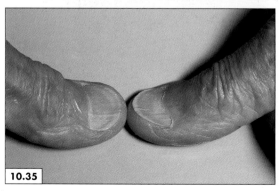
10.35

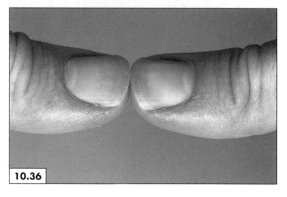
10.36

10.31
Congenital koilonychia

10.32
Acquired koilonychia (spoon nails)

10.33
Koilonychia with concave nail plates and everted edges

10.34
Koilonychia. Note the unspilled water drop on the concave nail of the index finger

10.35
Koilonychia

10.36
Normal nails

In some forms of **congenital koilonychia**, the nails tend to be thin and underdeveloped (10.37). In acquired koilonychia, the nails may be thin or thickened (10.38), there may be longitudinal ridging (10.39), the underlying tissue may be healthy, or there may be subungual hyperkeratosis, which is easily seen at the free margin.

In **pachyonychia congenita**, the nails are very hard and yellowish-brown in colour (10.40). At the free edge there is a hard keratinized mass. All nails are affected and vulnerable to recurrent paronychia.

Epidermal and dental abnormalities are associated in two groups of **ectodermal dysplasia**; one of these has defective sweat glands (**anhidrotic**) and is transmitted through a sex-linked recessive gene; the other is autosomal dominant and associated with normal sweating (**hidrotic ectodermal dysplasia**). In the latter, the hair is sparse, thin and brittle (10.41) and the nails are discoloured and dystrophic (10.42). Unlike the anhidrotic variety, the teeth and sweating are normal but the nails and hair (10.43) are almost always involved. In the

10.37
Congenital koilonychia with poorly developed nails. Note the fleshy fingertips uncovered by nails

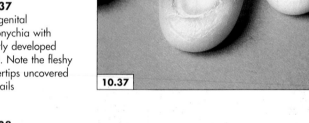

10.38
Thickened nail plate with distal hyperkeratosis

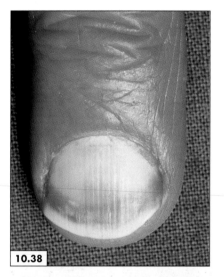

10.39
Congenital koilonychia with longitudinal ridging

10.40
Congenital pachyonychia with deficient, thickened, yellowish-brown nails

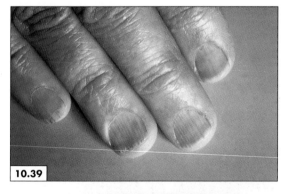

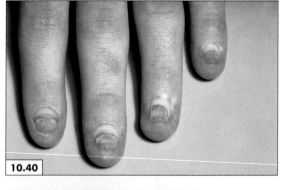

10.41 and 10.42
Ectodermal dysplasia: sparse, thin, spindly hair and thin, discoloured nails with inverted edges

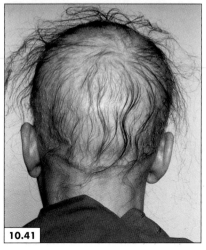

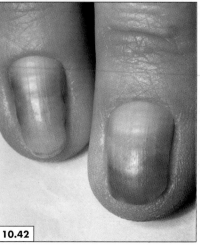

anhidrotic form the teeth, sweating, hair and skin all tend to be abnormal.

Clubbing of the fingers, which is often subjected to clinical compromise, has been referred to in the preceding section. It will be considered here only for its relevance to the shape of the nail plates. There is longitudinal, as well as transverse, convex curvature of the nail plate (10.44) and an *enlargement of the soft tissues of the nail bed* (10.45). A critical comparison of this resulting deformity (10.45) with the profile of a normal finger (10.46) will show that the angle between the proximal nailfold and the curved nail plate (Lovibond's 'profile sign') is increased from the normal 160° to over 180°. In the normal finger, the distal phalanx forms an almost straight line with the middle phalanx, whereas in the clubbed finger this angle is reduced to around 160° (Curth's modified 'profile sign').

It cannot be overstressed that these angles are used to measure the degree of deformity caused by swelling of the nail bed, and should not be used if the only abnormality observed is an increased curvature of the nail plate. Mistakes in diagnosing *false* clubbing can be avoided if the fingers are viewed in profile from the radial side, looking for the presence of swelling of the nail bed (10.47). If there is associated cyanosis of the *warm* fingers, as was the case in this patient with **fibrosing alveolitis** (10.48), or periun-

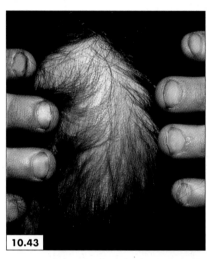

10.43

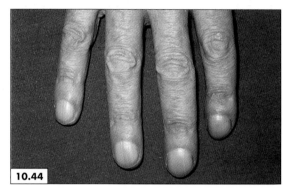

10.44

10.43
Ectodermal dysplasia: sparse hair and thin, somewhat concave nails

10.44
Clubbing of the fingers

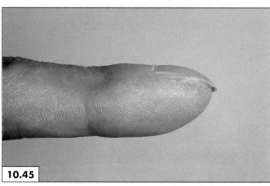

10.45

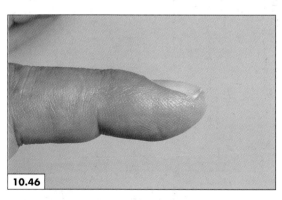

10.46

10.45
Clubbing with thickened nail bed giving the fingertips a bulbous appearance

10.46
Normal nail bed

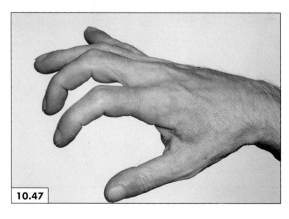

10.47

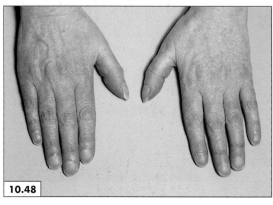

10.48

10.47
Clubbing of the fingers viewed laterally

10.48
Clubbing with cyanosis of the fingers

gual erythema (10.49), then these can provide additional support for a confident diagnosis. Nevertheless, the diagnosis of clubbing should be a primary event (based on the *appearance* of the fingers) as it should be for all *fundamental* signs.

Congenital clubbing (10.50) may be indistinguishable from the acquired form but there is often a history available that shows that the peculiar shape of the nails was noted during early childhood.

As stated earlier, some general but very important conclusions can be drawn from the appearance of the nails. Overgrown nails (**onychogryphosis**) on dry and unwashed toes (10.51) say a lot more than is said by the relatives about the patient being a cynosure of a caring and loving family. In these cases, as in the occasional congenital form,

the big toe is usually involved and the nail may look like a buffalo's horn (10.52). The surface of the overgrown nail is marked by transverse striations. Fungal infection may occur and further distort the nails.

Nicotine staining is seen as a brown discolouration with a yellowish tint on the fingertips and nails (10.53). For staining to occur the fingers need to be exposed to a colouring agent, which comes from nicotine (usually 20 or more cigarettes a day), in the presence of moisture provided by sweating in patients of anxious disposition. However, nicotine staining can also occur in subjects who are not habitually anxious. Recurrent friction by cigarettes may cause callous formation as seen on the dorsum of the middle finger (10.53); the associated clubbing of the fingers tells its own tale in this patient with a **bronchogenic carcinoma**.

10.49
Clubbing with periungual erythema

10.50
Congenital clubbing of the fingers

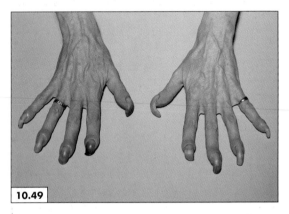

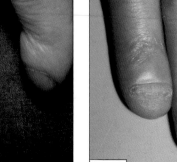

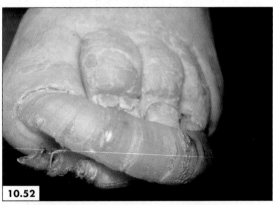

10.51 and 10.52
Onychogryphosis: overgrown nails with poor local hygiene. Note the transverse ridging

10.53
Nicotine-stained nails and fingers. Note the associated clubbing

10.54
Onychophagia: habitual nail biting

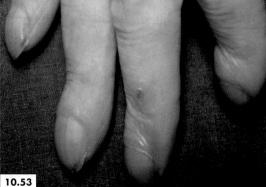

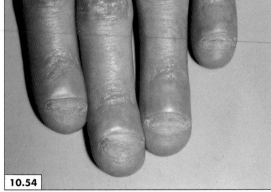

Nail biting, or *onychophagia* (10.54), is thought to be a manifestation of an anxious personality *among the subjects seeking medical advice*. The nail growth is increased as a result of this but it does not keep pace with the frequent biting during periods of stress, thus resulting in short and overcut nails in all fingers (10.55). A close examination will often reveal teeth marks on the short and thin, free edge (10.56).

In the general population there are many nail-biting children and adults who are normal and do not have any evidence of psychiatric disease. However, spells of anxiety, boredom, mental concentration, stress, contemplation and depression are all associated with an increased tendency to nail biting. Some subjects devour the nail and cuticle of only one or two selected fingers (10.57).

Splinter haemorrhages are assiduously looked for by medical practitioners when examining the nails and, when not found, are often mentioned as a negative sign in the final MB and higher examinations. In fact, they are neither specific for, nor very common in, **infective endocarditis** (less than 5%). It is often said that proximal splinter haemorrhages have more diagnostic validity but there is no evidence to support this. Most splinter haemorrhages (from any cause) occur in the distal one-third of the nail (10.58) where they originate from the special, spirally wound capillary, which can be seen as a pink line through the nail about 4mm proximal to the tip of the nail.

A discrete haemorrhage in that area seen under a healthy and nontraumatized nail (10.59) should always arouse suspicion about an associated disorder, as was the case in this patient with **infective endocarditis**. In this condition, splinter haemorrhages are thought to be embolic in

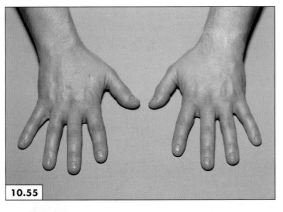

10.57

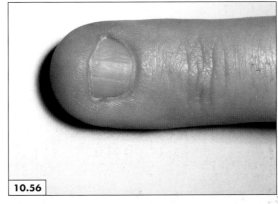

10.55

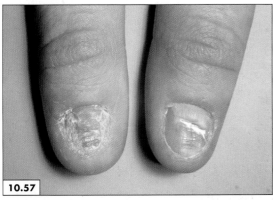

10.59

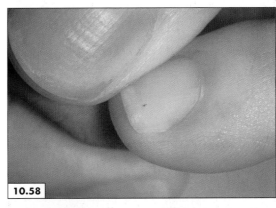

10.58

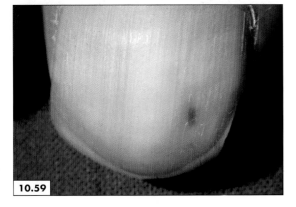

10.59

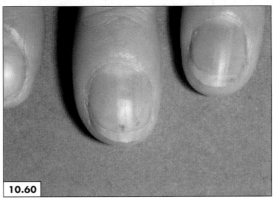

10.60

10.55
Onychophagia: short and overcut nails

10.56
Overcut nail with teeth marks on the free edge

10.57
Onychophagia: the disfigured nails suggest that the entire nail plates of these two fingers are habitually attacked

10.58
Splinter haemorrhage

10.59
Splinter haemorrhage

10.60
Traumatic splinter haemorrhages. Note the whitish streaks caused by trauma

origin and, sometimes, there may be several and in more than one finger. Distal splinter haemorrhages close to the free edge with some evidence of trauma (10.60) are easy to distinguish from those of a sinister origin. Occasionally, there may be a *subungual haematoma* and the capillaries of the fingertip may also be involved (10.61). Splinter haemorrhages have been reported in many conditions, but they are most frequently seen after **trauma** to a nail (10.60) and in **psoriasis** (10.62; see also 10.8). The conditions associated with splinter haemorrhages may be summarized as follows:

- Trauma (e.g. occupational hazard);
- Septicaemia (e.g. infective endocarditis);
- Skin diseases (e.g. psoriasis, onychomycosis, Behçet's disease);
- Metabolic (e.g. porphyrias, haemochromatosis, haemodialysis);
- Vascular (e.g. vasculitides, Buerger's disease, hypertension, cryoglobulinaemia, Raynaud's disease).

A *subungual haematoma* may be spontaneous as in **infective endocarditis** (10.61) or may appear acutely after **trauma**, and may involve the nails of the fingers or toes (10.63). The accumulated blood under the nail plate usually produces pain and needs to be drained. Successful treatment prevents secondary dystrophy of the nail plate and encourages its normal regrowth. A casual glance might confuse a **naevus** (10.64) with a subungual haematoma; however, the former is *painless*, is present from birth and has a sharper violaceous hue that does not change with time.

The **median nail dystrophy** consists of a symmetrical longitudinal defect of the nails of the thumbs (10.65) although sometimes it may involve other fingers. It may be associated with an enlarged lunula. The aetiology is unknown; familial cases have been reported and, in some cases, it may be caused by self-induced trauma.

In the **yellow nail syndrome**, the characteristic appearance of the nails (10.66) is often accompanied by *lymphoedema* and *pleural effusions*. The clinical triad consists of yellow and dystrophic nails, lymphatic abnormalities

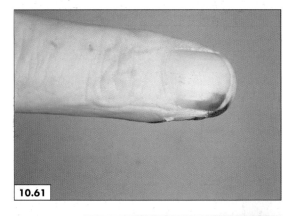

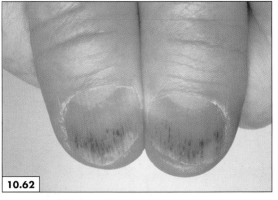

10.61
Subungual haematoma in a patient with infective endocarditis

10.62
Psoriasis with multiple splinter haemorrhages

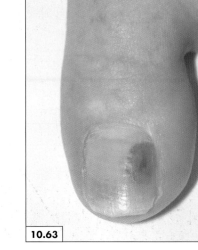

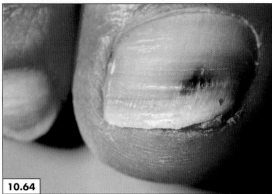

10.63
Subungual haematoma caused by trauma

10.64
Congenital naevus with violaceous streaks

(e.g. aplasia, ectasia, lymphangitis, lymphoedema) and systemic illness (e.g. pleural effusion, bronchiectasis) or a malignancy (e.g. Hodgkin's lymphoma, melanoma). The nails are extremely slow growing, thickened and excessively curved from side to side (10.67), leaving spare fleshy lateral nailfolds and fingertips beyond the stunted nails (10.68). The colour is usually pale yellow but may be brown or green with a yellowish tint (10.69, 10.70).

The nychial changes are specific to the diagnosis but may lag behind or even precede the other manifestations. Unexplained ankle oedema (often asymmetrical) and recurrent unexplained pleural effusions may occur before the development of the characteristic nail changes. Alternatively, lymphoedema and a pleural effusion may not be seen for years after the nail changes, even though the abnormal nails are thought to be the result of defective lymphatic drainage. Atresia and hypoplasia of the peripheral lymphatics have been demonstrated in many patients. Occasionally, the syndrome may be associated with bronchiectasis, thyroid disorders, increased susceptibility to skin infections and asymmetrical breasts.

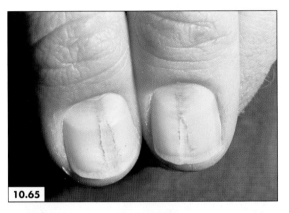

10.65

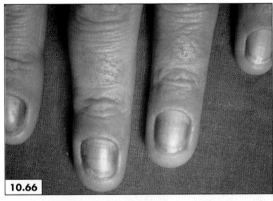

10.66

10.65
Median dystrophy with large lunulae

10.66
The yellow nail syndrome: yellowish-dark undergrown nails

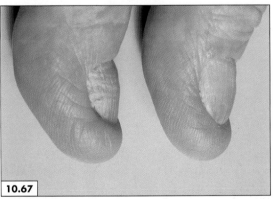

10.67

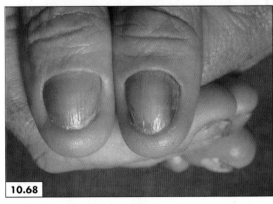

10.68

10.67 and 10.68
The yellow nail syndrome: yellowish-dark, stunted nails with fleshy, bulbous fingertips

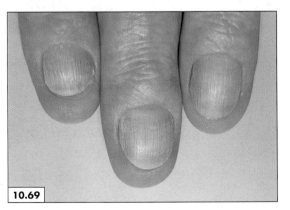

10.69

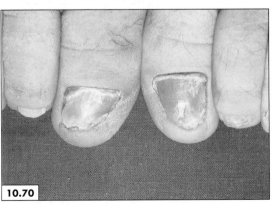

10.70

10.69 and 10.70
The yellow nail syndrome: yellowish-green, dystrophic nails

The **nail–patella syndrome (osteo-onycho-dysplasia)** is characterized by an absent patella (90%) and thin, fragile, deficient or absent nails. The changes are most marked in the thumbs (10.71, 10.72). The lunula may be absent (10.71) or V-shaped (10.72, 10.73). Other associated features are a small head of the radius, *iliac crest exostosis* and developmental abnormalities in the eyes and kidneys.

The *white nails* of **hepatic cirrhosis** exhibit a uniform opaqueness extending from the base of the nail curtaining over and obscuring the lunula. It stops short a few millimetres from the distal border of the nail, leaving a normal pink zone. The changes tend to be more marked in the thumb and index finger though all fingers may be equally affected (10.74). The appearance of the nails in 10.75 is called the 'half-and-half' nail (also known as Terry's nail). The distal half to one-third is pink and sharply demarcated from the proximal two-thirds, which is dull and white and obliterates the lunula. It may be a manifestation of hypoalbuminaemia associated with hepatic cirrhosis. Half-and-half nails are found in 10% of patients with the uraemia of chronic renal failure.

Striate leuconychia, transversely (10.76) or longitudinally (10.77), may occur in one or more fingernails. This whitening resembles that seen in superficial onychomycosis but no fungi are isolated in culture. One-quarter of patients with **systemic lupus erythematosus** show a variety

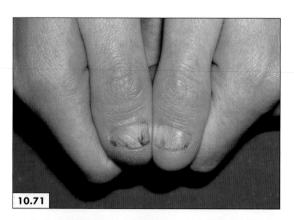

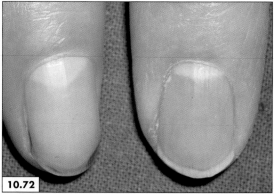

10.71 and 10.72
Osteo-onychodysplasia: thin, fragile nails. Note absent lunulae in 10.71

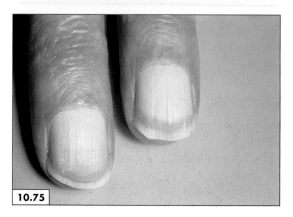

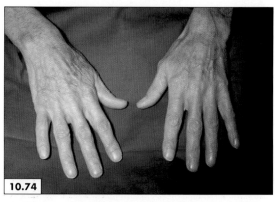

10.73
Osteo-onychodysplasia: thin nails with V-shaped lunulae

10.74
Leuconychia

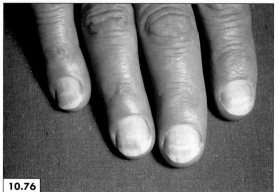

10.75
'Half-and-half' nails

10.76 and 10.77
Striate leuconychia: transverse and longitudinal whitish striations in a patient with systemic lupus erythematosus

of nail changes, including striate or longitudinal leucony-chia, pitting, ridging, onycholysis, splinter haemorrhages, nailfold telangiectasis and infarcts (10.78).

Transverse sulci, or *Beau's lines*, affecting the surface of all the nails at corresponding levels (10.79) represent a transient arrest of nail growth caused by an illness. As the growth rate is around 0.1 mm a day, it is possible to esti-mate the approximate time of the previous illness that has marked the nails (5 months in 10.79).

Perionychial tissues (nailfolds and cuticles) are subject to both trauma and the extreme variations of temperature and hydration caused by their exposure to the elements. Painful cracks occur in the nailfolds and cuticle (10.80) as

a result of exposure to cold and frosty winds. The trauma may be self-inflicted, causing erosions of the nailfolds in association with neurosis and depression. This may be an important consideration when assessing the other symp-toms of a patient. Some systemic disorders are also asso-ciated with abnormalities in the perionychial tissues.

In **dermatomyositis**, characteristic nailfold erythema, telangiectasia and infarcts are seen (10.81, 10.82). The cuticle is rough, thickened and irregular, and there are dilated capillary loops on the proximal nailfold. These changes are specific and show remissions and exacerba-tions in keeping with the severity of the disease process elsewhere in the body.

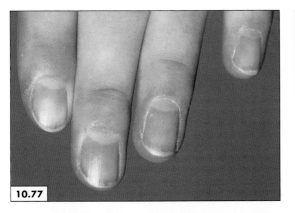

10.77

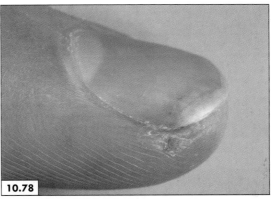

10.78

10.78
Systemic lupus erythematosus: an ulcerated nailfold infarct

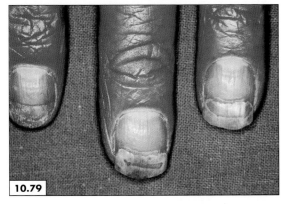

10.79

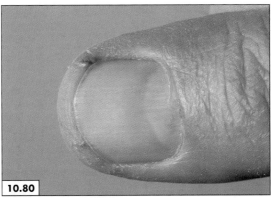

10.80

10.79
Beau's lines

10.80
Fissuring of the nailfold caused by exposure to cold

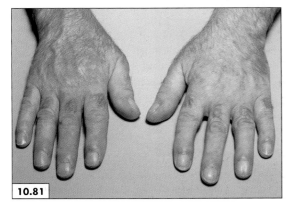

10.81

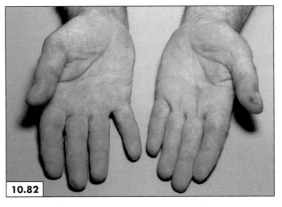

10.82

10.81 and 10.82
Dermatomyositis: periungal erythema, nailfold infarct (left thumb) and fading Gottron's papules on the interphalangeal joints

Palmar and periungual erythema and nailfold infarcts are common in patients with **rheumatoid arthritis** (see also 9.12–9.14; p. **159**). Digital arteritis causes obliteration of the vessels resulting in small infarcts in the nailfolds (10.83, 10.84). Nailfold infarcts occur more frequently on the radial border of the index finger and the ulnar aspect of the thumb (10.84). There is a close correlation between pressure areas and vasculitis; lesions can be seen on top of the cutaneous nodules, especially at the elbow (see 9.43; p. **165**).

A large variety of abnormalities including onycholysis, longitudinal striations, absent lunulae and periungual in-farcts have all been reported in **systemic sclerosis** and **mixed connective tissue disease** (see also 9.82–9.93; p. **173–5**). Nailfold infarcts and ulcers on the terminal digits (10.85, 10.86) are a frequent occurrence in these two conditions. Digital ischaemia may cause dystrophy of the nails (10.87).

Discolouration of the nails, onycholysis and absent lunulae (10.88, 10.89) can occur in **porphyria cutanea tarda**, as well as in other forms of porphyria. Transverse leuconychia on brownish nails is seen in erythropoietic protoporphyria. Koilonychia can also occur and may precede any of the other cutaneous manifestations. Bullae,

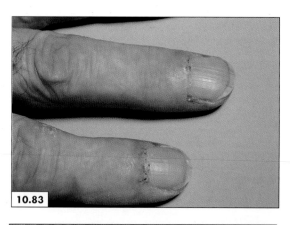

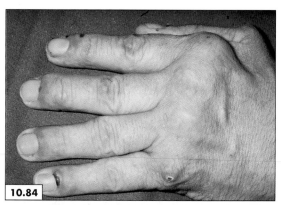

10.83 and 10.84
Rheumatoid arthritis: periungal erythema and nailfold infarcts

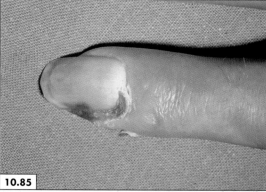

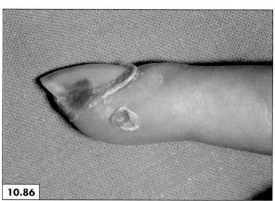

10.85 and 10.86
Systemic sclerosis: nailfold infarcts and ulcers

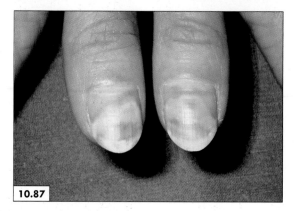

10.87
Onychodystrophy

the hallmark of porphyria, may occur underneath the nail plate and these may become infected.

A bluish discolouration of the normally white lunula suggests chronic cyanosis as in this patient with **Eisenmenger's syndrome** who also has cyanosis and clubbing of the fingers (10.90). Darker blue lunulae are sometimes found in patients on antimalarial drugs or minocycline. They are also associated with haemochromatosis, Wilson's disease and ochronosis.

Muehrcke's nails (10.91) are characterized by paired, narrow, horizontal white bands, separated by normal, pink bands; both of these remain immobile as the nail grows.

These nails are seen mostly in patients with *hypoalbuminaemia* associated with **nephrotic syndrome**. Curiously, their presence correlates with low serum albumin levels but the mechanism of this relationship is not known.

Periungual and *subungual fibromas* (Koenen's tumours) (10.92, 10.93) usually appear after puberty in **tuberous sclerosis (epiloia)**. These fibromas are an important marker of epiloia and usually arise in the periungual groove, as grain-shaped growths, which then extend over the nail plate. They are said to occur as frequently as renal hamartomas in this condition. In some patients a periungual fibroma may be the only sign of the disease.

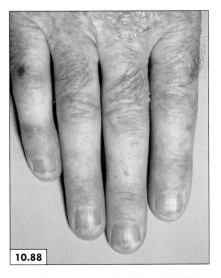

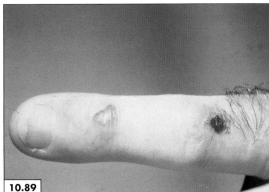

10.88 and 10.89
Porphyria cutanea tarda: fragile, thin skin, ruptured blisters and transverse leuconychia. Note absent lunulae

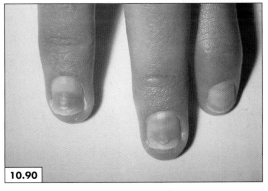

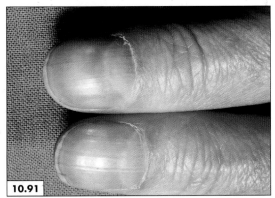

10.90
Blue nails

10.91
Muehrcke's nails: well-demarcated horizontal pink and white bands

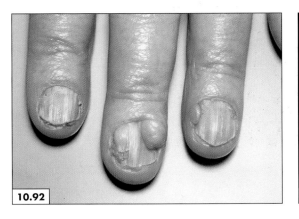

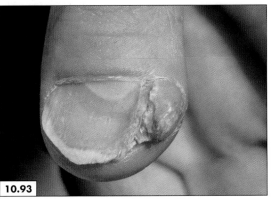

10.92
Proximal periungual fibromata

10.93
Lateral periungual fibroma eroding the nail plate

In **superior vena caval obstruction** and **congestive cardiac failure**, the veins on the dorsum of the hands become engorged and static, with the resulting *cold*, or peripheral, cyanosis of the fingertips and suffusion of the periungual tissues (10.94). The lunulae lose their paleness and may become suffused. In both these conditions, the lunulae may sometimes become red; however, this phenomenon is not specific and may also occur in psoriasis, alopecia areata and in connective tissue diseases (10.95).

A large variety of tumours can occur under the nail but these are rare. A **malignant melanoma** occasionally arises under the nail plate (10.96) as it does elsewhere. *Spreading pigmentation* (*Hutchinson's sign*) is a pathognomonic feature of malignant melanoma that can result in complete destruction of the nail plate.

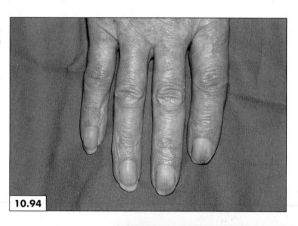

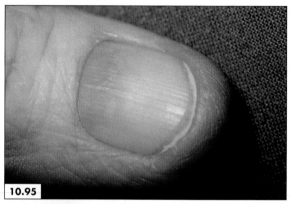

10.94
Periungual suffusion and cyanosis of the fingers

10.95
Red lunulae with longitudinal ridging

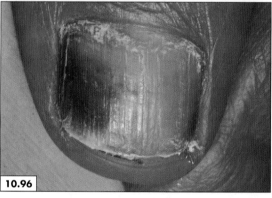

10.96
Malignant melanoma: variegated colour from faint pinkish to purplish brown

11 THE LEGS

The inspection of the legs is usually carried out during the initial *scalp-to-sole visual scan* of the patient, and forms an essential, although often in practice a cursory, part of the general examination. It is not unusual for medical students to hear their tutor say, 'Finally, as you conclude the inspection, have a *quick* look at the legs to see if there is any abnormality'. This approach is unfortunate as it plants a misconception in the mind of the student, that the examination of the legs is not very rewarding, and that it does not contribute much to the synthesis of the final diagnosis.

A look at the face and the hands usually yields positive signs more often than a look at the legs. However, those signs likely to be found on the legs have more *diagnostic power*, since over 80% of them are *fundamental signs* and therefore have a specific link to one or more diseases. Unilateral lower limb swelling (11.1), inflammation and swelling of the first metatarsophalangeal joint (11.2), bowing of the legs (11.3), erythema nodosum (11.4),

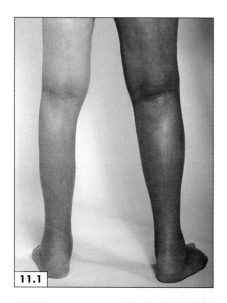

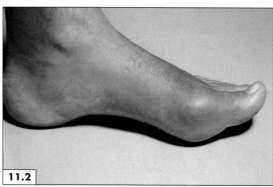

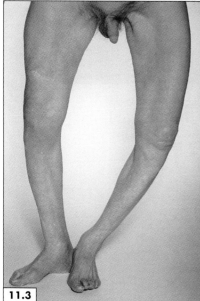

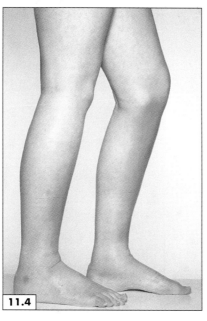

11.1
Deep venous thrombosis: diffuse swelling of the right leg

11.2
Acute gout: swollen, inflamed first metatarsophalangeal joint

11.3
Paget's disease with marked curvature of the legs

11.4
Subcutaneous nodules with erythema of the overlying skin

erythema ab igne (11.5), necrobiosis lipoidica diabeticorum (11.6) and pyoderma gangrenosum (11.7) are but a few examples of the signs predominantly found on the lower limbs, which either provide the diagnosis, or present a specific clue for a line of further investigation.

In real life, clinicians make a detailed examination of the legs only after they have formed a tentative diagnosis from the history and systemic examination. Some physicians look at the legs and feel the peripheral pulses when they are testing tendon reflexes. Experienced clinicians often have a good idea of what they are looking for in the legs after they have completed the rest of the examination. Alternatively, an initial thoughtful inspection might provide a crucial clue that can help the entire process of making a diagnosis. What follows in this section has been presented keeping both these approaches in perspective.

Only an experienced physician who is able to identify the system at fault, and who has a good knowledge of the possible clinical signs in the legs related to each system (Table 11.1), can use the first approach mentioned above. For example, when assessing a diabetic patient, such a physician will take extra care in palpating all the pulses in the legs, checking the integrity of both tissue perfusion and the peripheral nerves, assessing foot hygiene and pressure points, and looking for the presence of any cutaneous lesions such as a diabetic dermopathy or necrobiosis lipoidica.

A beginner will use the approach outlined in Table 11.2, although it is also applied by astute clinicians. In practice, a combination of both these methods is unlikely to miss anything. A detailed *visual survey* of the whole patient should identify an abnormality on the legs, and a return to this area after the systemic examination should assign it to the correct system. For most signs in the legs, it is possible

11.5
Ill-defined, reddish-brown, reticular pattern caused by chronic exposure to local heat

11.6
Large, yellow-orange plaques with raised, irregular borders

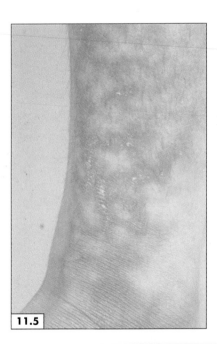

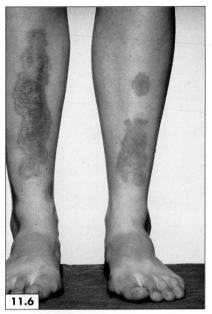

11.7
Ulcers with raised bullous, undermined borders and a haemorrhagic discharge

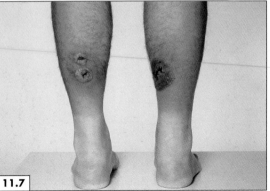

to relate them to the appropriate system at the initial scan. It is therefore profitable to present the various abnormalities likely to be found on the legs under their systems.

Endocrine disorders

Of all the endocrine diseases, **diabetes mellitus** is the one with the most abnormalities that can occur on the lower limbs. It affects adversely all the individual components of the legs (e.g. skin, muscles, nerves, blood vessels and bones), and the maxim, 'look at the diabetic's feet first then at their face', highlights aptly the chief concern of senior physicians who have seen the pedal ravages of this condition. In a large survey of a diabetic population, the amputation rate was halved after the introduction of a simple outpatient programme of foot inspection at every visit.

The breakdown of the diabetic foot is caused by a combination of dryness, neuropathy, infection, vascular maldistribution and inadequate foot care. The **neuropathic ulcer** (also called a trophic, perforating or pressure ulcer) characteristically occurs on the plantar surface (11.8) and at the base of the big toe (11.9). *Neuropathy* is an essential predisposing factor and is often, but not always, characterized by marked *loss of vibration*, pain and temperature sensations and absent ankle jerks. There is weakness and atrophy of the intrinsic muscles with simultaneous contraction of the long flexors and extensors producing '*claw toes*' (dorsiflexion at the metatarsophalangeal joints and plantarflexion at the interphalangeal joints) (11.9).

Table 11.1 Clinical signs in the legs	
System	*Signs*
Endocrine	Necrobiosis lipoidica diabeticorum, granuloma annulare, pretibial myxoedema, etc.
Locomotor	Arthritides – gout, osteoarthrosis, etc.
Neurological	Wasting, deformity
Cardiovascular	Oedema, pallor, cyanosis, phlebothrombosis
Skin lesions	Macules, papules, nodules, tumours, vesicles, blisters, bullae, urticaria, purpura, ulcers

Table 11.2 Visual scan of the legs	
Signs	*Possibilities*
Joint swelling/ deformity	Arthritides – osteoarthrosis, septic, Charcot's, gout, rheumatoid, etc.
Deformity of leg/thigh or foot	Paget's disease, sabre shin (syphilis), Charcot–Marie–Tooth disease
Swelling of leg	Congestive cardiac failure, phlebothrombosis, ruptured Baker's cyst, etc.
Wasting	Old polio, muscular dystrophy, myopathy
Skin lesion	Dermatoses, systemic disorders

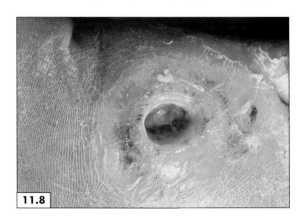

11.8

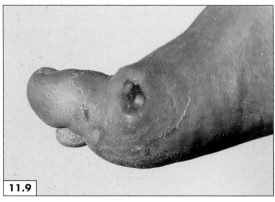

11.9

11.8
Deep ulcer crater, reaching the muscle, with nonhealing, callous, undermined edge

11.9
Ulcer with well-defined, undermined edge penetrating to subcutaneous tissues

The ulcer is characteristically punched out, circular and surrounded by callous (11.8–11.10). The foot is usually warm with palpable pulses and the ulcer is often painless. At the outset there may be only a mild degree of impaired perception of vibration and pain sensations. Recurrent ulcers result in loss of the toes (11.11). The neuropathy causes disarticulation producing a **Charcot joint** and neuropathic ulcers can also develop at proximal pressure areas (11.12). Other conditions causing neuropathic ulcers include tabes dorsalis, leprosy, syringomyelia and hereditary sensory neuropathy.

Nowadays diabetes mellitus is the commonest cause of **Charcot's arthropathy**. Other principal causes are tabes dorsalis (affecting knee joints), syringomyelia and leprosy (affecting upper limb joints). In diabetes mellitus, the midtarsal joints are involved with gross destructive changes, new bone formation, joint instability and deformity (11.13). These changes can sometimes develop at an alarming speed, as in this patient (11.14) whose problem started with a nail injury to the instep, which led to a septic arthritis even before the diagnosis of diabetes mellitus was made.

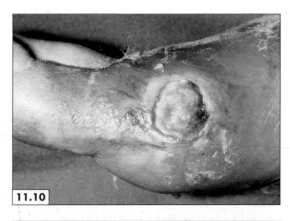

11.10
Ulcer with slough on the base and an erythematous edge surrounded by callous

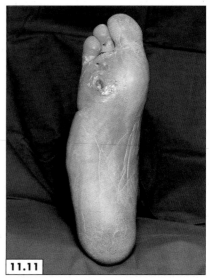

11.11
Loss of two lateral toes and an ulcer on the sole

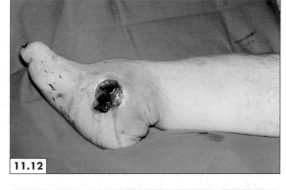

11.12
Charcot's ankle with a punched-out ulcer

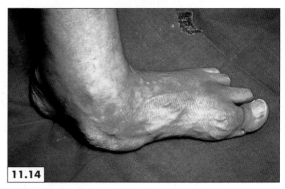

11.13 and 11.14
Charcot's arthropathy with grossly deformed feet

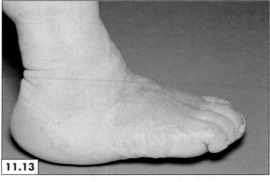

Peripheral vascular disease, gangrene and **amputation** occur more frequently in diabetic patients, and equally in both sexes, than in nondiabetic subjects. In addition to accelerated atherosclerosis, diabetic patients also have multiple small vessel occlusions. This patchy involvement of the small arteries is illustrated by the presence of gangrene in one part, and palpable pulses with a good circulation in another part of the same foot. The heel of the diabetic patient is particularly vulnerable to pressure ischaemia, which leads to gangrenous changes (11.15, 11.16). This is because the heel and the lateral border of the foot are subjected to high pressure, which may render a marginally adequate blood supply inadequate. Often secondary infection supervenes with disastrous consequences.

The nondiabetic is more likely to have atherosclerotic changes in the big vessels (e.g. aorta, iliac and femoral vessels), whereas the diabetic patient tends to have these changes in the more distal vessels such as the tibial and peroneal arteries (11.17). The ischaemic process is often slowly progressive and less advanced in these smaller vessels. This explains the presence of a palpable dorsalis pedis and/or anterior tibial pulse in the foot that has severe peripheral vascular disease with patchy gangrene of the toes (11.18). Autonomic neuropathy sometimes contributes to this vascular maldistribution. Venous stasis, which also results in ulcers (11.19), often compounds the problem caused by the arterial insufficiency.

Diabetic dermopathy (*shin spots*) is the commonest cutaneous manifestation of diabetes mellitus. The spots start as multiple, discrete dull red papules (11.20). They occur mostly on the extensor surfaces of the legs but may also be found on the thighs and forearms. Male diabetic patients predominate over females in a ratio of 2:1.

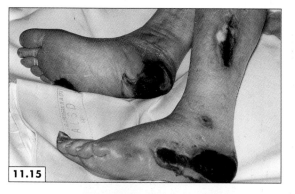
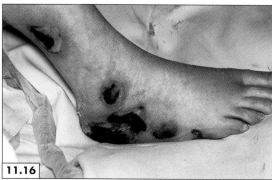

11.15 and 11.16 Gangrenous ulcers with black slough on oedematous feet

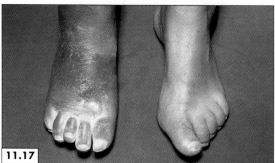
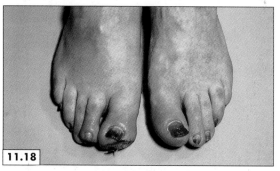

11.17 Peripheral vascular insufficiency with oedema and cyanosis of the worse affected foot

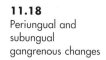

11.18 Periungual and subungual gangrenous changes

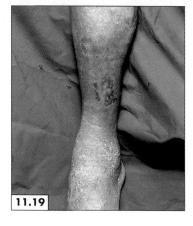
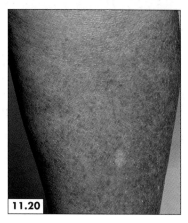

11.19 Venous stasis ulcer with pigmentation of atrophic skin

11.20 Multiple, dark red and brown maculopapular spots

Necrobiosis lipoidica diabeticorum (11.21, 11.22) is an uncommon cutaneous lesion in diabetic patients (approximately 0.2%) but it is strongly associated with the disease. It may even occur in those who only have impaired carbohydrate tolerance or a positive family history of diabetes mellitus. Most of the patients are less than 40 years of age and females predominate over males (ratio 3:1). Diabetes usually has been present for over 1 year, although in some patients (approximately 15%) the lesion may be present before the diagnosis of diabetes is made. Note the progressive changes of Charcot's arthropathy (clawing of toes, falling arches and drooping malleoli) in Figures 11.21 and 11.22.

Necrobiosis lipoidica is often bilateral but not necessarily symmetrical (11.23). The legs are affected in approximately 85% of patients and in the remaining 15% the lesions may develop on the arms, head or abdomen. The initial lesion is a reddish fleshy plaque, somewhat round or oval in shape (11.24), with sharply defined and elevated borders. It extends outwards in an annular fashion, the

11.21 and 11.22
Multiple, serpiginous plaques with central atrophy. Note flat feet with clawing of the toes

11.23
Necrobiosis lipoidica diabeticorum: large, dusky red plaques with well-demarcated, irregular margins and central atrophy

11.24
A dark red plaque with irregular margin. Note multiple scattered macules and papules (diabetic dermopathy)

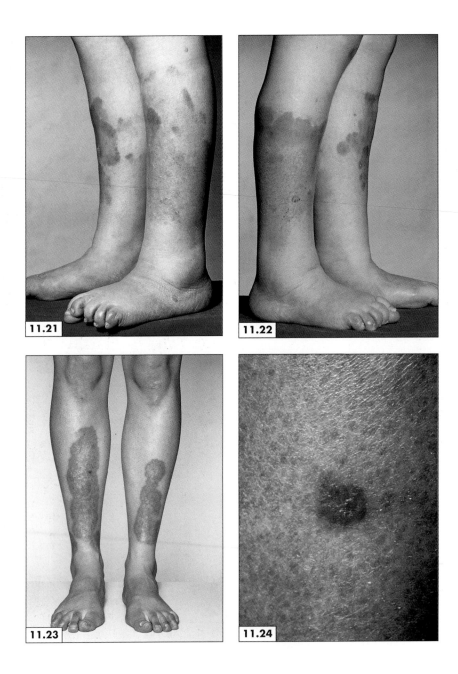

borders becoming irregular but often remaining elevated and erythematous, while the centre becomes depressed from atrophy of the epidermis, which looks transparent and takes a yellowish hue (11.25, 11.26). Occasionally, the atrophic epidermis breaks down and ulcerates. Good control of the diabetes does not appear to influence the lesions which remain persistent in most patients. In a few patients, the lesions clear spontaneously over many years.

Recurrent injection of high doses of insulin at the same site can cause *lipoatrophy*, with loss of the subcutaneous fat (11.27). The condition was commoner in females before the introduction of monocomponent and human insulins.

Granuloma annulare has been observed in diabetic patients but this association is rather weak as it develops frequently in patients with a normal glucose tolerance. The lesions occur characteristically on the dorsum of the hands and fingers, the extensor surfaces of the elbows and knees, on the dorsal surface of the foot (11.28) and around the ankles (11.29). It starts as a flesh-coloured dermal papule

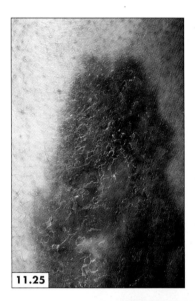

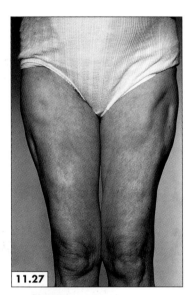

11.25 and 11.26
Necrobiosis lipoidica diabeticorum: large, waxy plaques with raised, irregular margins. Note a depressed scar in the middle in 11.25

11.27
Lipoatrophy causing depression of the skin at injection sites

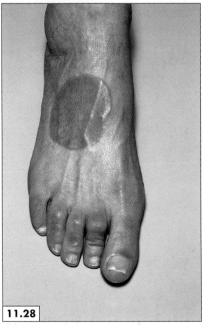

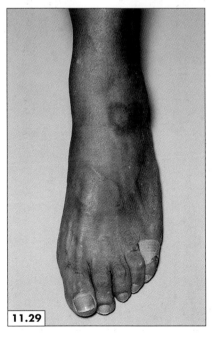

11.28
Granuloma annulare: large, annular, reddish-brown plaque with well-defined margin

11.29
A dark red plaque with central clearing

coalescing in a circular ring of 1–5 cm diameter (11.30). The lesions may occur at any age, even in children. A disseminated form of granuloma annulare is thought to be related to overt or latent diabetes mellitus (see 9.159; p. **188**). Approximately one-half of the lesions clear up spontaneously over a period of 2–3 years.

Diabetic bullae (*bullosis diabeticorum*), which resemble but are not caused by burns (11.31), occur in long-standing diabetics *with neuropathy*. The bullae are of rapid onset and are sometimes first discovered when getting out of bed in the morning. They may be unilateral or bilateral and usually appear on the toes, plantar and dorsal surfaces of the foot, and on the fingers (see also 9.158–9.162; pp. **187–8**). The blisters are tense, containing serous but sometimes haemorrhagic fluid, and their base and the adjoining skin are not inflamed.

Diabetic amyotrophy (proximal lower extremity motor neuropathy) usually involves the muscles supplied by the femoral nerve, principally the quadriceps group. It results in a progressive, painful, bilateral and usually asymmetrical, weakness and wasting of the thigh muscles (11.32, 11.33), with loss of the knee jerk but with very little sensory impairment. The syndrome mostly affects poorly controlled diabetic patients in their middle age, is heralded by recent weight loss, and is slowly reversible.

The classic cutaneous lesion of a **glucagonoma** (*necrolytic migratory erythema*) begins as erythema of the skin, becomes indurated and develops central blistering, which bursts and leaves a crust (11.34). The rash is most prominent on the perineum, along intertriginous folds (11.35, 11.36), around the mouth and on the tongue (see 2.74; p. **81**). The characteristic waxing and waning skin rash is considered to be the hallmark of the syndrome but only occurs in approximately two-thirds of patients. The other features of the syndrome are diabetes, hypoaminoacidaemia, weight loss and anaemia.

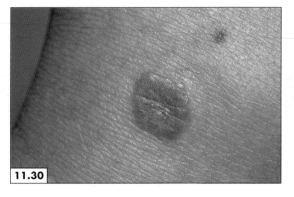

11.30
A reddish dermal plaque with well-defined margin

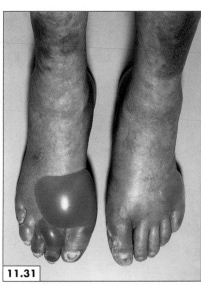

11.31
Diabetic bullae. Note necrobiosis lipoidica diabeticorum

11.32 and 11.33
Diabetic amyotrophy with asymmetrical flattening of thigh muscles

11.34
Migratory necrolytic erythema: erythematous plaques with irregular margins and central crusting

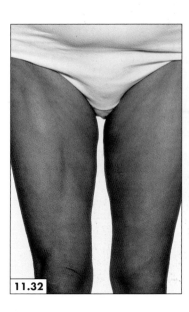

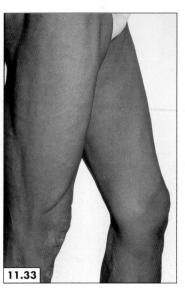

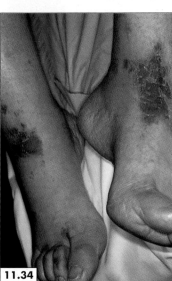

Approximately 5% of patients with **Graves' disease** develop localized myxoedema (often after being rendered euthyroid or hypothyroid with treatment), usually affecting the anterior aspect of the leg (*pretibial myxoedema*). Sometimes the hands or face may be involved, particularly if the affected area is subjected to constant trauma. The skin is thickened, raised, nontender and violaceous with coarse hair and nonpitting oedema (11.37).

In **Cushing's syndrome** *purple striae* can be found on the abdomen, buttocks (11.38) and on the thighs (11.39). The phenomenon is caused by thinning of the skin, which looks parched and transparent. There is usually underlying muscular weakness and wasting particularly affecting the lower limb-girdle muscles.

The feet are enlarged, broad and bulky (11.40, 11.41) in **acromegaly**. The increase in the size of the feet affects both

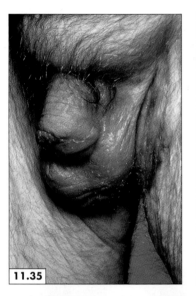
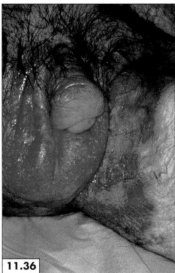
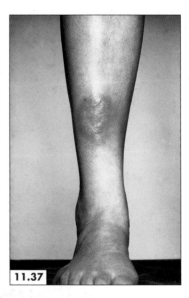

11.35 and 11.36
Glucagonoma syndrome: erythematous, inflammatory plaques of the scrotum, penile shaft and intertriginous area

11.37
Pretibial myxoedema: a raised, reddish plaque with irregular margins

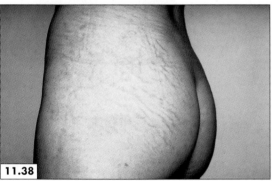

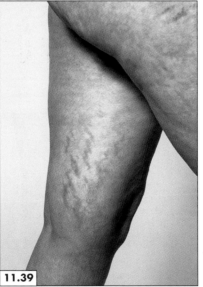

11.38
Cushing's syndrome: purplish striae

11.39
Scattered, purplish, streaky striae

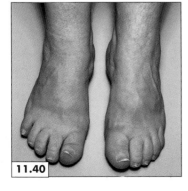

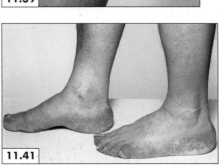

11.40 and 11.41
Acromegaly: large, square, bulky feet

the anteroposterior and transverse dimensions. It is caused by thickening of the skin and soft tissues, and is particularly noticeable over the heels and the lateral borders. Sometimes the pads of the feet are so thickened that the toes cannot be placed on the floor (11.42).

In **pseudohypoparathyroidism**, the short third, fourth and fifth metacarpals (see 9.145–9.147; pp. **184–5**) and metatarsals create dimples on the dorsum of the corre-

sponding hand and foot, with shortening of one or more fingers and toes (11.43, 11.44).

Polydactyly (11.45) is characteristically seen in the **Lawrence–Moon–Biedl syndrome** (see also 9.148; p. **185**).

The absence of hair and a reduced muscular bulk in the lower extremities of a male patient (11.46, 11.47) add substance to other features of **hypopituitarism** (see 1.96 and 1.99–1.102; p. **20**).

11.42
Acromegalic foot
with thickened sole
and heel

11.43
Pseudohypopara-
thyroidism: short
third, fourth and fifth
toes

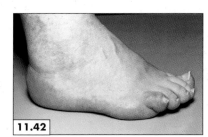

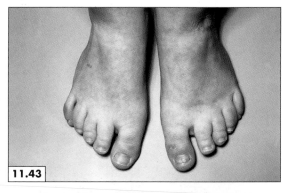

11.42

11.43

11.44
A short fourth toe due
to a corresponding
short metatarsal bone

11.45
Lawrence–Moon–Biedl
syndrome: polydactyly

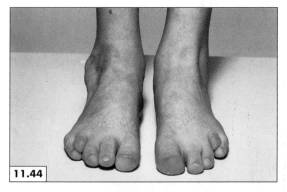

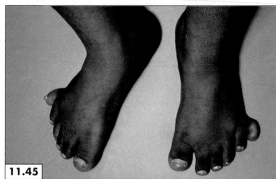

11.44

11.45

**11.46 and
11.47**
Hypopituitarism:
absent hair

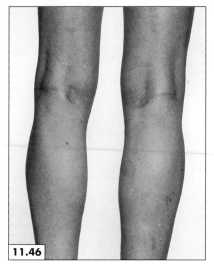

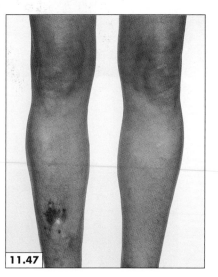

11.46

11.47

Locomotor problems

Spot diagnosis of a condition affecting the **locomotor system** of the lower limbs involves a visual scrutiny of the bones and joints and their dynamic behaviour on walking. By the time most clinicians look at the legs, they have already gained some diagnostic impressions from looking at the rest of the body. For example, this may be the time to add some final confirmatory touches to the diagnosis of **Marfan's syndrome**, by looking at the *tall* figure of the standing patient (11.48), by measuring the span *versus* the height (11.49), and by looking at the feet for the presence of *arachnodactyly* (11.50).

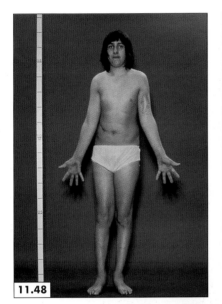

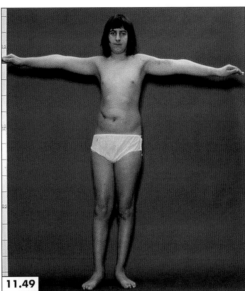

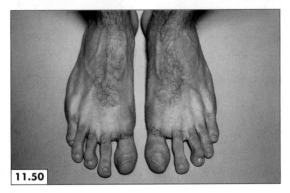

11.48 and 11.49
Marfan's syndrome: tall figure with long extremities

11.50
Arachnodactyly: long, webbed toes

Paget's disease of bone is a very common and visually arresting condition of the elderly. Part, or all of a bone or several bones may be involved. The affected tibia is often bent laterally (11.51) with bone destruction followed by excessive bone deposition, a high bone turnover, and an increased vascularity, which is often demonstrable by *warmness* of the overlying skin. The condition is often symptomless but may produce intractable pain. An **osteogenic sarcoma** is a rare complication. Paget's disease of the leg should be distinguished from the *sabre tibia* (11.52) of **late congenital syphilis**, which is caused by

osteoperiostitis with laying down of new bone over the tibia. The middle third of the tibia becomes wide with palpable irregularities along the anterior shin.

Osteoarthrosis of the knee joint often produces swelling and distortion of the surface markings of the joint (11.53, 11.54). The knee joint is the largest superficial joint in the body, and its swelling can be appreciated readily by inspection. For this purpose, the joint can be conveniently divided into two parts: the main femorotibial articulation and the patellofemoral compartment. The latter includes the suprapatellar extension of the synovial cavity and some-

11.51
Paget's tibia

11.52
Sabre tibia: a wider left leg with irregular anterior shin margin

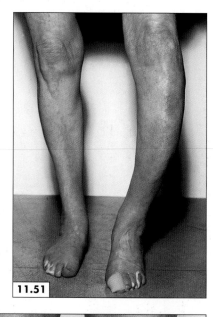

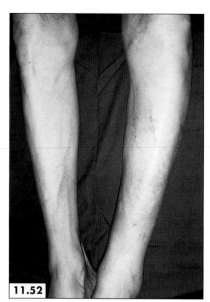

11.53
Osteoarthrosis: irregular, bulging outline

11.54
Osteoarthrosis with effusion of the knee joints

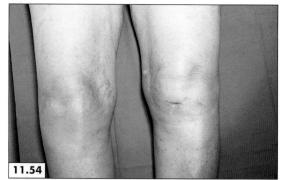

11.55 and 11.56
Advanced osteoarthrosis with effusion of the suprapatellar pouches

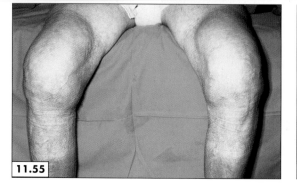

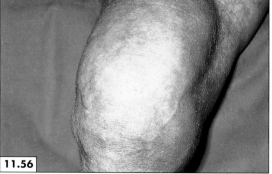

times it is this that bears the brunt of osteoarthrosis (11.55, 11.56). In such cases, a horseshoe-shaped swelling extends from the large suprapatellar pouch to the inferior border of the patella, filling in the depressions on either side of the patellar ligament.

The joint is usually painful and with the associated limited mobility there is rapid wasting of the quadriceps. With advanced damage the joint becomes unstable and may develop a varus (11.57) or a valgus deformity (11.58).

When there is also an effusion with osteoarthrosis the joint tends to be warm although less so than in **septic arthritis** (11.59), **gout, pseudogout** (11.60), **haemarthrosis** (usually in a **haemophiliac patient**) (11.61) and in **rheumatoid arthritis** (11.62). Since all these conditions raise differing management implications, the cause of the effusion, which has been detected clinically by palpation (*fluctuation*), should be established by aspiration, microscopy and culture.

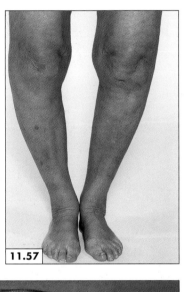

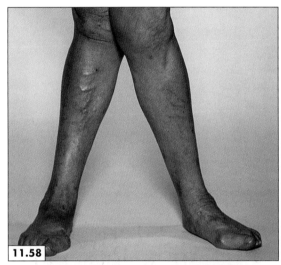

11.57
Osteoarthrosis: genu varus

11.58
Osteoarthrosis: genu valgum

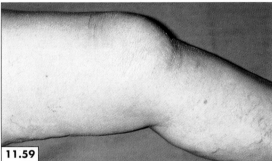

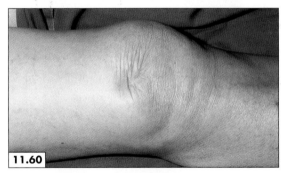

11.59
Acute monoarthritis with effusion: swollen joint with loss of surface markings

11.60
Pseudogout

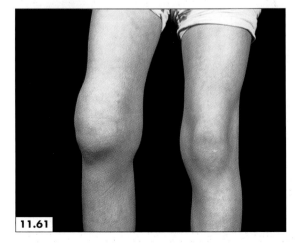

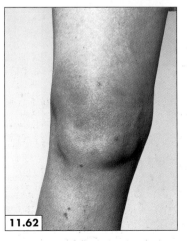

11.61
Acute effusion of the right knee joint (haemarthrosis)

11.62
Effusion of the knee joint in a patient with rheumatoid arthritis

Osteoarthrosis results when there is an imbalance between the mechanical demands and the joint stability, as happens often from excessive mechanical pressure associated with obesity. Nevertheless, marked joint laxity in the **Ehlers–Danlos syndrome** with a normal degree of mechanical pressure can achieve the same result (11.63). Note the 'cigarette-paper' scars on the skin overlying the joint.

Septic arthritis usually has an acute onset with malaise, toxaemia and fever. The affected ankle (11.64) or knee joint is painful, swollen, warm, tender and semiflexed to relieve the pressure on the capsule (11.65). Acute effusions should always be regarded with suspicion and the safe rule is *always to aspirate such joints for bacteriological investigation*. The objective is early treatment and prevention of pus formation.

The knee is among the most commonly affected weight-bearing joints to be involved in **rheumatoid arthritis** with synovial hypertrophy and often with effusion (11.66). The

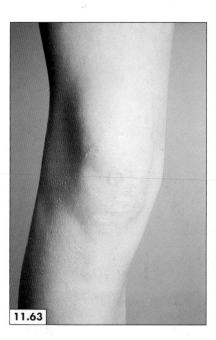

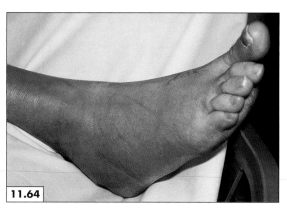

11.63
Ehlers–Danlos syndrome: osteoarthrosis of the knee joint with thin, whitish, papery scars ('papyraceous' scars) in the skin

11.64
Acute swelling of the ankle joint with erythematous overlying skin

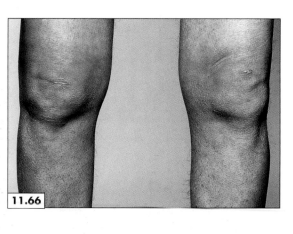

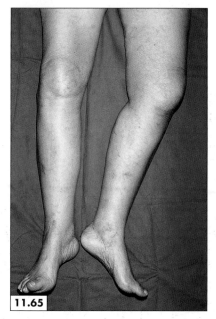

11.65
Septic arthritis of the left knee joint

11.66
Rheumatoid arthritis: thickened synovium causing bulging skin folds

diagnosis may be made by association with the relevant abnormalities elsewhere and by aspiration (11.67, 11.68). The enlargement of the semimembranous bursa into the popliteal space (*Baker's cyst*), and its rupture producing swelling of the leg, may mimic acute phlebothrombosis (11.69, 11.70). In either case, the patient presents with an acute, painful swelling of the calf. An effusion of the knee joint confirmed by aspiration favours rheumatoid arthritis as the aetiology of the swelling. An ultrasonogram and arthrography will help confirm the diagnosis.

As in the fingers, digital arteritis may result in an infarction of a toe (11.71, 11.72). Larger areas of ischaemia

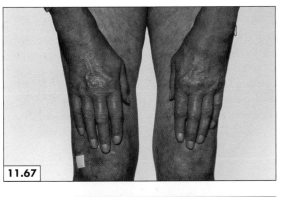
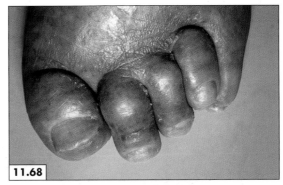

11.67 and 11.68 Rheumatoid arthritis of the hands, knees and toes

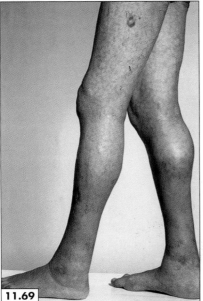
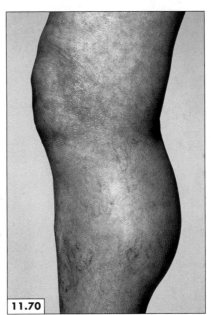

11.69 and 11.70 Ruptured Baker's cyst: swelling confined to the upper compartment of the leg

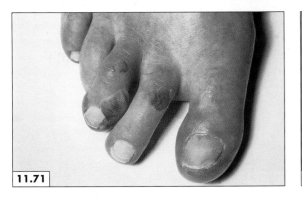
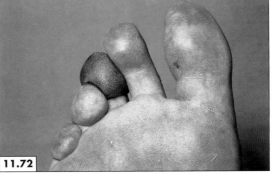

11.71 and 11.72 Rheumatoid arthritis with digital arteritis: infarction of the third toe

may occur in the lower extremities, with the development of ulcers over the malleoli (11.73). These ulcers are often covered with slough (11.74) and are difficult to heal. Rheumatoid vasculitis is frequently associated with a systemic disturbance (e.g., malaise, anaemia, fever, toxaemia).

Gout is the commonest form of **crystal arthropathy**. An attack of **acute gouty arthritis** classically involves the first metatarsophalangeal joint with pain, oedema and intense inflammation (11.75, 11.76). *Exquisite tenderness* is a prominent clinical feature and the patient, who often wakes up with the attack, cannot bear the weight of the bedclothes on the affected foot. Movements are very painful and the patient is unable to dorsiflex the big toe (11.77). Most such patients have had *asymptomatic hyperuricaemia* for many years, before the urate crystals accumulated in the joint and provoked an acute attack. During the acute episode, the serum uric acid level may be normal. The diagnosis depends on the characteristic clinical presentation and also on the demonstration of negatively birefringent needle-shaped urate crystals in the aspirated fluid, seen under polarized light microscopy.

11.73 and 11.74
Infarction ulcers with well-defined, raised margins and slough in the base

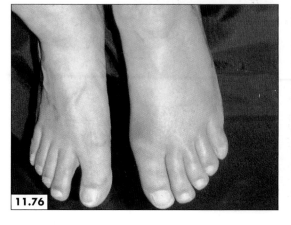

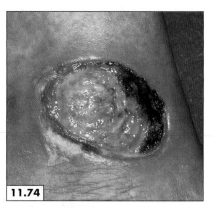

11.75
Swollen, inflamed first metatarsophalangeal joint

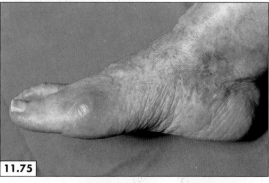

11.76 and 11.77
Acute gouty arthritis: erythematous skin over the first metatarsophalangeal joint and loss of dorsiflexion

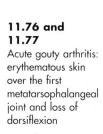

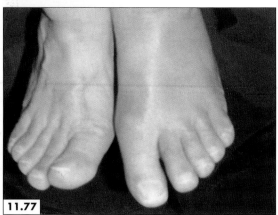

Recurrent attacks and tophaceous deposits of urate produce swelling and distortion of the affected toes (11.78, 11.79). These deposits sometimes invade the bone and ulcerate through the skin, giving rise to a punched-out ulcer on the head of the first metatarsal (11.80; see also 9.19–9.25; pp. **160–1**).

Pyrophosphate arthropathy (chondrocalcinosis, pseudogout) is a progressive degenerative joint disease that results from the deposition of calcium pyrophosphate crystals in the joints. Like gout, acute attacks may occur with pain, effusion and a systemic reaction but, unlike gout, both sexes are involved and larger joints such as the shoulders and knees are commonly affected (11.81).

Sometimes the diagnosis is made incidentally in an elderly patient whose radiograph of the knee joint shows a rim of calcification in the articular cartilage. More often gout is suspected in a swollen and painful knee joint (11.82). The correct diagnosis is made when pleomorphic pyrophosphate crystals are discovered in the aspirated fluid, which show weakly positive birefringence on polarized light microscopy. In a few patients, the condition

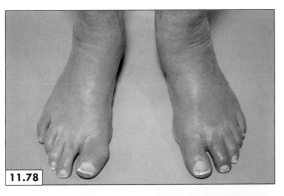

11.78

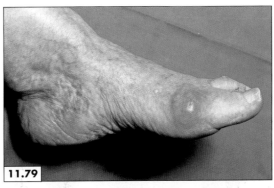

11.79

11.78 and 11.79
Recurrent gouty arthritis: tophaceous deposits with overlying shiny skin

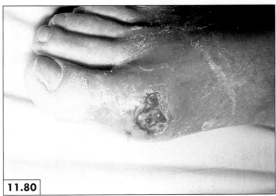

11.80

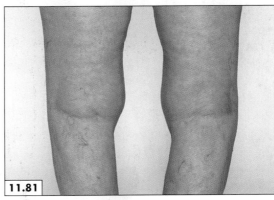

11.81

11.80
An ulcerated tophus

11.81
Recurrent attacks of pseudogout in the knees with pre-existing osteoarthrosis

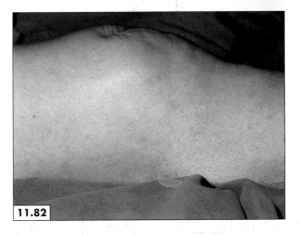

11.82

11.82
Acute monoarthritis: pseudogout

is associated with hyperparathyroidism, haemochromatosis, hypophosphatasia, gout, diabetes mellitus, acromegaly or Wilson's disease.

Charcot's (neuropathic) arthropathy characteristically involves the hip or knee joints (11.83, 11.84) in **tabes dorsalis**, which is a condition of syphilitic aetiology, and is so named because of the loss of the posterior column. As a result of the massive destructive changes, the joint is grossly misshapen (11.85) with joint instability and abnormal movements.

Neuromuscular disorders

There are only a few *visually static* signs in the lower extremities (e.g. wasting, burns, ulcers, deformity) that suggest the presence of a neurological disorder. Even when one takes account of the *visually dynamic* signs such as fasciculation, dyskinetic movements and abnormalities of the gait, inspection plays a relatively small part in the neurological evaluation of the lower limbs. Nonetheless, whenever a neurologically *relevant* sign is present, it is mostly unmistakable, visually arresting and highly specific. For example, *pes cavus* and *clawing of the toes* may be present without any neurological disorder, but there is also a high degree of association with one of the **hereditary ataxias** or **Charcot–Marie–Tooth disease** (hereditary motor and sensory neuropathy), as seen in these two patients (11.86, 11.87). There is distal wasting and the feet are slightly inverted, suggesting a weakness of the peroneal muscles. When considered with the other findings, the diagnosis can be made by inspection alone.

Foot drop (loss of eversion and dorsiflexion) with wasting of the anterior tibial and peroneal muscles, usually occurs when **the common peroneal nerve is injured at the head of the fibula** (from a fracture or compression). It is superficial here as it winds around the neck of the bone to divide into the superficial and deep peroneal nerves. Thin

11.83
Charcot's arthropathy in tabes dorsalis: a disarticulated left knee joint

11.84
Charcot's knee joint

11.85
A misshapen, disarticulated knee joint

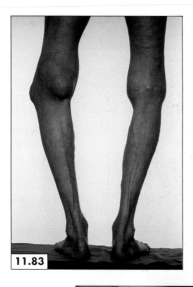

11.83

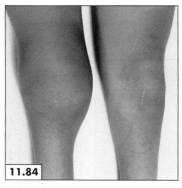

11.84

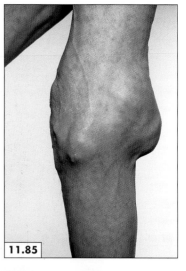

11.85

11.86 and 11.87
Charcot–Marie–Tooth disease: bilateral club feet with clawing of the toes. The toes are so clawed that they can only touch the ground if the heels are elevated

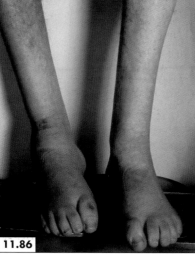

11.86

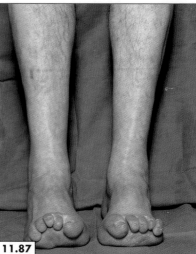

11.87

and undernourished patients and some healthy subjects are susceptible to pressure palsy of the nerve, sometimes induced by sitting with the legs crossed for prolonged periods. Such patients are unable to evert and dorsiflex the toes at the metatarsophalangeal joints (11.88). Sensory loss depends on the level and the extent of the lesion. The patient can stand on the toes but not on the heel of the affected leg. The ankle jerk is preserved. Preservation of inversion of the ankle (tibialis posterior) distinguishes a lesion of the common peroneal nerve from that of L4/5 root.

Compression or injury to the nerve before the division, or to the superficial peroneal nerve, will result in loss of sensation over the front and lateral aspects of the leg and over the dorsum of the foot (11.89).

Spastic foot drop (11.90) can occur if the lesion is in the spinal cord, as in this patient with **syringomyelia**. Such a

patient may have kyphoscoliosis, wasting of the small muscles of the hands, absent reflexes in the upper limbs, brisk reflexes in the legs, dissociated sensory loss (loss of temperature and pain with the retention of touch, position and vibration sensations) and extensor plantars.

Wasting and a lack of prominence of the muscles in one limb compared with its fellow in a standing patient (11.91) suggests **old poliomyelitis**. The affected leg tends to be shorter because of growth impairment from early childhood when the disease was contracted.

Gross muscle wasting affecting both limbs with foot drop (11.92) can represent a part of generalized muscle wasting that is characteristic of **progressive muscular atrophy (motor neurone disease)**. However, cord compression, syphilitic amyotrophy and old poliomyelitis are among the conditions that should be excluded when considering such a diagnosis.

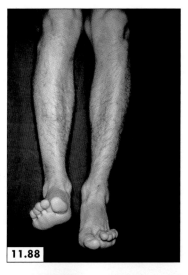

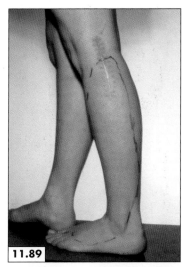

11.88 and 11.89
Left common peroneal nerve palsy: loss of dorsiflexion and eversion. Note the marked area of sensory loss

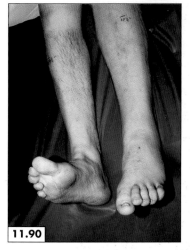

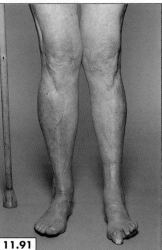

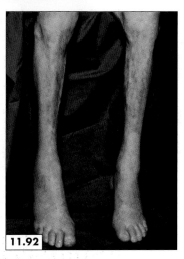

11.90
Foot drop

11.91
Old poliomyelitis of the left leg

11.92
Motor neurone disease: generalized muscle wasting and bilateral foot drop

Vascular and other systemic disorders

After having looked for some familiar examples of endocrine, locomotor and neurological disorders, there remains a group of signs that is always associated with the legs, and has a great relevance to some specific systemic disorders. Since the lower limbs contain a large network of vessels, there are quite a few vascular disorders that develop in the legs with their various manifestations. As a part of the inspection routine, the clinician should specifically check for signs of:

- Oedema (11.93);
- Phlebothrombosis (11.94);
- Peripheral vascular insufficiency (11.95);
- Vasculitis (11.96).

Oedema of the legs can point to a variety of underlying disorders such as congestive cardiac failure, hepatic failure, venous obstruction and severe hypoalbuminaemia, but it is not specific to any one of them. Apart from ascertaining whether the swelling is solid, as in myxoedema or lymphoedema (11.97), or is caused by fluid and hence pits on pressure (11.98), one can get very little insight into the underlying disorder without a proper clinical assessment of all the systems.

11.93
Oedema

11.94
Deep venous thrombosis: a bulky right leg with oedema and obscured articular features of the knee joint

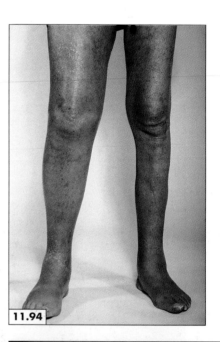

11.95
Arterial insufficiency with cyanosis and erythema

11.96
Necrotizing vasculitis with 'palpable purpura' and crusted sites of cutaneous infarction

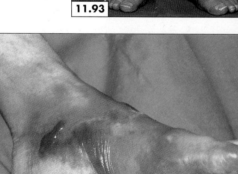

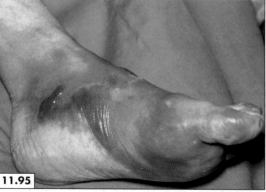

Deep venous thrombosis produces oedema and induration of the surrounding tissues increasing the girth of the affected leg (11.99), and the thigh if extending to the femoral vein (11.94), with shiny, inflamed and tender overlying skin. As already stated, the legs should be inspected routinely for signs of phlebothrombosis, since this major source of potentially lethal emboli is asymptomatic in approximately one-half of the cases.

Deep vein thrombosis should be distinguished from **superficial thrombophlebitis**, which is painful and visually startling (11.100) but does not cause embolic complications. It occurs frequently after pregnancy and in patients with varicose veins. A migratory form of superficial thrombophlebitis (11.101) occurs in thromboangiitis obliterans and autoimmune haemolytic anaemia.

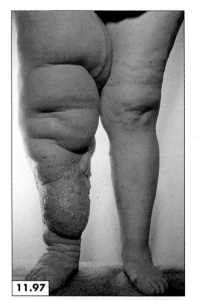

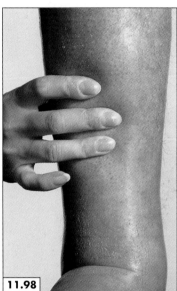

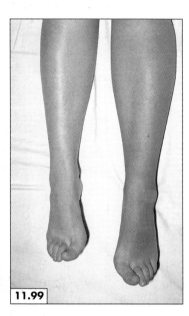

11.97
Lymphoedema: solid, nonpitting, deforming swelling

11.98
Pitting oedema of fluid retention

11.99
Phlebothrombosis

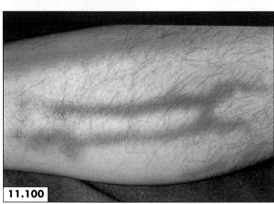

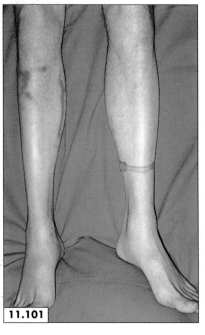

11.100
Thrombophlebitis: red, inflamed streaks along the course of veins

11.101
Thrombophlebitis of superficial veins

11.102
Varicose veins: tortuous, engorged superficial veins

11.103
Diffuse varicosities along the course of veins

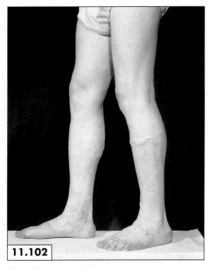

11.102

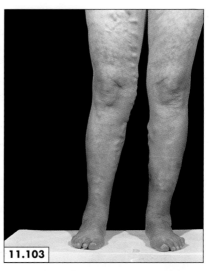

11.103

11.104
Chronic arterial insufficiency: wasting, cyanosis and microinfarcts

11.105
Arterial insufficiency with cyanosis of the forefoot and toes

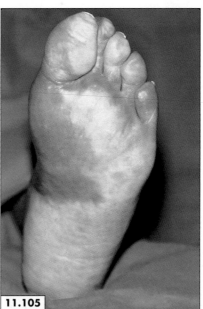

11.104

11.105

11.106
Ischaemia with erythema over pressure points at the base and tip of the big toe

11.107
Ischaemia with superimposed cellulitis

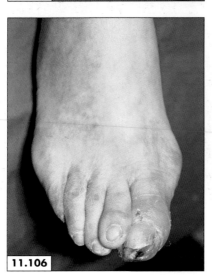

11.106

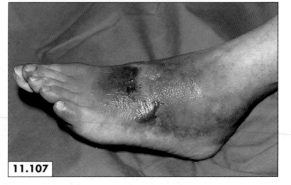

11.107

Varicose veins are abnormally distended, tortuous and easily visible in an ambulant subject (11.102). The condition is slowly progressive with advancing age leading to gross distension of veins on the legs and thighs (11.103). Pregnancy, ascites and congenitally absent or defective valves may be the cause in some cases, but in most patients no clearly identifiable reason can be found.

Peripheral arterial insufficiency produces profound changes in the appearance of the legs. Often there is pallor of the legs, cyanosis of the *cold* feet from stagnation and desaturation of the blood, muscular wasting in long-standing cases and small areas of infarction (11.104). The arterial pulses are absent. The rate of restoration of a pink colour, after skin blanching on digital pressure, on the pads of toes is delayed. More commonly, one or more cutaneous ulcers may appear on the leg as the first telling sign of the circulatory disorder.

In severe cases of **atherosclerosis obliterans** one or more toes or a portion of the foot may become dusky (11.105). The skin is usually cold, dry and puckered over the pads of the toes owing to atrophy of the underlying soft tissues. Ulceration and gangrene may form on the terminal parts of the toes, usually around the nails (11.106) and, in time,

these can become loose and slough off from their bases. The tips of the nails are vulnerable from the normal pressure of the shoes in ordinary walking. The process is worse in the other foot of this patient because of a combination of ischaemia and cellulitis (11.107).

Even trivial mechanical or thermal trauma, unnoticed by the patient, may set up the ulceration and the gangrenous process at the tips of toes (11.108). Ischaemic ulcers tend to have a somewhat pale base and dry margins (11.109). These lesions seldom cause systemic effects with toxaemia unless secondary infection supervenes and spreading cellulitis develops. Unlike neuropathic ulcers, which are often painless, ischaemic ulcers usually cause severe pain, especially on elevation of the leg. Gangrene also develops on other pressure areas such as the heels, malleoli and the first and fifth metatarsal heads.

Infarctive (Martorell's) ulceration characteristically affects the lower legs of hypertensive patients (posterolaterally or medially) (11.110), especially in those who also have diabetes. These ulcers are caused by avascular necrosis of the skin, they develop rapidly with severe pain, do not appear on pressure areas and are single and large with a red base (11.111).

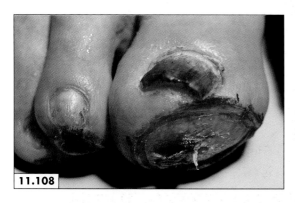

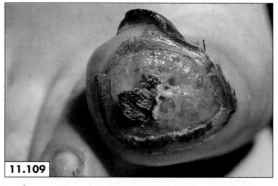

11.108 and 11.109
Inflamed, gangrenous toe tips with an ulcer and haemorrhagic crusts

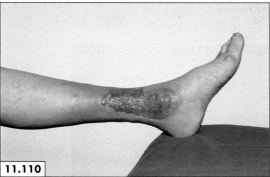

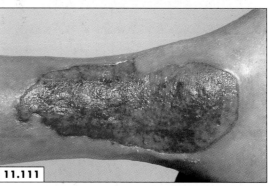

11.110 and 11.111
Martorell's ulcer: punched-out, sharply demarcated ulcer with a haemorrhagic base and an erythematous halo around it

Large single ulcers on the legs, as described above, should be distinguished from the ulcers of **pyoderma gangrenosum**, which have oedematous undermined edges (11.112). These can occur anywhere on the body but are often seen on the thighs and legs where they may be confused with ischaemic ulcers (11.111). Pyoderma gangrenosum is associated characteristically with **chronic ulcerative colitis** and occurs in approximately 10% of patients with the disease. Approximately one-half of the patients with these ulcers are found to have ulcerative colitis, Crohn's disease, rheumatoid arthritis, dysproteinaemias, leukaemias and lymphomas. In the remaining half no cause is found.

The initial lesion is an erythematous plaque in which pustules develop (11.113). These small ulcers coalesce to form a large ulcer, with a bluish, oedematous, undermined edge and necrotic areas on the red base (11.114). The ulcer usually relates to the severity of the bowel disease and sometimes is a presenting feature.

Thromboangiitis obliterans (Buerger's disease) occurs predominantly in young (25–40 years of age), male smokers of *all* races and occupations. Pain in its various forms (intermittent claudication, rest pain in the digits and, in the later stages, pain of ischaemic neuropathy, ulceration and osteoporosis) is the outstanding symptom. Ulceration and gangrene develop early, usually in one extremity at a time (11.115), most frequently in the distal half of the digits around the margins of the nails (11.116). This suggests that the pressure on the nails from shoes during walking may be enough to cause necrosis of the skin and tissues, which have impaired blood supply.

11.112
Pyoderma gangrenosum with raised undermined borders and haemorrhagic exudate

11.113
A haemorrhagic pustule

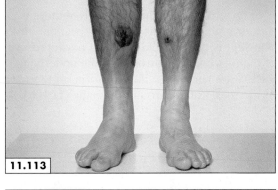

11.114
Pyoderma gangrenosum: erythematous, irregular margin and necrotic ulcer

11.115
Thromboangiitis obliterans: gangrene and loss of terminal digits

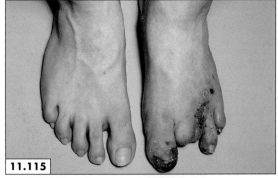

11.116
Thromboangiitis obliterans with recurrent gangrene of the toes

11.117
Thromboangiitis obliterans with segmental thrombophlebitis

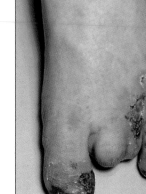

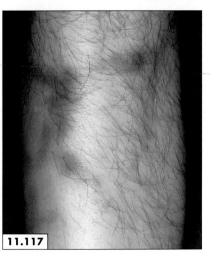

Segmental thrombophlebitis of small and medium-sized veins (11.117) occurs at some stage in well over one-third of cases. The lesions usually develop acutely as red, raised and tender cords, 0.5–4 cm in length. When seen in association with occlusive arterial disease, the diagnosis of thromboangiitis obliterans must be considered.

Digital arteritis leading to gangrene of the toes is a well-known complication of **rheumatoid arthritis**. As in thromboangiitis obliterans, the pressure areas around the nails are vulnerable (11.118), but the changes of arterial occlusion usually affect the sides of the digits and then involve the entire toe (11.119). The proximal arteries in the feet and legs are palpable unless there is a coexistent atherosclerosis obliterans. Moreover, the articular changes of rheumatoid arthritis make the diagnosis comparatively easy.

Vasculitis, or inflammatory and proliferative changes of small arteries and arterioles, occurs in many heterogeneous systemic disorders (see p. **56**). The vasculocutaneous manifestations of these diseases are not always specific to any particular entity but point to a group of well-known conditions and are therefore regarded as *fundamental signs*.

Erythema nodosum is by far the commonest vasculocutaneous disorder characterized by the acute appearance of inflammatory, nonsuppurative, tender cutaneous and subcutaneous nodules on the extremities (11.120) and, less frequently, on the trunk. It occurs most commonly on the shins of young females (female:male ratio of 5:1), and is often associated with an arthralgia, malaise, fever and sometimes lymphadenopathy. The rash often appears 2–3 weeks after an upper respiratory tract infection.

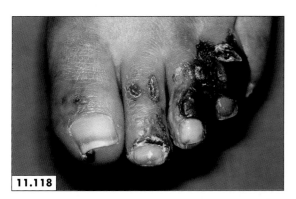

11.118

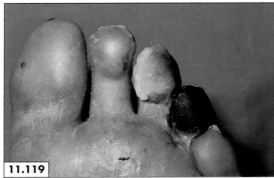

11.119

11.118 and 11.119
Rheumatoid arthritis with digital arteritis and gangrene of the toes

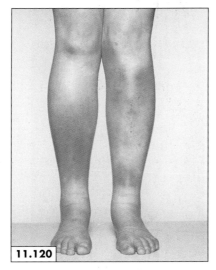

11.120

11.120
Erythema nodosum: ill-defined cutaneous nodules with erythema of the overlying skin

Dusky red, elevated, painful lesions, 2–6 cm in size with indistinct margins (11.121), appear particularly on the shins where they may merge with one another (11.122, 11.123). Over a week or so they develop a bruised appearance (11.124) and are sometimes followed by fresh lesions. The diagnosis is usually easy although sometimes, in the early stages, it may be difficult to distinguish it from cellulitis (11.125) and **nodular panniculitis** (see 9.187, 9.188; p. **193**). Streptococcal pharyngitis and sarcoidosis are among the principal underlying disorders (Table 11.3).

A careful initial inspection of the legs of a young patient brought in with a 2-day history of malaise, fever, chills, headaches, myalgia and arthralgia may prove life-saving, by revealing the cutaneous hallmark (11.126) of a potentially lethal infectious disease such as **meningococcaemia**. The cutaneous lesions are red macules accompanied by petechiae, purpura and sometimes ecchymoses (11.127). There may be red pustules with necrotic grey centres (11.128), usually suggestive of fulminant meningococcaemia with a grave prognosis. Sadly, this malignant variety has occasionally been mistaken for chicken pox!

When contemplating the diagnosis of **infective endocarditis**, the legs sould get their due share of the clinician's attention for the search for *Osler's nodes* on the toes and soles (11.129, 11.130), and for *Janeway lesions* (11.131). Figure 11.129 shows an Osler node on the big toe which was *palpable* and *tender*. Janeway lesions, in contrast, are nontender, small macules, approximately 1–4 mm in diameter, which develop on the palms, soles, ankles, ears, flanks and forearms. They are common in **acute bacterial endocarditis** and seldom occur in bacteraemia without endocarditis.

Wegener's granulomatosis is characterized by focal necrotizing lesions in the upper respiratory tract (lethal midline granuloma) and lungs, and vasculitis in the lungs, kidneys and skin. Destructive granulomas develop in the nose (see also 1.284, 1.285; p. **56**) and sinuses. Although some patients do not complain of any symptoms, direct

Table 11.3 Causes of erythema nodosum	
Bacterial	Streptococcal throat infection, primary tuberculosis, syphilis, leprosy, salmonella
Acute sarcoidosis	
Viruses and chlamydiae	Lymphogranuloma venereum, cat scratch disease, hepatitis B, infectious mononucleosis, psittacosis, etc.
Inflammatory bowel disease	
Yersinia infections	
Mycoses	
Drugs	Sulphonamides, penicillin, gold, salicylates, codeine, barbiturates, oral contraceptives, etc.
Malignant disorders	Leukaemias, Hodgkin's disease, lymphomas
Idiopathic	

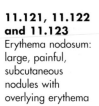

11.121, 11.122 and 11.123 Erythema nodosum: large, painful, subcutaneous nodules with overlying erythema

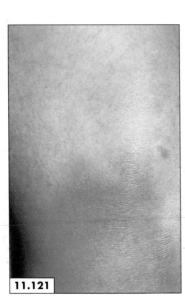

11.121

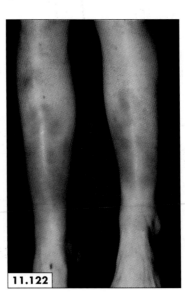

11.122

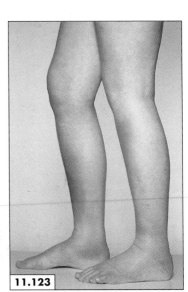

11.123

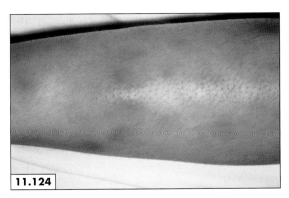

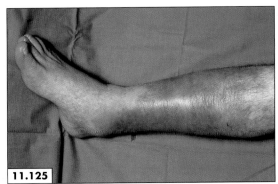

11.124
Erythema nodosum with bluish discolouration of age of the lesion

11.125
Cellulitis: diffuse swelling and erythema

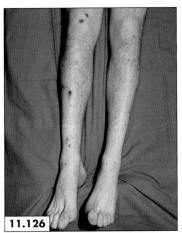

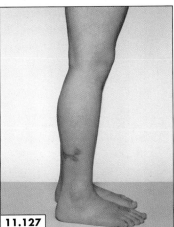

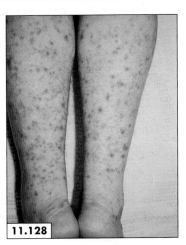

11.126, 11.127 and 11.128
Acute meningococcaemia: palpable purpura and purpura fulminans

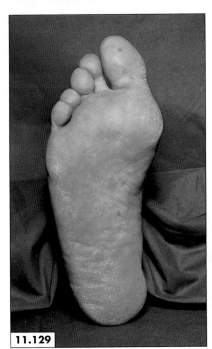

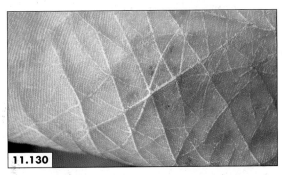

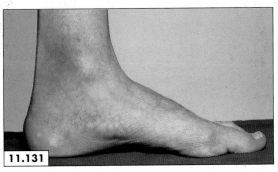

11.129
Osler's nodes: small, purplish, subcutaneous nodules on the sole and pulp of the great toe

11.130
Osler's nodes on the sole

11.131
Janeway lesions: haemorrhagic, infarcted macules and papules

questioning often reveals a recent history of catarrh, cough and pain in the region of sinuses. The cutaneous changes are of macules, papules, ulcerating purpuric nodules and pustules (11.132, 11.133). The usual course is a local spread of the granulomas in the nasopharynx, a generalized advance of the vasculitis in the kidneys and skin (11.134), and death within 2 years from renal failure. In a few cases, a limited form of this disorder has been reported in which the kidneys are not involved and the prognosis is good.

The **Henoch–Schönlein syndrome (anaphylactoid purpura)** is a form of *necrotizing vasculitis* of small vessels, affecting children and young adults, with involvement of the bowel, joints, skin and kidneys. The clinical manifestations include *palpable purpura* on the lower extremities (11.135, 11.136) and buttocks (11.137) from a leucocytoclastic vasculitis of the dermal vessels, arthralgia of large joints (usually knees and ankles), and gastrointestinal involvement with colic, haemorrhage and intussusception.

11.132
Wegener's granulomatosis with palpable purpura and crusted, infarcted lesions

11.133
Necrotizing vasculitis with haemorrhagic bullae

11.134
Vasculitis with diffuse 'palpable purpura'

11.135 and 11.136
Henoch–Schönlein syndrome with 'palpable purpura' on the legs

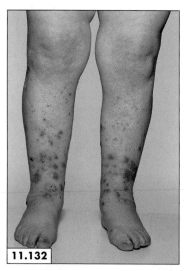

11.132

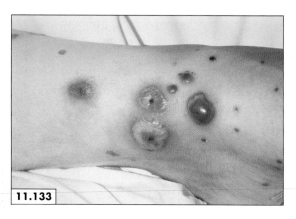

11.133

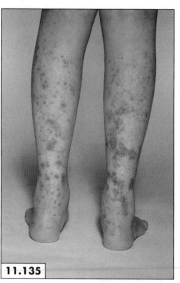

11.134

11.135

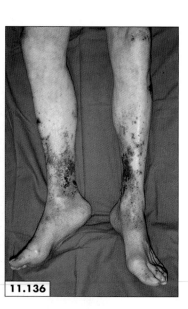

11.136

The most serious association is nephritis, which resembles IgA nephropathy and occurs in approximately 30% of patients. The disorder follows some 2 weeks after an upper respiratory tract infection. After a short prodromal phase, the rash appears initially as macules, which rapidly become purpuric (11.138), sometimes with central necrosis (11.139). A confident clinical diagnosis can be made if a young patient (aged 20 years or less) develops palpable purpura, mostly on the legs and buttocks, and he or she also has some symptoms of bowel angina (diffuse abdominal pain, worse after meals, often with bloody diarrhoea).

Livido reticularis, or a bluish-red mottling of the skin (11.140), related to small vessel occlusion, may occur as a result of vasculitis in association with **polyarteritis nodosa** and **systemic lupus erythematosus**. In some cases there may be no associated disease, while in others it may be the result of impaired perfusion, as in **atherosclerosis obliterans** and in cholesterol embolization, or due to *hyperviscosity*, as in **cryoglobulinaemia** and hyperglobulinaemia. In systemic lupus erythematosus there may be nailfold infarcts (11.141) and a variety of other cutaneous lesions (see 9.80, 9.81, 10.76–10.78; pp. **173**, **210–11**).

Indurated, smooth, red or plum-coloured nodules or plaques (11.142) occur in **B-cell lymphoma**. The lesions are firm, nontender, fixed subcutaneous masses.

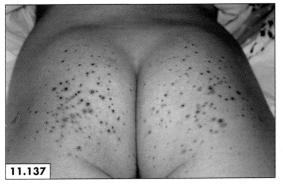

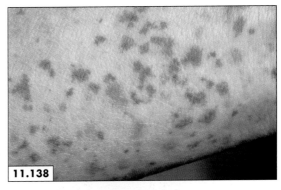

11.137 and 11.138 Palpable purpura with crusted, haemorrhagic infarcts

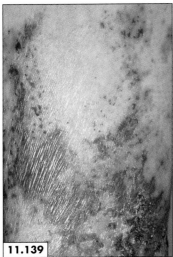

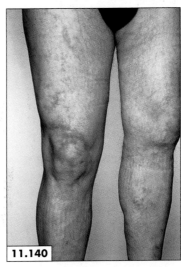

11.139 Crusted, multiple cutaneous infarcts

11.140 Polyarteritis nodosa: bluish-red mottling of the skin and multiple, reddish dermal nodules

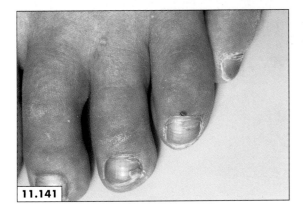

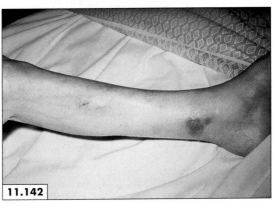

11.141 Systemic lupus erythematosus: nailfold infarcts

11.142 B-cell lymphoma: confluent, violaceous nodules

Skin lesions

The separation of this section from the preceding sections that also refer to conditions with cutaneous manifestations is not entirely arbitrary. Some commonly seen skin lesions such as purpura and petechiae have been referred to in the section on vasculitis because these are only a pointer to an underlying disorder. The conditions described here are mostly of dermatological interest in which the diagnosis does not begin, as in the previous section, but may end with the cutaneous lesion. Most of these disorders have been described in other chapters, and will be mentioned here briefly in as much as they affect the lower limbs.

As suggested elsewhere (see pp. **58** and **166** and Tables 1.5, 9.1), the diagnosis of skin lesions depends on the char-acteristics of a single as well as a group of lesions, their distribution, and on the associated features. An expert dermatologist will recognize **ringworm** infection at first sight (11.143) but a beginner will also reach the diagnosis by looking closely at the red, scaly, macular lesions that have spread peripherally, forming a somewhat circular patch (hence the name ringworm). This patient also had fungal involvement of the soles (tinea pedis) with fine, silvery scaling, fissuring and erythema (11.144).

Sharply marginated, round or oval macules varying in size and colour occur in **tinea versicolor (pityriasis versicolor)** (11.145, 11.146). The colour of the macules tends to contrast with that of the surrounding skin, either brown or white, and the usual site of predilection is the trunk (11.147). Sometimes the legs are predominantly involved and the macules may be white, brown or reddish-brown (11.148).

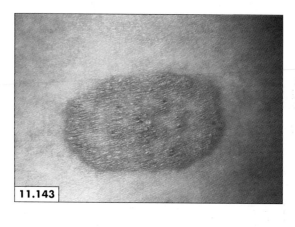

11.143
Ringworm: sharply marginated plaque with scaling

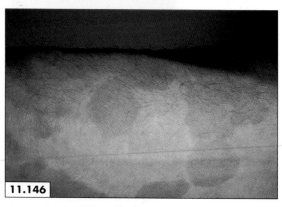

11.144
Tinea pedis: diffuse erythema with scaling and fissuring

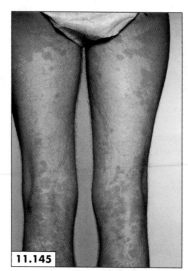

11.145
Tinea versicolor: confluent, darkish pink macules

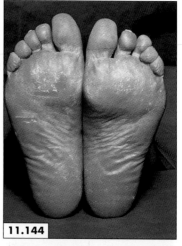

11.146
Tinea versicolor: sharply marginated, large, pinkish macules

The diagnosis of **psoriasis** is easy when erythematous patches covered with thick, silvery-white keratotic plaques are localized to the extensor surface of the knees (11.149). However, difficulty may be experienced in the generalized form when sharply marginated red plaques are distributed on both legs (11.150, 11.151). Often a careful look will reveal silvery-white scales over some of the plaques. Furthermore, an examination of the hairline, the elbows and the nails should remove any remaining anxiety. In lichen planus and psoriasis typical lesions sometimes appear along the line of traumatized skin (*Koebner phenomenon*), damaged by scratching (11.152) or surgery.

Erythematous papules and small haemorrhagic vesicles distributed in *groups* (11.153) and associated with severe itching suggest a diagnosis of **dermatitis herpetiformis**. The

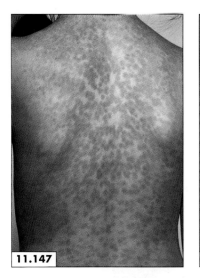

11.147

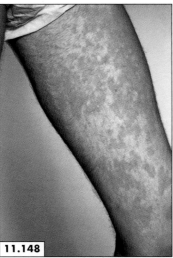

11.148

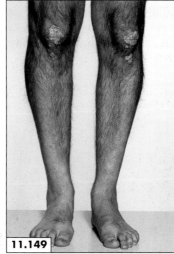

11.149

11.147
Sharply marginated, brown and pinkish-brown macules

11.148
Brownish-red macules on pale skin

11.149
Psoriasis: plaques covered with silvery scales

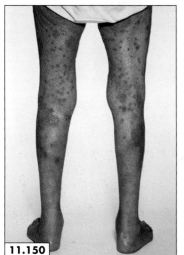

11.150

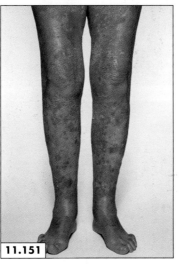

11.151

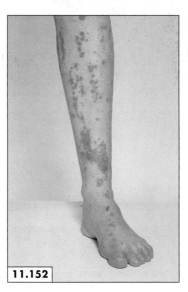

11.152

11.150 and 11.151
Psoriasis: sharply marginated, erythematous papules and plaques, some with fine silvery scales

11.152
Koebner phenomenon: linear eruption of psoriatic lesion over the scratch marks

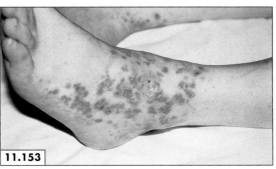

11.153

11.153
Dermatitis herpetiformis: crops of papules and ruptured vesicles around the ankle

lesions tend to be in groups but may be of variable size and shape (11.154). The vesicles may have collapsed leaving behind a denuded red base and, in some cases, the collapsed roof may form a crust over the base (11.155). In approximately one-fifth of patients, erythematous blotches, looking like urticarial weals, may appear in a linear pattern with IgA deposition (11.156).

Apart from dermatitis herpetiformis, there are two other common conditions, **pemphigus** and **pemphigoid**, which are characterized by the presence of blisters. In **pemphigus**, the bullae are initially skin-coloured and contain serous fluid (11.157). They arise on normal skin, are round or oval, and are distributed throughout the body in a random pattern. Since these bullae are intraepidermal they rupture easily and leave raw areas, which are tender to touch and are spread over a large area of the skin (11.158).

Pemphigus occurs most commonly in patients between the ages of 40 and 60 years and affects women more than men. The mucous membrane of the mouth is almost always involved. In contrast, **pemphigoid** is a bullous disease of the aged in which large, tense and sometimes haemorrhagic blisters arise on normal or erythematous skin (11.159, 11.160). The diseae only occasionally involves the mucous membrane and may remain localized to the legs, but often becomes widespread.

11.154 and 11.155
Dermatitis herpetiformis: collapsed blisters with denuded, red bases

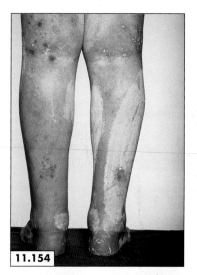

11.154

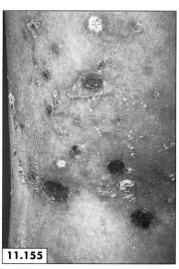

11.155

11.156
Dermatitis herpetiformis: urticarial weals with erythematous skin

11.157
Pemphigus: thin blisters containing serous fluid

11.158
Pemphigus: ruptured blisters with red areas

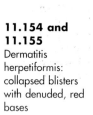

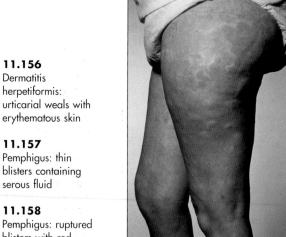

11.156

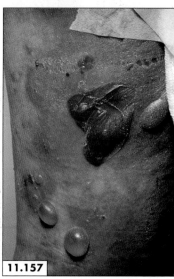

11.157

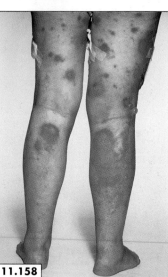

11.158

Discoid (nummular) eczema has a predilection for the hands and lower legs of older males where groups of small papules and vesicles appear on an erythematous base (11.161). The lesions may coalesce into rounded or coin-shaped (Latin *'nummularis'* – 'like a coin') plaques, 4–6 cm in diameter, and have an erythematous base with an indistinct border. Crusts and excoriations are present. The skin over the hands and lower legs tends to become dry, particularly during the winter months. The patient often scratches, setting up an inflammatory base on which the vesicles and papules arise.

Nodular prurigo occurs in anxious patients who com-pulsively dig the fingernails into the skin of any accessible area. These patients usually admit that the lesions are self-inflicted but say that they are unable to stop themselves, for reasons of chronic itching, irritation, or for no reason at all. The lesions are nodules or slightly elevated papules, some covered with a blood crust and some, in which the crusts have fallen off, with a depigmented top (11.162, 11.163). Although many such patients have *neurodermatitis (neurotic itch)*, sometimes with delusions of parasitophobia, occasionally there may be a serious underlying disorder such as a lymphoma.

Drug eruptions can be caused by almost any drug and

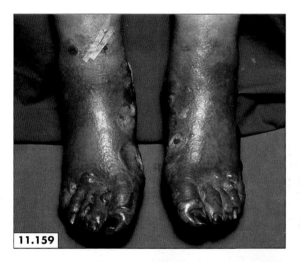

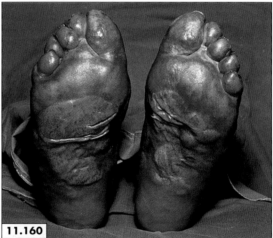

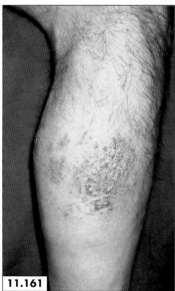

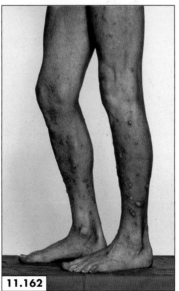

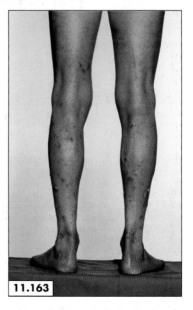

11.159 and 11.160 Pemphigoid: diffuse erythematous skin with ruptured and intact blisters

11.161 Nummular eczema: a round nummular plaque with erythema, scales and crusts and some satellite lesions

11.162 and 11.163 Nodular prurigo: papules and nodules scattered in the legs, some with depigmented tops

can mimic virtually any morphological expression in dermatology. A pleomorphic rash containing pinpoint-sized to large macules and papules, some discrete/some confluent forming erythematous patches, and some lichenified, appear symmetrically on the trunk and extremities as in this patient (11.164) who was taking nitrazepam. A drug rash must occupy the first place in the differential diagnosis of the appearance of a sudden, itchy, symmetrical eruption.

The **penicillin rash** is one of the commonest exanthemata, sometimes with urticaria (11.165), encountered in clinical practice. Sometimes urticarial weals (11.166) appear on the face, upper and lower extremities (11.167) and the trunk (11.168) in patients on penicillin, salicylates or erythromycin.

Repeated exposure to heat from a fire causes a reddish-brown reticular discolouration on the legs referred to as

11.164
Drug eruption: diffuse maculopapular lesions

11.165
Penicillin rash: diffuse urticaria

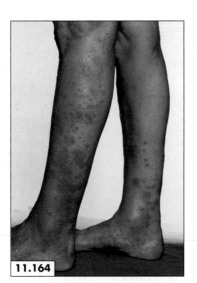

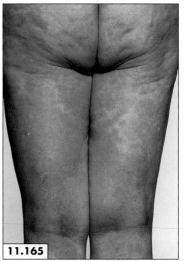

11.166
Urticaria: raised, reddish weals

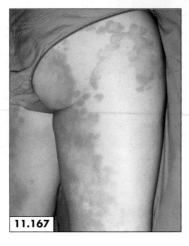

11.167 and 11.168
Urticaria: maculopapular lesions with urticarial weals

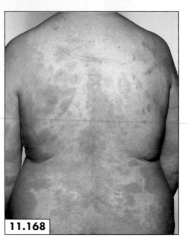

erythema ab igne (11.169). Chronic exposure of the skin to heat produces a heavy deposit of melanin in the basal layer of the epidermis over the capillary network, forming the dark brown reticulation (11.170). In some cases, with recurrent exposure to a high intensity of heat, abrasions and ulcerations are formed, which heal with depigmentation (11.171). There are two main clinical implications of erythema ab igne. First, there may be an underlying disorder of cold-intolerance such as **hypothyroidism**. Second, continual thermal damage may lead to **cutaneous malignancy**.

Palmoplantar hyperkeratosis (tylosis) occurs on the palms (see 9.107; p. **177**) but it is often more marked on the soles (11.172, 11.173).

Carotenaemia, which has been referred to in Chapter 9 (see 9.185; p. **193**), may be easily recognizable by looking at the soles (11.174).

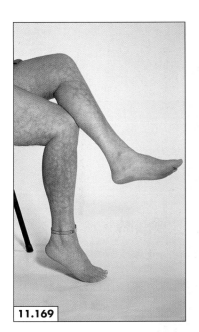
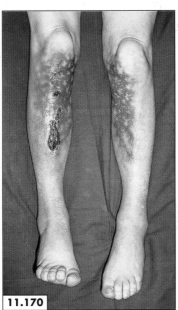
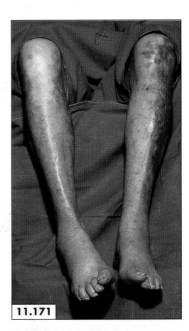

11.169, 11.170 and 11.171
Progressive erythema ab igne leading to ulceration and disordered pigmentation

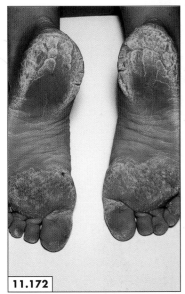
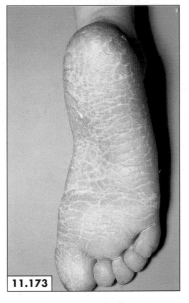
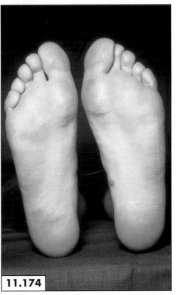

11.172 and 11.173
Tylosis: thickened skin with hyperkeratosis and fissuring

11.174
Carotenaemia: yellowish skin

Kaposi's sarcoma usually begins on the leg as a collection of bluish-red macules and papules that gradually coalesce to form larger lesions (11.175). Spread then occurs to other parts of the skin and to almost every organ, especially the gastrointestinal tract. Kaposi's sarcoma is frequently associated with the **acquired immunodeficiency syndrome** and with some cases of **lymphoma**.

Hyperlipidaemias produce a variety of cutaneous lesions on the legs. *Eruptive xanthomas* (11.176) occur in uncontrolled insulin-dependent diabetes mellitus in association with hypertriglyceridaemia. These are small, yellow papules, 1–5 mm in diameter, surrounded by a rim of erythema, and appear over the extensor surfaces, particularly over the joints of the limbs and buttocks. Although the lesions present most often in diabetes with an associated rapid rise in serum triglycerides, they can occur in any form of hypertriglyceridaemia. The serum is milky-white in such patients.

Tuberous xanthomas are yellowish nodules of varying size and occur on the elbows, buttocks and knees (11.177).

Tendinous xanthomas, from diffuse infiltration of the tendons with cholesterol, occur mainly on the extensor tendons (11.178, 11.179). These lesions are strongly suggestive of **familial hypercholesterolaemia**. Table 11.4 shows the relationship of various types of xanthomata with the various lipoprotein disorders.

11.175
Kaposi's sarcoma: a bluish-red papule surrounded by a yellowish-green halo

11.176
Papular eruptive xanthomata: multiple, discrete yellowish-pink papules

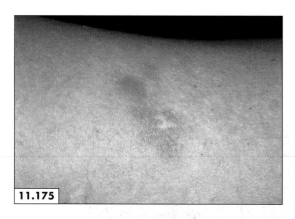

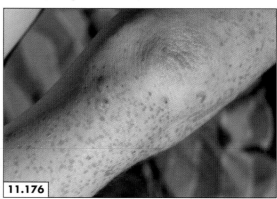

11.177
Yellowish papules and nodules

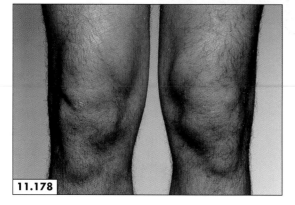

11.178 and 11.179
Tendinous xanthomata: subcutaneous nodules attached to tendons

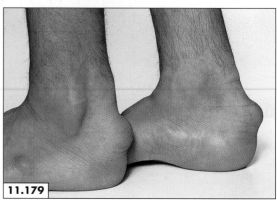

Table 11.4 Relationship of the type of xanthomata to the various types of lipoprotein disorder

Xanthomata	Lipoprotein disorder
Xanthelasmata	Normolipaemia or familial hypercholesterolaemia/ dyslipoproteinaemia
Tendon xanthomata	Type IIa familial hypercholesterolaemia
Tuberous xanthomata	Familial dyslipoproteinaemia/ hypertriglyceridaemia, familial (homozygous) hypercholesterolaemia (types IIa, III, IV)
Eruptive papular xanthomata	Familial dyslipoproteinaemia/ hypertriglyceridaemia, familial lipoprotein lipase deficiency (types I, II, IV, V), diabetes mellitus
Palmar xanthomata	Familial dyslipoproteinaemia (type III)

A **capillary haemangioma** (*port-wine stain*) can occasionally occur on the lower extremities. It is present at birth, is not raised above the level of the skin, and varies from a few centimetres in size to an extensive sheet but does not cross the midline (11.180).

Haemochromatosis may be recognized by the characteristic slate-grey pigmentation (11.181), which is the result of the deposition of haemosiderin and melanin in the skin. Such a patient may also have hepatosplenomegaly from an associated cirrhosis.

Although *clubbing* may have been noticed already in the fingers of a patient, it may be more florid in the toes (11.182).

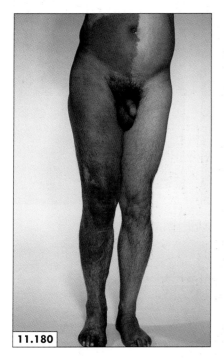

11.180

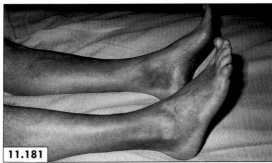

11.181

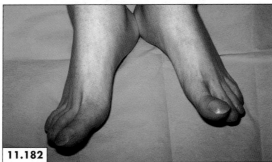

11.182

11.180
Port-wine stain

11.181
Grey and dark-brown pigmentation of sun-exposed areas

11.182
Clubbing and cyanosis of the toes

Scurvy is not as rare in the Western hemisphere as is generally supposed. The condition is caused by a dietary *deficiency of ascorbic acid*. It occurs in children who do not get citrus fruit and in old people who do not eat fruit, vegetables or salads. The disorder is characterized by anaemia, ecchymoses and *perifollicular purpura* on the skin (11.183), haemorrhages into the periostium in children, intramuscular and articular haemorrhages (11.184) and bleeding gums. The most characteristic cutaneous manifestation is seen on the calves as follicular hyperkeratotic papules with haemorrhages (11.185).

Solar dermatitis occurs on the legs as it does on other exposed parts of the body (see 1.299, 5.9, 9.68; pp. **59**, **124**, **170**). The skin is brown with a reddish tinge and excessive folds and there may be warty or reddish papules (11.186).

Keratoderma blennorrhagica (11.187) is a characteristic finding in **Reiter's syndrome** though a similar appearance is seen in **pustular psoriasis**. The lesions start as macules, papules or vesicles, which increase in size and develop pus-

tules in the centre. The surface becomes hyperkeratotic and crusted. *Subungual pustules* (11.188) result in onycholysis and hyperkeratosis. Apart from the cutaneous lesions the syndrome consists of an episode of *arthritis* (11.189), *urethritis* and *genital lesions* (11.190).

In **secondary syphilis**, papular lesions occur characteristically on the palms (see 9.205; p. **196**) and soles (11.191).

Larva migrans (*creeping eruption*) is an infection by a larval nematode (mostly *Ankylostoma caninum*) that wanders through the subcutaneous tissues (11.192). The skin overlying the larvae develops an erythematous, serpiginous, papular rash associated with *intense itching*.

Malignant melanoma (11.193) accounts for approximately 5% of all skin cancers and occurs overwhelmingly in white-skinned people. The developed lesion is usually about 8–15 mm in diameter, dark brown or black, with a pink or bluish hue and marked variegation (11.194).

11.183
Perifollicular purpura. Note keratin plugging of some follicles (perifollicular hyperkeratosis)

11.184
Scurvy: haemarthrosis

11.185
Follicular hyperkeratotic papules

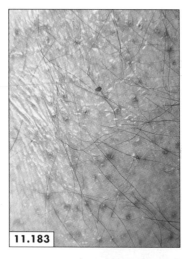

11.183

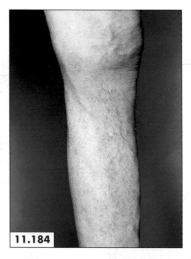

11.184

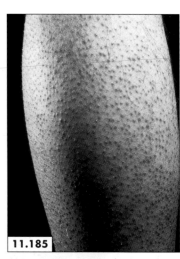

11.185

11.186
Solar dermatitis: brown, tanned skin with reddish-brown papules and excessive wrinkling

11.187
Keratoderma blennorrhagica: diffuse erythema, pustules with erosion and hyperkeratotic crusting

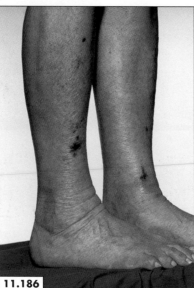

11.186

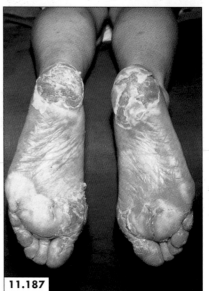

11.187

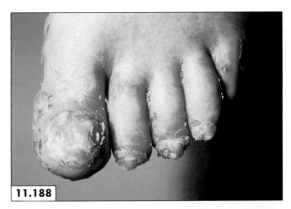

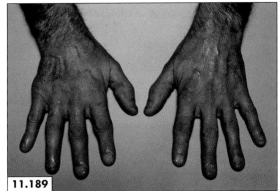

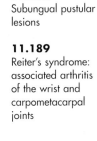

11.188
Subungual pustular
lesions

11.189
Reiter's syndrome:
associated arthritis
of the wrist and
carpometacarpal
joints

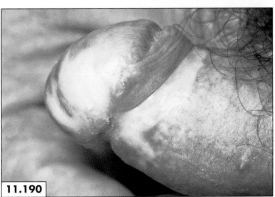

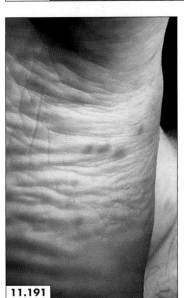

11.190
Erosions and
pustular lesions on
the glans and the
penile shaft

11.191
Secondary syphilis:
multiple, rosy-red
papules

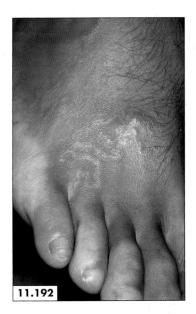

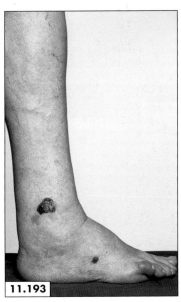

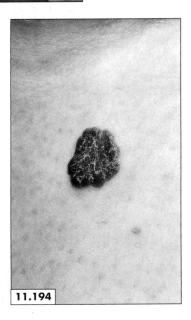

11.192
Larva migrans:
circuitous tunnel
routes

**11.193 and
11.194**
Malignant
melanoma:
variegated, purplish
plaque with well-
defined, irregular
border

Warts occur frequently on the feet. The common wart, from the human papilloma virus infection, is a large, firm papule with a rough hyperkeratotic surface (11.195). The plantar wart occurs on the plantar surface of the foot, where it is constantly pressed against the shoe by the weight of the body and does not project much above the skin surface (11.196). Unlike corns, which represent a thickening of the horny layer of the skin, warts contain blood vessels which may bleed and, in time, give the wart a darkish brown colour (11.197).

11.195
A verrucous, skin-coloured nodule

11.196
Flat-topped, blackish (thrombosed capillaries with haemorrhage) nodule

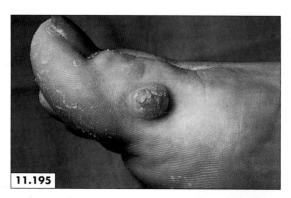

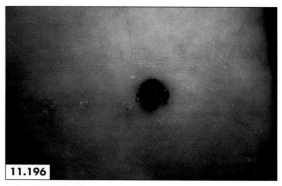

11.197
Verruca plantaris: multiple, skin-coloured, verrucous, confluent keratotic nodules, two with thrombosed capillaries and old haemorrhage (brownish-black tops)

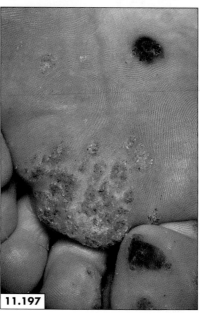

Index

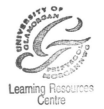